Reasoning against Madness

Rochester Studies in Medical History

Senior Editor: Theodore M. Brown
Professor of History and Preventive Medicine
University of Rochester

Additional Titles of Interest

Infections, Chronic Disease, and the Epidemiological Transition: A New Perspective
Alexander Mercer

Save the Babies: American Public Health Reform and the Prevention of Infant Mortality, 1850–1929
Richard A. Meckel

Intrusive Interventions: Public Health, Domestic Space, and Infectious Disease Surveillance in England, 1840–1914
Graham Mooney

The Antivaccine Heresy: "Jacobson v. Massachusetts" and the Troubled History of Compulsory Vaccination in the United States
Karen L. Walloch

Healthy Boundaries: Property, Law, and Public Health in England and Wales, 1815–1872
James G. Hanley

Psychiatry and Racial Liberalism in Harlem, 1936–1968
Dennis A. Doyle

Childbirth, Maternity, and Medical Pluralism in French Colonial Vietnam, 1880–1945
Thuy Linh Nguyen

Setting Nutritional Standards: Theory, Policies, Practices
Edited by Elizabeth Neswald, David F. Smith, and Ulrike Thoms

Technological Change in Modern Surgery: Historical Perspectives on Innovation
Edited by Thomas Schlich and Christopher Crenner

The History of the Brain and Mind Sciences: Technique, Technology, Therapy
Edited by Stephen T. Casper and Delia Gavrus

A complete list of titles in the Rochester Studies in Medical History series may be found on our website, www.urpress.com.

Reasoning against Madness

Psychiatry and the State in Rio de Janeiro, 1830–1944

Manuella Meyer

University of Rochester Press

The University of Rochester Press gratefully acknowledges generous support from the University of Richmond.

First published 2017

University of Rochester Press
668 Mt. Hope Avenue, Rochester, NY 14620, USA
www.urpress.com
and Boydell & Brewer Limited
PO Box 9, Woodbridge, Suffolk IP12 3DF, UK
www.boydellandbrewer.com

ISBN-13: 978-1-58046-578-6
ISSN: 1526-2715

Library of Congress Cataloging-in-Publication Data

Names: Meyer, Manuella, author.
Title: Reasoning against madness : psychiatry and the state in Rio de Janeiro, 1830–1944 / Manuella Meyer.
Description: Rochester, NY : University of Rochester Press, 2017. | Series: Rochester studies in medical history, ISSN 1526-2715 ; v. 41 | Includes bibliographical references and index.
Identifiers: LCCN 2017014092 | ISBN 9781580465786 (hardcover : alk. paper)
Subjects: LCSH: Psychiatry—Brazil—Rio de Janeiro—History—19th century. | Psychiatry—Brazil—Rio de Janeiro—History—20th century.
Classification: LCC RC451.B62 R657 2017 | DDC 362.1968900981/53—dc23 LC record available at https://lccn.loc.gov/2017014092

A catalogue record for this title is available from the British Library.

This publication is printed on acid-free paper.

Printed and bound in Great Britain by TJ International Ltd, Padstow, Cornwall

In Loving Memory of Reynold Meyer

Contents

Acknowledgments

It is a great pleasure to acknowledge the many people who have supported me throughout this project. I owe an enormous debt of gratitude to Stuart B. Schwartz, Gilbert M. Joseph, Alondra K. Nelson, and John Harley Warner, my advisers at Yale University. They've guided my work wisely and generously while inspiring me through their writing and teaching.

In recent years, my University of Richmond colleagues David Brandenberger, Joanna Drell, John Gordon, Robert Kenzer, Tze Loo, David Routt, Nicole Sackley, Carol L. Summers, John Treadway, Sydney Watts, Hugh West, Yücel Yanikdağ, and Eric Yellin have provided me with an intellectually enriching and nurturing environment. Deborah Govoruhk, the most thoughtful and supportive department administrative assistant one could ever hope for, deserves special mention. She provided me with endless technical support, useful advice, and kindness.

The staffs of libraries and archives in the United States and Brazil guided me through the challenges of the research process. In the United States, I would like to thank César Rodriguez at Yale and the staff of the Hispanic Division at the Library of Congress. In addition, Mary Lou Reker, Jason Steinhauer, and Carolyn Brown at the John W. Kluge Center of the Library of Congress, along with Jeannine Keefer, visual resource librarian at the University of Richmond, provided critical support and encouragement during the last stage of research.

Individuals too numerous to list assisted me in my research in Brazil, including the amazing staff of the Arquivo Nacional, the Arquivo Geral da Cidade do Rio de Janeiro, the Biblioteca Nacional, and the Arquivo Público do Estado do Rio de Janeiro. The staff at Oswaldo Cruz Foundation (Fiocruz) and the Academia Nacional de Medicina proved indispensable to the project. Moreover, they always welcomed me warmly and enthusiastically. Cátia Mathias, the head librarian at the Psychiatry Institute of the Federal University of Rio de Janeiro, and Cristiana Facchinetti, scholar extraordinaire of the history of Brazilian psychiatry, were also invaluable to this project. I am very grateful for their help.

My research would not have been possible without support from the Jacob K. Javits Fellowship, Fulbright-Hayes Fellowship, Yale University Graduate

School, Yale Council on International and Area Studies, Yale Department of History Mellon Research Grant, the Yale Latin American Studies Mellon Fund, and the Ann Plato Fellowship program at Trinity College. The David K. Larson Fellowship in Health and Spirituality through the John W. Kluge Center at the Library of Congress and the Faculty Research Committee at the University of Richmond funded my final forays into the archive.

En route to becoming a part of this volume, an earlier version of chapter 1 appeared as "Sanity in the South Atlantic: The Mythos of Philippe Pinel and the Asylum Movement in Nineteenth-Century Rio de Janeiro," *Atlantic Studies* 7, no. 4 (2010): 473–92. An earlier version of chapter 2 appeared as "'Of Grand Intentions' and 'Opaque Structures': Managing the Hospício Pedro II during Brazil's Second Empire (1852–90)," *Bulletin of the History of Medicine* 89, no. 4 (Winter 2015): 733–60, © 2015 by the Johns Hopkins University Press. I wish to thank the publishers of these works for their kind permission to reprint.

Ted Brown, series editor of the Rochester Studies in Medical History, and the anonymous readers vastly improved this book with their many insightful suggestions. A particular note of thanks to Ted for believing in this project and patiently teaching this novice author about the process of producing a book. Sonia Kane and Ryan Peterson at the University of Rochester Press shepherded this book through its various stages.

Friends have provided deep support over the years and across continents. I owe my most enthusiastic thanks for solidarity, friendship, and intellectual support to Louise Walker, Ryan D. Crewe, Amy Chazkel, Brandi Hughes, Alison Bruey, Jay Driskell, Emmanuel Raymundo, Martine Jean, Kari Zimmerman, Melissa Stuckey, Emily Musil, Vijay Prashad, Okezi Otovo, Colin Jones, Marc Hertzman, Sonia Song-Ha Lee, and Tara Tappert. As I type out the letters of your names, I picture conversations over coffee, walks to restaurants, chats in office hallways, and email exchanges offering productive criticism on a chapter draft or advice on book preparation. I hope that you each read between the lines your important individual contributions to this book.

The idea of this book most likely began when I was five years old in Port-au-Prince, Haiti. My mentally ill uncle Raynold and I talked to each other for hours on end. While many failed to fully comprehend my most reliable and dear confidante, he was always intelligible to me. In more ways than one, this project begins and ends with him. Bearing witness to the ways in which my grandmother and father cared for him left an indelible imprint on my mind about resilience, courage, and love. Both my mother and father have given me so many things for which I am grateful, especially their insistence that I pursue my passions and their unwavering support. I would also like to acknowledge my supportive siblings, Natacha and Hans Karl, along with my in-laws on all sides of the family.

Last but certainly not least, I would like to thank my son, Miles, and my husband, Will Machin. Miles bore the brunt of the time I put into finishing this book with grace and good humor. Will, my critic, editor, mentor, and best friend, has been with this project and in my life through its inception, development, and conclusion. I am grateful for his support, love, and patience.

Note on Brazilian Orthography and Terminology

The Brazilian Portuguese language had not yet been orthographically standardized in the nineteenth and early twentieth centuries. For all proper names of persons, I used the spelling that most frequently appeared in the contemporaneous documentation. I spelled all proper names of places according to present-day conventions. For all other words, I hew to today's standard.

The translation of racial labels from Brazilian Portuguese to English is a difficult task. The terms that denote some form of African ancestry (e.g., *negro, preto, pardo, mulato,* etc.) do not have clear equivalents in English. Racial categories and labels in any language are messy and problematic as racial categories in and of themselves can be. In the pages that follow, I frequently use "Afro-Brazilian" and "black," familiar terms to most US readers and others with accessible Brazilian Portuguese equivalents such as negro or preto. In addition, I use "African-descended," "men and women of color," and so on. As much as possible, I have preserved these, and other, labels in direct quotations, and in my own prose, I have attempted to use terms that establish a balance between Brazilian and US conventions. However, it is important to note that English terms do not represent a pristine reproduction of the language used by the men and women that appear in this book.

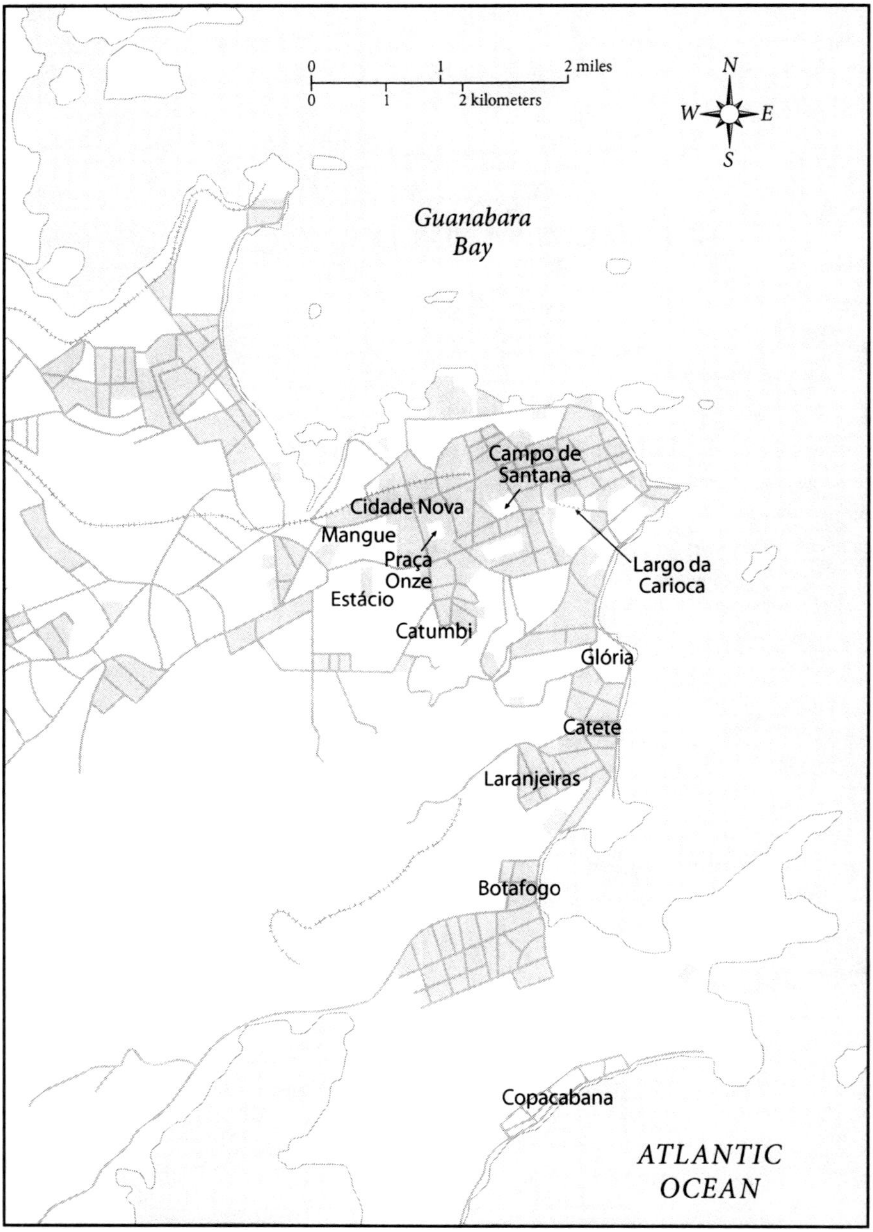

Rio de Janeiro, ca. 1890. The map here represents a general spatial overview of the city's key neighborhoods and landmarks. Map by Bruno Carvalho and Bert Barickman, in Marc A. Hertzman, *Making Samba: A New History of Race and Music in Brazil* (Durham, NC: Duke University Press, 2013), 16. © Duke University Press. Reproduce by permission.

Introduction

On December 5, 1852, doctors, Catholic officials, Emperor Dom Pedro I, and other members of the royal court celebrated the inauguration of the first national public mental asylum, the Hospício Dom Pedro II, in Rio de Janeiro. The lavish ceremony was seemingly a success as the press touted the institution "a great triumph of philanthropic ideas" that placed the city on the "path of material progress," marking "a notable era in the civilization of the country."[1] Prior to the second half of the nineteenth century, the mentally ill were treated according to their means. The wealthy, if relatively tranquil, were treated at home and sometimes sent to Europe by their families under the advisement of doctors. Their poor and working-class counterparts were placed under the care of their families or housed in one of the multifunctional jails or poorhouses that held societal castoffs such as beggars, prostitutes, orphans, and vagrants. The mad were treated much the same as other marginalized sectors of Brazilian society.

By the mid-nineteenth century, however, the insane were sharply distinguished from other "problem populations." They were incarcerated in a state-supported asylum system that isolated them both physically and symbolically from the larger society. The Hospício de Dom Pedro II contained only the mentally ill with the aim of medically treating and rehabilitating them through methods that affected the psyche. Over the course of the mid-nineteenth and early twentieth centuries, a new set of experts, the alienists, later known as psychiatrists, introduced the Brazilian public to a series of treatments and initiatives to treat the mad. They also hoped to instill sound mental hygiene practices among their fellow citizens. How and why, then, did an asylum, the first in Latin America, come about? How did psychiatrists emerge to become one of the primary knowledge experts to manage the presumed mentally ill? Explaining these remarkable shifts is the central task of this book. This project investigates how professional psychiatry emerged in Rio de Janeiro. A seemingly innocuous protest led by doctors over the spread of a mysterious "fever" outside Rio de Janeiro in 1830 paved the way for a larger critique of public health institutions and measures. By undermining the legitimacy of existing state institutions that purported to care for the mentally ill, and by extension, the constitutional monarchy's inability to secure the health of its citizens-subjects, doctors compelled state officials to authorize the creation of an asylum lest these officials confirm the state's tenuous obligation to its population during a critical time of state formation. Unlike the wave of independence movements finding success throughout Spanish America during the early nineteenth century, the political leadership in Brazil followed its own peculiar path when Emperor Pedro I formally broke with Portugal in 1822. In one of its many points of divergence with its Spanish American counterparts, Brazil became the only Latin American country to gain independence by imperial decree and to establish itself as a constitutional monarchy until the declaration of the republic in 1889. Many historians of Brazil noted that the fear of democratic revolution after independence ushered in a political process wherein politicians chose to reconcile differences and conflicts as a means to safeguard the political system from supposed unpredictable forces. As the politics of conciliation became a hallmark of Brazilian political culture during the latter half of the nineteenth and early twentieth centuries, its complex, uneasy, and sometimes unwieldy workings could prominently be seen through the professionalization of psychiatry.

The emergence of psychiatry in Brazil as a discrete medical specialty can be situated within the processes of bureaucratization and secularization. The professionalization of medicine and the application of more stringent standards in teaching and practice, the priorities of state building, the construction of national identities, the centralization of state power, and the reduction of the role of the church in public life were dominant themes in the medicalization of madness and the emergence of psychiatry.[2] But the particular way that madness was modernized in Brazil highlights several previously unexplored social and political dimensions of Brazilian psychiatry. The professionalization processes of numerous occupational groups in the latter half of the nineteenth century had much in common with that of psychiatrists. They, like lawyers, journalists, and businessmen, among others, sought to prove their professional legitimacy in the public sphere by virtue of their possession of a specific form of expertise. However, among the multitude of medical specialties that became institutionalized, Brazilian psychiatry distinguished itself as its professionals stressed the existence of a public under threat from explicit and implicit mental ailments. This study then, reconstructs how, after having garnered a certain level of professional legitimacy, psychiatrists sought more influence by focusing on efforts to project a psychological mindset onto the Brazilian public in order to produce a disciplined and a mentally hygienic citizenry. A therapeutic society was not thrust upon Cariocas, as residents of Rio de Janeiro are called, by a conspiracy of medical experts who hid behind a screen of technical jargon. Psychiatrists did attempt to expand their sphere of influence, but they were often encouraged to do so by jurists, senators, and others who guided society and culture.

This book thus traces the kinds of sociopolitical arrangements that allowed for the identification and transformation of the problem of mental illness into a dilemma of postcolonial governance. In doing so, it examines the rise of psychiatry as a distinct medical specialty in mid-nineteenth and early twentieth century Rio de Janeiro, primarily through the trials, tribulations, maneuverings, and actions of its practitioners. The book chronicles their battles over the causes, management, and treatments of madness with competing knowledge experts while seeking to obtain legitimacy for psychiatry as a medical field and public utility. The thread of this narrative connects a cast of varied characters in an unstable context: psychiatrists, Catholic officials, candomblé healers,[3] Kardecist spiritists,[4] politicians, and the mentally ill in the shifting landscape of modern state formation. As medical training and education were being reformed after the declaration of the republic in 1890, doctors began to insert themselves more consciously into the public sphere as both shapers and enforcers of public policies. Psychiatrists understood insanity not only as an illness but as a socially destabilizing force that threatened the progress and prosperity of the capital city and, by extension, the nation.

As a sociopolitical history of psychiatry, *Reasoning against Madness: Psychiatry and the State in Rio de Janeiro, 1830–1944* argues that an early twentieth-century Brazilian psychiatry, marked by a new focus on the collective and the social environment, both transformed liberal politics alongside notions of mental hygiene and, crucially, forged new connections between the two. It describes the processes through which doctors transformed madness from an unremarkable, if troubling, dimension of human experience into a serious sociopolitical problem; a public health dilemma; an intellectual conundrum; and, above all, a problem that medicine promised, and failed, to solve. As doctors, Catholic officials, Kardecist spiritists, and candomblé healers with competing visions of the causes and treatments for insanity each sought to wrest interpretive control from the others as well as from their subjects, psychiatric assertions of authority over mental illness failed to achieve broad assent.

When nineteenth-century Brazilian doctors turned their attention to madness in all its forms—from mild neuroses to full-blown insanity, from depression to hysteria, from trying to fathom the motives of murderers and suicides—they became deeply implicated in governmentality by "producing new forms of knowledge, inventing new notions and concepts that contributed to the 'government' of new domains of regulation and intervention."[5] The operation of governmentality in Rio de Janeiro that began in the early nineteenth century with the implementation of reforms orchestrated under the arrival of the Portuguese court observed by many historians continued exponentially over the course of the early twentieth century.[6] Reforms aimed at transforming personal behaviors were intended to reorient personal conduct damaging to individual and public health. Drinking, gambling, prostitution, forms of public leisure and entertainment, and an unsanitary urban milieu became objects of concern because of their presumed harmful effects. These behaviors not only damaged individual health but threatened Brazil's social progress and restrained its economic prosperity. As people had to be trained or taught that they had an obligation to care for themselves, part of being a responsible and productive subject required "self-care" and entailed "shifting responsibility for social risks, illness, unemployment, poverty into a domain of individual choice and responsibility for the self."[7] The creation of a public in need of care that necessitated considerable medical and state intervention did not preclude the public's acceptance of public health and medical reforms. Indeed, it is not at all clear that psychiatrists achieved a great deal of success training individuals in self-governance. The effects of psychiatric thought are difficult to measure and assess, but the view from the asylums and outpatient mental hygiene clinics alongside the ways in which doctors wrote about mental illness and its causes strongly suggest that while psychiatric ideas were influential in shaping specific public policies, they had limited effects in their diffusion and acceptance.

Focusing upon the complex social and political status of psychiatrists leads me to not overestimate their roles as been acknowledged in Brazil and elsewhere. Where it has been considered at all by historians of Brazil, mental illness has usually been treated in relation to or as a variation on the state's concern with maintaining social order, providing more efficient policing of the city and enforcing new laws on disruptive public behavior, especially drunkenness, violence and prostitution. The mad have been portrayed as little more than criminals, deviants, and of concern to authorities only because of the threat they posed to social order. This study takes a slightly different perspective, focusing less on the role of the insane and more on the role that psychiatrists played in structuring relationships between themselves, patients, the public, and the state.

I do not showcase the perspectives and experiences of the mentally ill. Mental illness was real, terrifying, and destructive for its sufferers. However, I faced a paucity of sources on the perspectives of the mentally ill, finding few that would lend themselves to an analysis that would truly shed light on their experiences. Although this book understands madness both as a medical fact and a personal reality, it concentrates on the intellectual and cultural construction of madness as a field of knowledge, thereby making psychiatrists the subjects under the academic gaze.

My methodology draws on works propelling sociopolitical and cultural discursive analyses that lie in the intersections of history, political theory, and anthropology and aims to oppose the disaggregating of medicine from politics, society, and culture. In this manner, I make extensive use of a wide variety of sources that include asylum records, medical journals, government documents, fiction, chronicles, travelogues, and newspapers, among others. Newspapers proved a particularly invaluable resource as forums of public debate that included critiques of psychiatrists and their responses. As historian Jeremy Popkin observes in relation to the French Revolution, newspapers operated as both "purveyors of information and ideology" and as important sites for the construction of sociopolitical and cultural identities in Brazil in the period the book addresses.[8] Following Popkin, I treat newspapers as an interactive literature of reform during Brazil's "long nineteenth century" (from political independence in the 1820s to the rise of nationalist challenges to liberalism in the 1930s), as readers of the period became participants in state matters through this forum.

This book makes an important scholarly intervention in Brazilian historiography by tracing the complex professionalization of psychiatrists through a long period of national modernization. Few historical studies have traversed the conventional periodization of Brazilian history when looking at the state within the context of social assistance. Many historians of Brazil who focus on modernization processes tend to concentrate on the Old or First Republic (1889–1930) period. Specifically, historians such as Teresa Meade, Dain Borges, and Jeffrey D. Needell suggest that class and racial prejudices imbued an array of political and urban professional campaigns' attempts to moralize and modernize Brazilian cities (specifically Rio de Janeiro) by regulating and sanitizing public and private spaces.[9] Moreover, the public policies these notions inspired seldom sought to eliminate social hierarchies. In actuality, the claims of liberal nation builders compounded and exaggerated racial, class, and gender cleavages among different social groups and individuals. By following the maturation of psychiatry through the demarcations of Imperial Rule (1822–89), the Old Republic (1889–1930), and the era of President Getúlio Vargas (1930–45), this study allows for a richer and a deeper understanding of psychiatry's emergence and its bureaucracies of care. I aim to add nuance to the insightful appraisals of the Old Republic and provide a bridge between them and the emerging historical studies of social assistance in both earlier and later time periods.

In that vein, this study engages a variety of disciplines and historiographies. First, it speaks to histories of psychiatry that understand the asylum as a fountainhead of professionalization in the Anglophone Atlantic. As a mainstay of the history of psychiatry, the asylum has been a useful and yet limiting point of focus with which to examine madness and psychiatry since the institution has provided the greatest historical record with which to trace the treatment of insanity. However, inherent in conventional histories of the asylum is the notion that psychiatry was the only paradigm practiced inside. In many works, starting with Erwin Ackerknecht's and Gregory Zilboorg's classic texts and continuing with Roy Porter's monograph on the topic, historians of psychiatry and the mind sciences focused almost entirely on Western Europe and North America until the 1990s.[10] The notion that asylums and professional psychiatry were bastions of state power emerged from this Western bias. It was propagated by an entire generation of historians including Andrew Scull, who reinforced the notion of the asylum as an impenetrable and imposing prison, and David Rothman, who argued that the insane asylum was born in the same moment of institutional discipline as prisons and poorhouses in antebellum America.[11] Later scholars, such as Nancy Tomes, Gerald Grob, and Anne Digby, criticized the analytical lens with which these historians had framed the asylum and interrogated a broader array of primary sources that painted a more nuanced history of madness; however, the historiographical preoccupation with the Eurocentric asylum and professional psychiatry remained.[12] This book challenges this idea by building on the work of historians such as Megan Vaughan, Richard Keller, and Jonathan Sadowsky, who argue for a nuanced reading of the asylum in its colonial/postcolonial contexts.[13] Notably, Sadowsky's work illustrates how the total asylum made its way to Africa, importing colonial medicine as part of Western imperialism and interacting with local indigenous paradigms. He argues that medical services were a major rationale for colonial officials and that hospitals and clinics were typically most developed when and where there was a medical threat to the local workforce.[14] However, this book builds on his work by suggesting that Brazilian imperial and republican governments were also filled with moderate voices who on one hand argued that the state had an obligation to provide social services, but on the other hand harbored discriminatory thoughts about the marginalized populations in need of those services. Although my work draws strongly on that of Sadowsky, it nuances the social and political sensibilities of medical experts who had complex relationships with the people they sought to help.

This book has been greatly informed by the history of psychiatry in Latin America. However, in order to investigate the history of psychiatry, historians of the region (myself included) have used the lens of public health as an entry point from which to examine psychiatric notions of madness and attempts to manage it. Public health served as one of the most agile and expansive regulatory mechanisms in nineteenth-century Latin American cities. Although municipal public health institutions often had small budgets and staffs, they had considerable legal authority to regulate property and people's conduct in order to remove threats to the general population's longevity, health, and well-being. The public health mandate linked the condition and conduct of individuals with the vitality, strength, and prosperity of society overall. Earlier histories of public health in Latin America lauded the supposedly heroic efforts of local and international physicians and medical institutions for having tried to save the health of the inferior Latin American population from its supposed feeble constitutions. Yet by the mid-1990s, historian Marcos Cueto's contributions represented a fundamental shift in how scholars explored the relationship between medical science, public health, and nation-state building in the nineteenth and twentieth centuries. His work explored how disease, public health initiatives, and medical research intersected with the attempts of government officials to illustrate how important health and hygiene were to defining the modern nation and state. Cueto also demonstrated that public health policies and programs started by the government had ulterior motives regarding the health of lower-class citizens. Medical science, Cueto argued, allowed state officials and medical professionals to justify their characterizations of the lower classes by providing supposed empirical proof of their innate inferiority. State officials used medical science to create a narrative that required the segregation of lower-class citizens from middle- and upper-class citizens through measures such as housing and employment opportunities.[15] Extending the work of Cueto, scholarship on the history of Latin American nation-state building through public health and medical science began to emerge in the late 1990s and has continued to develop into a compelling area of research. In particular, this scholarship has unveiled unique and exciting ideas about how medical science was inextricably tied to nation-state building. Historian Christopher Abel has also nuanced the historiography of public health by identifying three major areas of convergence and divergence across Latin America during the late nineteenth and early twentieth centuries. In this manner, he has outlined three major thematic areas that he argues scholars in the field of public health should focus on: the complex reasons why late nineteenth-century state officials were concerned with the health of the citizens and hygienic conditions in major cities; how international groups, ranging from British philanthropists to the Rockefeller Foundation to the US government, sought to introduce innovative Western medical techniques to combat diseases such as yellow fever or malaria; and how marginalized racial and ethnic groups dealt with the introduction of medical efforts to improve their diets, health, and hygiene.[16] Greatly informed by these thematic structures, *Reasoning against Madness* frames the emergence of Brazilian psychiatry as a critical element of public health.

Whether or not lower-class citizens could become productive members of society was a question that reverberated throughout Latin America in the late nineteenth and early twentieth centuries as this issue became particularly salient in the psychological pathologization of racial and ethnic marginalized others. For example, historian Ann Zulawski explored how the Bolivian government chose to deal with improving public health despite having a considerable indigenous population. Liberal Bolivian physicians, psychiatrists, state officials, and elite citizens all agreed in principle that the country had to integrate the indigenous population into mainstream society in order to eliminate what this group called its "Indian problem." However, Zulawski concluded that unlike other Latin American countries that sought to incorporate the Indian at all costs, the Bolivian government, along with elite and middle-class citizens, decided to abandon any meaningful attempt to include indigenous populations into the body politic. Soon these elite groups began to define whiteness as the most important trait for becoming modern, thus eliminating the nonwhite citizens from joining the formal public sphere and its institutions.[17] Similarly, historian Cristina Rivera Garza has examined the ways in which socioeconomically marginalized groups during the reign of Porfirio Díaz (r. 1876–1911) were rendered dangerous by psychiatrists who adhered to an illiberal modernization program that undergirded the Porfiriato. These works and the idea of "liberal strategies of exclusion," to use political theorist Uday Mehta's felicitous expression, have provided influential hermeneutic keys for reading the history of liberal thought against the grain in republican Brazil.

A central theme of this book is the intersection of social assistance and its shift from philanthropy to welfare under the banner of liberalism. In liberal democracies, the concept of citizenship has established the meanings, expectations, and boundaries of full membership in society through claims of universal equality and access to political, economic, and social privileges, opportunities, and participation.[18] However, the emergence of a medical-legal state that sought to exercise control and authority over a fragmented and regionalized population in republican Brazil is rife with instances of citizenship deprived and of personal liberties denied to various groups on the basis of race, class, and gender. Any attempt to come to terms with how psychiatrists hoped to guide the modernization of Rio is confronted by this paradox of liberal professionals employing markedly illiberal means to carry out such a program.[19] At the core of this paradox is the notion that Brazilian psychiatry was afflicted by a persistent gap between the universal liberal values that the profession purported to represent and the historical fact of difference that such universal claims failed to accommodate.[20] It was this gap that authorized and justified the exclusion, marginalization, and derision that psychiatrists visited upon the presumed mentally ill who were either indigent, of African descent, or who frequented candomblé terreiros (ritual spaces of worship). Thick hierarchies often lurked beneath the surface of Brazilian social assistance programs' abstract language as liberalism's inclusive premises of moral equality often came riddled with perceptions of nonelites as fundamentally lacking the prerequisites for claiming the practical entailments of universal equality.

The historiography of psychiatry as it relates to public health and modernization in Argentina, by far, however, proves to be the most expansive counterpoint to Brazil, given the deep entrenchment of the psychiatric disciplines in Argentina.[21] Indeed, it has become a truism that of all the societies of Latin America, Argentina is the one in which the "psy" disciplines, and Freudian psychoanalysis, in particular, came to carry the most weight, not just in the building of state institutions but in broader cultural terms. For example, historian Mariano Ben Plotkin's seminal *Freud in the Pampas: The Emergence and Development of a Psychoanalytic Culture in Argentina* (2001) explores the early growth of psychoanalytic ideas in Argentina, the relationship of the analysts to the local medical culture, and the critical role of psychoanalytical "diffusers."[22] Critically, it also highlights the profound ways in which psychiatrists were already incorporating mental health paradigms in both public and private spheres by the late nineteenth century. While psychoanalysis in Brazil did not have the wide diffusion it did in Argentina, there has long been a Brazilian public psychiatric establishment, mostly supported by the state, which predates Argentina's.

Since *Reasoning against Madness* marries the interstices of political and medical histories, the works of historians Julia Rodriguez and Jonathan Ablard serve as complimentary counterpoints to Brazilian psychiatry. Rodriguez's *Civilizing Argentina: Science, Medicine, and the Modern State* (2006) explores the connective tissue between Argentine modernity, science, and medicine by specifically looking at how doctors (psychiatrists included) targeted women and men who threatened the public order and criminals as key rehabilitative groups. Ablard's *Madness in Buenos Aires: Patients, Psychiatrists, and the Argentine State, 1880–1983* (2008) looks at the waxing and waning of government support for psychiatry as the leitmotif running through the study is the failure of state structures to achieve psychiatric goals. Similar to *Reasoning against Madness*, both works use psychiatric institutions and initiatives as case studies from which to examine the political history of the state and the history of medicine.[23]

The growing body of work that examines the history of psychiatry and psychiatric professionalization in Brazil subscribes heavily to Foucault's understanding of madness as a social construct and the Great Confinement efforts of psychiatrists and the state.[24] Although insightful, these studies depict psychiatrists as almost exclusively agents of the state. While I view psychiatrists critically, I believe many of them genuinely wanted to aid the mentally ill and that even their bureaucratic goals were informed by their experiences as healers and often differed from those of state functionaries. Although they did sometimes overreach in diagnosing people as insane, they had no intention of confining the majority or even a large percentage of the populace into the asylum.[25] Rather, they intended to use the asylum primarily as a tool to maintain public order, to alleviate the burden of care for families with mentally ill members, and to practice their medical craft. Furthermore, psychiatrists envisioned the asylum as part of a dynamic network of institutions intended to mold modern productive citizens and to inculcate new modes of selfhood. In this manner, psychiatrists in Rio de Janeiro had much in common with their liberal professional counterparts in other parts of the Americas. For example, historian Silvia Arrom, in *Containing the Poor: The Mexico City Poor House, 1774–1871* (2000),[26] examines the ways which church and vice-regal reformers created the poorhouse as a radical program to not only eliminate poverty and promote economic development but to instill new modes of being.[27]

The book's point of departure is the asylum-construction campaign during the 1830s. Chapter 1 examines how proto-psychiatrists injected madness and mental health as critical matters of statecraft during a fragile political impasse.[28] Brazil's gradual modernization in the nineteenth century differed greatly from North American and European models; instead of growing within a bourgeois enclave, capitalism grew and developed within a dense network of patronage.[29] Throughout much of the country's colonial and early imperial history, a slave-owning, rural aristocracy maintained paternalistic sovereignty over the rest of the population. However, the political and economic culture that developed in the 1830s was in large part a consequence of the 1807–8 transfer of the Portuguese royal court that superseded the power of the rural aristocracy. The prince regent João VI and approximately fifteen thousand Portuguese nationals took up residence in a colonial port and dramatically transformed urban society. While local political and medical circumstances prompted medical reformers' call for an asylum, revolutionary intellectual currents in the Atlantic also influenced them. Of specific importance was the apocryphal story wherein French psychiatrist Philippe Pinel (1745–1826) breaks the chains of the confined and abused mentally ill at the height of the French Revolution sparking the institutionalization of a more humane medical regime for the insane. This became a grounding mythology from which Brazilian reformers advocated for the creation of the Hospício Dom Pedro II. The myth of Pinel as a chain breaker proved very useful, for it promoted an image of psychiatry that linked the incipient medical specialty to the ideals of revolution, emancipation, and humanism situating the psychiatrist as a liberator and a healer.

Chapter 2 chronicles contestations between the emergent psychiatrists and the Brazilian Santa Casa de Misericórdia Catholic lay brotherhood over the governance of the Hospício Pedro II. It investigates how psychiatrists, as apostles of professional rationality, developed their ideas about reason and bureaucratic power in a contested site of religious charity during Brazil's Second Empire. While these groups shared ideological ground about the need to seclude the insane in asylums, their divergent and entangled epistemologies about the constructions of madness, its treatment, and its bureaucratic governance shaped their conflicts. By the declaration of the republic in 1890, psychiatrists were able to wrest authority over the Hospício Pedro II, now called the National Insane Asylum, from the Santa Casa as religious actors were removed from key administrative positions. State officials would recognize psychiatrists as key experts on mental illness and endow them with professional and political authority as they drafted key legislative efforts related to the infrastructure of care for the mentally ill. Outside the asylum, Rio grew into an imperial capital city crucial to Brazil's export economy.[30] As the major Brazilian port of entry, approximately ten thousand enslaved men and women, taken mainly from Western and Central African sites, landed in Rio every year. In fact, the urbanization that transformed the colonial capital into a royal court and the expansion of Brazilian ports' involvement in foreign trade increased the demand for urban slave labor. The city's port economy and the gradualist approach to slave emancipation created a deeply international, multicultural, and multiracial kaleidoscope of workers that included African and Brazilian slaves in addition to multiclass European immigrant laborers.[31]

When the slave trade gradually ended during the late nineteenth century, members of the planter class began to shift their economic, political, and cultural weight to Rio de Janeiro, where they encountered a new urban population of liberal professionals, including psychiatrists. In the period immediately following the final abolition of slavery in 1888, Rio de Janeiro was not just the undisputed cultural and political capital of Brazil. It was a contradictory social landscape where poverty coexisted with manifestations of fantastic wealth and privilege as city residents grappled with the symbolic and empirical tenets of modernization.[32] The statesmen, public health officials, doctors, and scientists who comprised the urban elite sought to revitalize the nation as a model for, as the 1890 Brazilian flag would have it, "order and progress."[33] They began to regard the presumed mad that were scattered throughout the city and significantly marked by poverty and blackness as a threat to their ambitions for order. The elite and the emerging middle classes regarded black bodies, features, and behaviors as the visible embodiment of the danger that imperiled industrious cities and a disciplined citizenry. In particular, racist interpretations from abroad fueled elite anxieties about the country's racial identity. European intellectuals such as Henry Thomas Buckle, Benjamin Kidd, and Gustave Le Bon, who Brazilian elites avidly read, widely held up Brazil as a cautionary tale since the country's reputation as the world's largest importer of African slaves, and as a culture permissive of miscegenation, made it a prime example of tropical degeneration. According to these thinkers, promiscuous crossings characteristic of Brazil had produced degenerate, unstable individuals incapable of rational political, social, or economic development. As the monarchy came to a close with the deposition of Emperor Dom Pedro II by republican forces in 1889, Rio's psychiatrists, versed in the lexicons of criminology, eugenics, and degeneration theory, but still devoted to the idea of a triumphant Brazil, had a layered and complex set of responses to their Atlantic, and to a degree, internal Brazilian colleagues. While they also certainly held antiblack views of their fellow citizens, they rejected the deterministic pessimism that degeneration theories conveyed and their implications for emergent schemes of national modernization, in which Rio was to be the showcase. The growing strength of psychiatric belief and advocacy in Rio would be put behind a racial, and often racist optimism, in which psychiatrists saw themselves molding black and mixed-race citizens into a functional part of a great modern city.

Chapter 3 examines three key legislative decrees and their sociocultural underpinnings. By instigating Decree 206 (the establishment of Medical-Legal Assistance to the Alienated), Decree 791 (the authorization of the Professional School of Nurses), and Decree 1559 (the establishment of the Observation Pavilion), psychiatrists hoped to revolutionize the asylum into a monument of therapeutic care. These decrees reorganized both people and space, reflecting psychiatrists' understanding of the mentally ill, their medical collaborators, and themselves. Through a process of adding and removing bodies deemed inappropriate and the manipulation of the asylum's space, these measures sought to remedy problems such as inept and abusive nurses, overcrowding, and the pervasive presence of the chronically incurable. Psychiatrists invented and shaped complex relations between the inner and outer dimensions of asylum space that ultimately constituted the core of their narrative world-making. By focusing on how psychiatrists purported to improve and to expand care for the mentally ill, I argue that the racial, gender, and class biases of early Brazilian psychiatrists would both aid and hinder their work as they actively sought to undergird their profession to republican projects of modernism. Chapter 4 explores how denunciations of the asylum and its administration by various opponents of psychiatry, as well as rebuttals by the asylum's psychiatric administration, reveal the juxtaposition of a strong antirepublican tradition rooted in imperial nostalgia against secular bureaucracies of expertise. Nostalgia for imperial forms of social assistance in the late nineteenth and early twentieth-century Rio de Janeiro, represented by organizations such as the Santa Casa lay brotherhood, arose from the contested political significance of social assistance during the transition from empire to republic.

Chapters 5 and 6 take both a synchronic and diachronic approach to the examination of psychiatry in the public sphere during the early twentieth century. The chapters cover some of the same temporal ground but from separate thematic viewpoints. Chapter 5 addresses psychiatrists' invocation of a public whose claims required defense, focusing on 1903–37 period in which the interest of National Insane Asylum psychiatrists in serving a public outside of the asylum reached its apogee.

In Rio, as in other Latin American capitals, psychiatry was born and grew to maturity as part of larger modernizing projects. By the late nineteenth century, Rio de Janeiro was the most populated city in Brazil, containing more than half a million people in 1890 and over eight hundred thousand in 1906.[34] In the early decades of the twentieth century, Rio de Janeiro was reshaped by urban reforms constructed to create an image of a civilized cosmopolitanism. In a nation that was largely agricultural and dependent on coffee exports and ruled by oligarchic elites, Rio de Janeiro was not only the political and cultural center of the nation but was also the iconic city where new forms of socialization, consumption, and modernization were being debuted. Urban reforms sought to constitute a bourgeois ordering of public space by dictating to the public the norms of behavior, dress codes, and hygienic space. Aside from the infrastructural modernization and hygienic reasoning behind public works and public health measures, the norms and impositions of the municipality were also tinged by a desire to curtail popular culture and manifestations of "low culture" (read Afro-Brazilian) in an attempt to instill a model of Europeanized bourgeois civility that has led historian Jeffrey D. Needell to refer to the late nineteenth and early twentieth centuries as Rio's "Belle Epoque."[35] Inspired by French Prefect Georges-Eugène Haussmann's renovation of Paris, the city's urban planners began to eliminate configurations of public space dating from the colonial period and earlier, seeking to scrub away the "disorderly" working-class uses of the city.[36] As the city almost doubled in size between 1890 and 1906, it created modern systems of public service such as transportation, lighting, sanitation, and policing due to the efforts implemented by the energetic mayor Pereira Passos during his term from 1902 to 1906.[37] Dubbed the "tropical Haussmann," Passos, alongside federal government officials, sought to alter the image of Rio as a retrograde colonial port. He undertook infrastructure reforms that included the opening of new avenues and the improvement of public transportation. Allied with charismatic and tireless public health advocate Doctor Oswaldo Cruz, Passos promoted a veritable crusade to eradicate epidemic diseases to impose obligatory vaccination, and to reinforce hygienic methods. The search for the modernization of the city was conditioned not only by diverse mentalities but also by differing pacts between the municipal authorities, the central government, and the governing elites. In the early twentieth century, people throughout the Atlantic region began to consider sickness as an avoidable flaw rather than an inevitable condition of living. As public health officials considered the regulation of the body, conduct, and living environment as an increasingly crucial practice in guarding against the infiltration of disease, they developed a series of agencies founded upon notions of social hygiene.[38]

A north and south Atlantic professional trend had embraced mental hygiene, and a growing number of Brazilian psychiatrists began to understand the social and political environment as a key player in shaping human character. Describing the development of an individual's personality as connected to the interpersonal dynamics making up distinct cultures and societies, they began to figure psychiatry as the key to explaining, and even resolving, a wide range of related social and political problems. At this juncture, Brazilian psychiatrists, in particular, were at the forefront of public health campaigns as they used the discourses of epidemiology, population management, and prevention to define civic responsibilities and to promote a public psychiatry as part and parcel of state modernization. As a better established field of global reach, public health offered psychiatrists access to an expansive language of reform. Brazilian psychiatrists employed new categories of normal and deviant, which were dramatically defined and invigorated by race, class, and gender differences.[39] In the name of safeguarding the health of the entire population, public strategies of surveillance, documentation, and quarantine generated new concepts of individual behavior sometimes at odds with the existing and popular standards of social conduct. The growing construction of medical knowledge about mental illness, deviance, and danger emerged in the context of a fervent antipoor, antiblack, and patriarchal political culture generated by the social tumult of industrialization, rapid urbanization, and tremendous migration into Rio de Janeiro.

By the 1920s and 1930s, Brazilian mental health professionals showed a renewed interest in the relationship between the sociopolitical environment and mental health. As members of a Rio-centered reformist group within Brazil's elite class, they rejected a national narrative of racial pessimism and argued that improvements in health, culture, and most importantly, education, could mend degeneracy.[40] In pursuit of the belief that psychiatry itself could address both personal and social vices and errors, psychiatrists maintained control of the asylum they had fought so hard to hold but uncoupled the profession from asylum practice. They expanded the boundaries of the profession as they focused on the outpatient clinics and other urban facilities devoted to evaluation, short-term treatment, and prophylactic programs rather than indefinite custodial care that had first appeared at the end of the nineteenth century. These sites provided the basis for a psychiatry of everyday life, concerned less with insanity than with employment, marriage, sexual morality, and child rearing. By focusing on these domains, we can better appreciate the extent to which psychiatrists hoped to intertwine and to build both the institutional and cultural aspects of their project and assess the successes, failures, and unintended consequences of their efforts.

The last chapter looks at how psychiatrists responded to challenges from spiritism, which they characterized as a negative cynosure that functioned as a portmanteau representation of national degeneration. It specifically explores how psychiatrists pathologized both candomblé and Kardecist spiritism. It addresses these questions: Why did Brazilian psychiatrists render spiritism as both a form and cause of madness? Why did they assail its practitioners and followers? Spiritism's logics and logos fundamentally upset psychiatry's model of the self-possessed citizen and nation bound to the vicissitudes of time, materiality, and territoriality. Indeed, psychiatrists' inability to curtail spiritism's popularity reflected a failure to articulate a compelling politics of persuasion to the very Brazilians they hoped to assist. The abatement of psychiatry's vitriolic battles against spiritism during the early 1940s illustrates psychiatry's gradual and grudging acceptance of supernatural beliefs among a Brazilian populace that often blithely combined an enchanted worldview with modernity.

In many ways, Brazilian psychiatry was a movement built in the bureaucratic fissures of government infrastructures. Although psychiatrists sought to manage and serve the Brazilian masses, they remained most successful in the terrain in which they were born: the field of institution formation. They were ultimately largely unsuccessful in winning the hearts and minds of Brazilians for a number of reasons. Most critically, however, they would overreach their diagnostic power in the public sphere and have to cede cultural and institutional ground to Kardecist spiritism and candomblé. These alternative systems' espousal of ideological frameworks that identified the sources of mental illness and their cures proved more compelling to many Brazilians than psychiatry's messages of self-control, austerity, hierarchy, discipline, and secularity. Unlike in Argentina, psychiatry failed to become Brazil's state "religion-of-the-self." Instead, it gave over much of its momentum and legacy as an innovator of muscular programming to the state proper while it relinquished cultural space that it hoped to claim (and Argentinian psychiatry enjoyed) to more popularly grown, permeable, and resilient cultural institutions. Thus, by the 1940s a mature Brazilian psychiatry would manage the asylum, consult on state programs, and engage in private practice.

Ultimately, the professionalization of psychiatry mirrored the historical processes of political and socioeconomic upheaval. The closing of the National Insane Asylum in 1944, which was by that point one among many secular state institutions available to the mentally ill, would serve as perfunctory notice of the end of psychiatric leadership of public infrastructure development, technological innovation, liberal political reform, and moral regeneration. A new era would emerge in Brazilian psychiatry in which state institutions and programs would be overwhelmingly created and directed by state officials, sometimes in consultation with psychiatrists. Ultimately, this book explores how psychiatry in Brazil came into being as an adjunct utility to, among other institutions, the Santa Casa de Misericórdia, how it grew to become a key driver of Brazilian modernization, how it failed to become a popular culture-making force and how it then receded, arguably taking up its mature role in Brazil as an adjunct utility to the emergent secular state, which in turn took over responsibility for many of the structures and public roles that psychiatrists had created.

Chapter One

Sanity in the South Atlantic

The Myth of Philippe Pinel and the Asylum Campaign Movement, 1830–52

Nineteenth-century Brazilian doctors did not agree on the causes of insanity any more than they agreed on what insanity actually was. As a group, they believed that it grew from multiple roots. Some hypothesized physical causes, as yet unseen or unidentified by medical science, while others saw nonphysical triggers in play such as luxury, poverty, bad luck, or religious excitement. Civilization itself was also often cited as the underlying cause of many kinds of insanity, with some thinkers positing that the demands of urbanization detrimentally affected weak or fragile personalities, unable as they were to keep their feet within the polyglot whirlwind of an internationally emergent Atlantic metropolis like Rio. Despite the divergent views of the originating causes of insanity, a growing consensus stipulated that it was on the rise throughout the opening decades of the nineteenth century.[1] Even if doctors could not agree on what exactly insanity was, or what caused it, they agreed that the treatments employed in the premier public institution in the city, the Santa Casa de Misericórdia Hospital, were arcane and grossly inadequate.

Medical and state officials around the Atlantic world grew concerned that the mad haunted the cities for which they had such new and carefully designed plans. This concern, along with advances in medicine and the secularization of insanity, led to the proliferation of asylums in a number of countries and with it, the rise of psychiatry as a profession. In this, Brazil was no exception. This chapter chronicles the asylum-building campaign in mid-nineteenth-century Rio de Janeiro, with a focus on how the campaign was launched by medical doctors, some of whom would, with the forming of a discrete space for the treatment of mental illness, become Brazil's first psychiatrists. Although their call to construct an asylum was based on local political and medical circumstances, they drew their intellectual impetus from the Atlantic marketplace of ideas. Political and intellectual currents in France, in particular, electrified Brazilian medical doctors intent on transforming the management of madness. More specifically, the context from which French psychiatrist, Philippe Pinel (1745–1826) articulated a more humane medical treatment of the mentally ill, known as "the moral treatment," grounded an aspirational narrative with which reformers advocated for the construction of Brazil's first asylum. From before its birth as a physical space, the asylum was meant to encompass the creation and perfection of new treatment regimes for the mad. It will come as no surprise in subsequent chapters, then, to find that mandate growing to include the making of an entire profession of caregivers who excelled, as much as anything, in the creation of institutional cultures.

Close examination of the asylum campaign in Rio de Janeiro also sheds light on how often-overlooked asylum movements in disparate nations drew from one another. Emergent psychiatrists, sprinkled as they were around the vast nineteenth-century Atlantic shores, looked beyond their national boundaries to explore the etiology of madness, its management, and the potential roles of the psychiatrist. It helped that much of the European colonial diaspora, led by France, developed a preoccupation with madness during the 1800s. By 1870, while speaking before the Corps Legislative in Paris, French republican deputy Léon Gambetta would claim "madness seems to be the disease of the century," citing public concern over the increasing number of hospitalized lunatics and the inability of asylum psychiatrists to tame insanity.[2] One can look at the early nineteenth century as an Atlantic tipping point: urbanization, the continuing slave trade with its inherent rumors of abolition, the diminishing power of Christian authorities, the professionalization of medicine, and the establishment of the modern nation-state and its bureaucracies, most notably among them public health, led to a "psycho-cultural moment" in which new attempts to manage insanity became critical to both state and civil societies.

Examination of the construction of Latin America's first public asylum offers a unique opportunity given Brazil's political status during the nineteenth century. Having shed its colonial status, Brazil would claim an anomalous identity as an independent empire in 1822 while other Latin American countries were gaining independence from Spain and establishing republican rule during the same time period. This chapter is interested in the lateral flows of ideas and power that created the asylum movement.[3] It is from within this terrain that Brazilian psychiatry, and as importantly, the modernizing movement at whose center the profession would reach maturity, would be born. A critical appraisal of the intellectual architecture shared by the doctors who would become Brazil's first psychiatrists provides an opportunity to understand the specific ways that Brazilian medical and cultural reformers took the story of Philippe Pinel as an inspiration. Some scholars interpret the doctors' deployment of Pinel as an example of colonial mimicry in which European ideas were present as matter-out-of-place.[4] This borrowing is sometimes cited as a postindependence display of cultural inferiority or a natural function of the periphery coveting the cultural tradition of the metropole. While many Brazilian reformers were Francophiles, and while their relationships with French intellectual culture were certainly complex, I argue that they took the myth of Pinel the chain-breaker and used it to leverage social processes that would be instrumental in the creation of modern Brazilian political, public health, and welfare institutions. In turn, those constructions would become fundamental to the creation and maintenance of state legitimacy in Rio de Janeiro. Pinel, appropriated as figure and myth, became the charismatic lever that allowed Brazilian reformers the local cultural muscle to see the new asylum built.

The protopsychiatrists who became key organizers of the asylum campaign had been indelibly influenced by the social, economic, and political currents in early nineteenth-century Rio de Janeiro. Historians of psychiatry have long affirmed that environmental determinism, the notion that the environment shapes behavior, was of signal importance to the greater Atlantic asylum project. Authors including David Rothman, Edward Porter, and Andrew Scull have noted that changes wrought by the early modern period, and the fears engendered by increasingly diverse and modernized cities in Great Britain, Canada, and the United States alike, led doctors to the "discovery of the asylum."[5] Brazilian doctors, similar to their counterparts throughout the Atlantic world, shared common values about the potential of the asylum to function as a curative force within a city seen as a source of vice and contagion. Although an exhaustive analysis of the urban environment's influence on early nineteenth-century Brazilian protopsychiatrists is beyond the scope of this work, the first part of this chapter does offer a brief demographic profile of Rio de Janeiro to ground an exploration of the sociology of the city. In this context, the sociocultural and political contours of the urban landscape against which psychiatric hopes, dreams, and aspirations would emerge, will be fleshed out. The second part of this chapter then looks at the myth of Pinel in order to understand how incipient psychiatrists used the Pinelian myth as a narrative device to advocate for the construction of the asylum and a new understanding of treating madness.

The Sensate City

Before mental-health-preoccupied doctors gave rise to the psychiatrists who would come to professionally know and describe the city, they were advocating for the asylum against the already complex nation and its capital city. In the 1830s, when the asylum movement started, Rio was, as it had been and would continue to be, a city of disparate peoples enmeshed in unequal relations. Beginning in the 1530s and dwindling to a trickle after the 1850 Queiróz law that abolished the international slave trade to Brazil, slave traders took more slaves from Africa to Brazil than to any other destination in the New World. The slave trade to Brazil peaked between 1780 and 1850, a seventy-year period during which more than two million slaves (half the total number of slaves taken to Brazil) were brought to Brazil.[6] Even after 1830, when Brazil had officially submitted to English demands and legally declared all newly arrived Africans free, the slave ships arrived and sold their human cargo with relative immunity. International pressure and Brazilian law aside, Brazil was a committed slave state, at least until the mid-nineteenth century. In the last years of the slave trade, during the decade of 1840–50, nearly four hundred thousand slaves were successfully off-loaded, mostly in Rio.[7] The demand for slaves on plantations and mines was voracious and still expanding. After 1850, with the number of new arrivals dwindling, slaves were traded from areas of diminishing profitability, like the sugar regions of the north, to thriving coffee centers in Rio de Janeiro, São Paulo, and Minas Gerais.[8] Coffee, first planted in the state of Rio in the 1770s,[9] extended slavery's central place in Brazil's economy for another century, or until abolition on May 13, 1888. It is difficult to estimate the exact number of people enslaved under Brazilian slavery. Most records of slaving transactions were ordered destroyed by minister of finance Rui Barbosa with the stated aim of granting Brazil a new beginning during the first regime of the republic. However, even according to the most conservative estimates, around four million Africans were "legally" brought to Brazil between 1530 and 1850.[10]

As a destination for humans, both in chains and free, and a port busy with export, Rio emerged as a critical node in the Atlantic circulation of goods, people, and ideas. In the latter half of the eighteenth century, the city became a thriving site crucial to Brazil's export economy. Generally considered a "black city,"[11] Rio de Janeiro's demographic landscape was transformed by a series of sweeping ethnic, racial, and urban-rural shifts over the course of the nineteenth century. In 1780 half of the city's two hundred thousand inhabitants were enslaved while the other half included Portuguese- and Brazilian-born whites and free people of color. From 1790 to the end of the legal Atlantic slave trade in 1830, nearly seven hundred thousand enslaved Africans were off-loaded at its port. This number represents two-thirds of all imports into Brazil during the same time period, with 80 percent arriving from West Central Africa.[12] The slaves who lived in Rio through the entire period from 1808 to 1850 bore witness to the city's growth as it expanded from a colonial outpost to the center of the

Luso-Brazilian world. With the arrival of the Portuguese court in flight from Napoleon's armies in 1808, Rio transformed into the political, social, and cultural capital of the Portuguese Empire and then, when the court returned to Portugal, into that of an independent Brazil in 1822. They saw it grow into the chief port for the new coffee monoculture of the Paraiba Valley and for the influx of waves of immigrant coffee workers primarily from Europe but also from Africa and North America. The arrival of the royal court in 1808 increased the number of whites, as Brazilians would welcome not only Portuguese refugees of noble birth but also the likes of British merchants, peasants from the Azores, French artists, German and Irish mercenaries, Swiss colonists, and North American adventurers—among the global mix of others who sought a future in Rio. In addition to stimulating the growth of the white population who would require slaves, the arrival of the court increased the demand for slaves to build the new houses, palaces, and public buildings and to work as household servants. In spite of the arrival of white immigrants, the people of color (including free black Brazilians, as well as African-born and Afro-Brazilian slaves) were still in the majority as travelers of the period consistently estimated that two-thirds of the population of Rio were people of color.[13]

When one takes into consideration the intimacy of services that urban slaves rendered and were forced to render, including wet-nursing elite children, laundering clothes in the homes of the middle and upper classes, prostituting themselves on the streets and in extended quasi-familial "arrangements," the city's inextricable blackness (something that would confound race-preoccupied reformers later on) becomes evident. In asymmetrical ways, Africans in Rio were deeply involved with Europeans and European cultures while Europeans were also deeply involved with Africans and African cultures. The diffused presence of slaves in the city under the ganho system (earning system) led to their wide circulation in the public sphere as large numbers of African-descent peoples colonized informal and public spaces for improvisational practices including hawking, raising livestock, hairdressing, and most importantly for this study, healing. During the eighteenth and early nineteenth centuries, a range of popular healers—including midwives, homeopaths, and tooth pullers—practiced within the city's heterogenous landscape. African-born *curandeiros* (healers) or *feiticeiros* (sorcerers) were some of the highest-profile denizens of the urban informal economy of social services, and as Brazil's religious and public health cultures would mature over the next one hundred years, they were probably the most important. Apart from curing illness, they offered to facilitate the aversion of misfortune, the provision of security, and the safeguarding of property, dispensing advice and medicines for mental, physical, and spiritual maladies out of ritual places or temples on city streets. In fact, African lay healers were often the leaders of candomblé terreiros. They garnered respect from black and white, free and enslaved alike; however, increasingly over the course of the nineteenth and early twentieth centuries, they raised the suspicion of this chapter's doctor-turned-psychiatrist protagonists.

During the 1830s, Rio's boundaries were geographically and demographically permeable; thus, the city seemed to have no fixed parts and no completeness. Instead, it became an amalgam of disjointed circulatory processes. Although the city was filled with the informal practices of slaves, freed slaves and recently arrived European immigrants were certainly a very real source of motivational anxiety for doctors—so, too, were the formal structures of imperial society. While psychiatry would later become a significant state utility for a time, in the 1830s they were a small, incipient, modernist group of men looking to reform nearly every strata of imperial Brazil. They saw themselves becoming an insurgent reformist force representing an Atlantic-wide psychiatric movement for change; like their profession to be, their allies and their compromises in Rio had not been created yet.

In addition to lay healing, another traditional force that earned the antipathy of the doctors was the Santa Casa de Misericórdia, one of the most important institutions in the Portuguese Empire. As an extension of the Portuguese medieval brotherhood of the same name, the Santa Casa representatives from Lisbon created chapters in most of the significant urban centers of Brazil by the mid-sixteenth century.[14] Formal responsibilities loosely defined as "philanthropic" meant, in practical terms, that burying the dead, incarcerating prisoners, care and feeding of orphans, housing of unwed mothers and their children, and the confinement of the insane all fell within the domain of Santa Casa. As the organization expanded with the city, it received an increasing number of money-making concessions and municipal tax exemptions granted by the crown while providing, according to the medical doctors, insufficient and inadequate services.[15] It is against this backdrop that the men who advocated for the asylum would give rise to Brazil's first psychiatrists, and it is, in part, against these very processes that they were to build the modern medical service structures they believed their city needed.

Society of Medicine

The cadre of doctors who formed the nucleus of the nation's first professional medical organization, the Medical Society of Rio de Janeiro (Sociedade de Medicina do Rio de Janeiro), spearheaded the hygienist movement that was ultimately responsible for the asylum. The society was the brainchild of a first generation Brazilian named José Martins da Cruz Jobim. Deeply influenced by Paris's urban reform movement while he was there studying to be a doctor, upon his return he decided to organize Brazilian physicians in Rio to emulate the Medical Academy of Paris in their structure, and not coincidentally, in their progressive approaches to medicine as well. Once in Rio de Janeiro, he met an Italian immigrant named Luís Vicente de Simoni, the former chief physician in colonial Mozambique during the last years of the Joanine era and currently a physician at the Santa Casa de Misericórdia hospital. Simoni would later describe the hospital by writing, "The fights, beatings, and cries produced a constant and unbearable noise reminiscent of Dante Alighieri's hell in Canto III of *The Divine Comedy*:

> Languages diverse, horrible dialects,
> Accents of anger, words of agony,
> And voices high and hoarse, with sound of hands, Made up a tumult that goes whirling on
> For ever in that air.[16]

Still, the Santa Casa de Misericórdia, founded in Lisbon in 1498, was the most prestigious and privileged lay brotherhood at the time. Called the "Brotherhood of Our Lady, Mother of God, Virgin Mary of Mercy," the Santa Casa de Misericórdia assumed a large measure of responsibility for providing formal social welfare services in the city of Rio. Jobim began to work at the Santa Casa hospital alongside De Simoni. The head Santa Casa surgeon, Joaquim Soares de Meireles was a Brazilian mulatto, son of a barber-surgeon, and former chief surgeon of the navy; like Jobim, he was educated in Paris in the 1820s, and he developed close friendships with both men.

This internationalist group of three began meeting informally but quickly became formal enough that they extended "invitations to join" to two French immigrant physicians, José Francisco Xavier Sigaud and João Mauricio Faivre, both of whom promptly accepted. Sigaud would be responsible for the first journal of the Society of Medicine of Rio de Janeiro, *O Semanário de Saúde Pública*, published from 1831 until 1835, and for writing many of the society's statutes. These five founders would form the core of the newly minted Medical Society of Rio de Janeiro, quickly inviting a dozen other physicians and surgeons to join as charter members.[17] Its charter delineated the group's purpose: to promote the advancement of European-style scientific medicine in Rio. The society was "destined to promote the illustration, progress, and propagation of Medical Science, to treat free of charge with its knowledge and counsel the poor in its infirmaries, and generally to benefit humanity, favoring and guarding the preservation and improvement of Public Health—under the authorization and protection of the government."[18] The charter members' early careers had corresponded to the tumultuous and yet culturally fecund days of Brazilian independence. They were part of a generation that witnessed the political workings of both imperial politics and early state formation.[19]

The outbreak of what Rio's doctors would later call "intermittent fever" (malaria) during the hot summer months of 1828 and 1829 marked a critical turning point in the history of disease and health in and around Rio. The city's existing public health infrastructure, a thin network of imperial public health officers and Catholic priests supported by the Santa Casa's manpower if needed, largely failed to respond. When reports of a raging epidemic fever cutting through the nearby provincial hinterlands (namely a key town Macacú, located in the heart of the Paraíba Valley and Magé) first filtered back to the city of Rio, the outbreak was well underway. Officials at the highest levels of the imperial government became concerned. The former president of the senate, then minister of the interior, and future head of the Santa Casa (1838–54) José Clemente Pereira, became extremely alarmed by reports that provincial ecclesiastic personnel, the "timid priests," who were charged by the imperial government with the care of victims during emergencies, refused even to "visit the sick."[20] He took matters into his own hands both to calm local fears and to prevent the spread of the illness into the capital itself. He commissioned a group of doctors to venture out to the region with the mandate of calming an anxious rural population. Medical personnel, in turn, were enthusiastic about experimenting with novel medical treatments such as quarantine and antifebrile agents in an effort to ameliorate the situation. The commission was seen as a success. To the extent that doctors calmed the people's fears, the decision to send a commission to the provincial towns proved successful as Robert Walsh, a British clergyman who traveled extensively in Brazil in 1828 and 1829 observed: "Physicians were sent over . . . and a close examination and inspection took place, and their reports calmed the rising apprehensions" while the parish priests of the region "were severely reprimanded by their superiors, and one was sent out of the country."[21]

Efforts to combat the illness by the city's new, protomodernist medical community, at whose cultural center the Medical Society was forming, earned them unprecedented legitimacy. Upon their return, many of the doctors who had participated in the commission would join the five founders of the Medical Society as charter members. This caused multiple changes. First, it would more than triple the ranks of the society; second, it would channel the new medical legitimacy through the society's formal publications and public statements; and third, it would alter the society's demographics, making it more Brazilian and more closely tied both to the people of Rio and to state authorities. Over the next decade, the Medical Society would be entrusted to make critical reexaminations of the city's largely imperial and Catholic public health institutions, starting one of the trends critical to the rise of medical and psychiatric modernity in Rio: the voluble public and bureaucratic critique of the institutions of rival ideologies. As such, one of the largest results of the malaria outbreaks was perhaps the first critical reappraisal of the city's Santa Casa hospital and its usefulness as a potential therapeutic center.

The Magé-Macacú epidemic experience left a lasting imprint on the minds of Medical Society doctors who worried about possible epidemics in Rio itself. The outbreak in provincial Rio underscored the significance of maintaining medical authority in the eyes of the laboring classes. Doctors worried that, in the event of an urban epidemic like cholera, Rio could be torn apart by mass panic. With Asiatic cholera spreading quickly from India into Europe at that time,[22] many society doctors had all-but-concluded that an urban epidemic was inevitable in the capital city. They doubted that Rio's imperial and municipal authorities were prepared to lead the city through such a crisis, and they were deeply concerned about the consequences, both medical and social, that might result from a void of leadership at such a time. The doctors felt that if they themselves prepared Rio in advance for the crisis and managed it effectively, they could not only serve the city's vulnerable populace but also enhance their own credibility and undermine the Santa Casa de Misericórdia's lay practitioners, whom the Medical Society members believed were in fact a threat to the city's health with their "arcane" methods.[23]

Pinel's myth could hardly have found more fertile ground, at least in terms of institution building. The doctors of the Medical Society had it fresh in their minds that organized, connected men with a cause and a service to offer could transform the workings of their government and their city. They appropriated the narrative of Pinel and took it upon themselves to transform what they saw as the dire state of medicine and public health in the city.

The Myth of the Chainbreaker

At the center of the myth of broken chains lie the actual changes in treatment credited to Pinel and advocated for by Atlantic Pinelists. Called "the moral treatment,"[24] this system of therapeutic care based on nonrestraint was the hallmark of progressive secular asylums. Moral treatment referenced a benevolent approach to treating mental illness and caretaking the mentally ill wherein reformers were to help patients develop self-control in order to restore their reason. The moral treatment rested on the premise that those suffering from mental illness could find their way to recovery if treated kindly and in ways that appealed to the parts of their minds that remained rational. It repudiated the use of harsh restraints and long periods of isolation that had been used to manage the most destructive behaviors of mentally ill individuals. It depended instead on specially constructed hospitals that provided quiet, secluded, and peaceful settings; opportunities for meaningful work and recreation; a system of privileges and rewards for rational behaviors; and gentler kinds of restraints used for shorter periods. In these early manifestations of what would become part of a relatively robust program of social assistance, these secular reforms were originally implemented within a dense ecology of religious caregivers. Historian Ann Goldberg notes that in France, Pinel "incorporated the pastoral care of the [Catholic] Church" by retaining nuns as caregivers, but he limited the participation of priests and secularized the rationale for treatment, turning it, even in the hands of dedicated nuns, "into a tool to wrest medical jurisdiction and expertise of madness from the Church in a campaign to exclude the religious orders from the care of the insane."[25]

Pinel was (and to a degree still is) believed to have released the inmates from their chains at the Bicêtre and Salpêtrière hospitals in Paris at the height of the French Revolution. He was immortalized in countless books and paintings, most notably by Tony Robert-Fleury in his famous 1876 painting, *Pinel Freeing the Insane*, where the doctor is portrayed as a stoic force, standing resolutely with a young woman kneeling almost kissing his right hand, while an attendant unlocks the chains of a madwoman in a courtyard occupied by the desolate mentally ill. Though captivating, scholars have discredited what has become known as "Pinel's Gesture," or the unlocking of chains, through documentary evidence. In another story presented to the Royal Academy of Medicine in 1836, Pinel confronts Georges Couthon, a member of the autocratic Committee of Public Safety, who had come to inspect the situation of the mad at the Bicêtre hospital. Pinel confronts Couthon and demands that all the inhumanely restrained madmen be instantly freed. In defying the powerful Jacobin, Pinel risks his life in defense of the mad. Nothing in Couthon's biography, Pinel's writings, or contemporaneous accounts corroborate the visit between the two men. Moreover, it seems that Couthon was out of town during the supposed encounter. Despite the fallacy of these stories, they endure as foundational fictions.[26] Certainly during the mid-nineteenth century, the veracity of Pinel's gesture was not highly contested, and although there were other contemporaneous figures who also advocated a more humane treatment of the mad, none came with a narrative that so aptly captured the Atlantic zeitgeist: the triumph of liberty, freedom, and individuality over repression.

What was unique about Pinel's cultural presence in the Atlantic world was the volatile political context embedded in his myth. To a large extent, he symbolized the ideas of the French Revolution. In the age of democratic Atlantic revolutions, the French Revolution exemplified the central principles of democratic liberalism: liberty and equality that foresaw the end of man's enslavement and exploitation. Pinel's gesture (the cutting of the chains), though fiction, symbolized the idea that every human being, however maligned, discriminated against, enslaved, deprived, or alienated was entitled to just and fair treatment by public authorities. The mythopoetic power of the gesture would resonate throughout the Atlantic and would cast Pinel, a shy but political provincial intellectual outsider in Paris, as a champion of the disenfranchised and dispossessed. In other words, Pinel came to exemplify the great nineteenth-century Atlantic politicization of mental, and to a degree, public health care. This transatlantic political movement would become nothing less than "the first modern attempt to grapple with the daunting problem of providing health care for an entire needy population."[27] When incipient public health and psychiatric professional communities linked capacious abstract concepts such as freedom to mental health and public health, they inaugurated the development of a new Brazilian social contract based on medical citizenship. Within the state-subject/citizen contract, doctors, in their role as experts, framed themselves as the defenders of the "people." This set of ideas would become as much of a guiding principle for emergent Brazilian psychiatry as the moral treatment itself.

Pinel the Reformer

Born in southern France, Pinel studied medicine in Toulouse and Montpellier. When he arrived in Paris in 1778, he hoped to practice as a doctor. However, he found that due to restrictive regulations, the Paris faculty would not recognize his provincial degree. An outsider, he spent approximately fifteen years earning his living as a writer, translator, and editor. During this same time, he developed an interest in mental illness and began to study the topic intensely. Pinel was particularly interested in the causes and treatments of mental disorders. By the late eighteenth century, Pinel would make impressive strides in the field of mental health. A series of patrons and fortuitous friendships enabled him to become a physician at the Bicêtre hospital in 1793. Under the tutelage of the hospital superintendent Jean-Baptiste Pussin and his wife, Pinel witnessed firsthand the tenets of the moral treatment. In 1795 Pinel was transferred from Bicêtre to its counterpart for women, the Salpétrière. There he progressively refined his approach to mental illness, publishing his notable *Nosographie Philosophique, ou Méthode de l'Analyse* in 1798. Over the next few years, influenced by the work of Scottish physician William Cullen, he published several important "mémoires" that eventually formed the core of his major oeuvre, *Traité Médico-Philosophique sur l'Aliénation Mentale ou la Manie* (1801).[28] These texts show that Pinel's moral treatment called for establishing a personal and intimate relationship between staff and patient not based on violence but on trust and empathy in order to instill faith and hope in the patient on the assumption that insanity, writ large, would be curable.

While Pinel's clinical achievements were notable, they were not novel. Many clinicians in France and elsewhere were experimenting with various manifestations of the moral treatment. Pinel never claimed to be the absolute creator of the moral treatment. From his earliest published references to it, he acknowledged the derivative nature of the concept. He routinely assigned its distant origins to ancient practitioners and credited its contemporaneous English doctors with its use. What Pinel *did* claim was that he was the first to explicate the moral treatment fully. He asserted that "the English rivals perversely touted it while keeping it, for all practical purposes, impenetrably veiled." He also claimed that he was the first to place the technique on a scientific (and accessible) footing.[29] Perhaps the moral treatment's most lasting contribution has been the commitment to isolate, identify, and classify mental diseases, something that Pinel championed. This became the originative psychiatric paradigm, allowing for the progressive creation of an international professional psychiatric community.[30]

Asylum Campaign Movement

Before Pedro I went back to Portugal in 1831, municipal authorities, in an alliance with Medical Society members, began to scrutinize Rio with the deliberate intent of systematically documenting the medical deficiencies of the city as a means to attack the power of the Santa Casa de Misericórdia. In a groundbreaking but characteristically bureaucratic move, the society established six permanent commissions comprising members who advised and wrote reports on issues concerning various urban health matters, engaging—as critics, and on paper—with the perceived pathologies of the city. In 1830 they published a Sanitary Commission Report that indicted hospitals that housed the insane. Often filthy and overcrowded, these places served as mere holding pens. Once the cells were teeming with bodies unable to move, some of the interned would be released onto the streets, only to be later picked up by the police and placed back in a hospital. They reserved their most virulent critiques for the Hospital of the Santa Casa de Misericórdia, the oldest lay religious organization in the city.[31] According to the Sanitary Commission, the mentally ill interned at this institution received "barbaric treatment that not only failed to alleviate their maladies, but aggravated their already disturbed states."[32] The cold baths, whippings, and darkened cells used to control the mad were considered ineffective and outdated practices. Moreover, lumping together patients with mental afflictions that ranged from melancholy to psychotic rage in overcrowded cells was believed to be inhumane and bad medical practice. They argued that the situation was so bad that "many times (commissioners) lost the courage to represent all that was observed, preferring instead to propose the only possible serious reform: destroy the old establishments construct new ones in their place."[33] Given the zealous approach taken by municipal/medical representatives, the Santa Casa and other institutions employed defensive measures to counter a possible takeover. They stressed that the 1828 Law of Municipalities, which authorized the commissions, did not mandate municipal investigations of the internal administrative practices of charity-run institutions because that remained the private domain of individual brotherhoods.[34] Therefore, while the commission could freely inspect the physical structures and spaces of various hospital facilities, it could not inspect the records of specific establishments to examine how resources were accumulated or spent. For Jobim and other Medical Society doctors, the lack of managerial information was particularly vexing, given that his educational experience in Paris impressed upon him the significance of sound management. Preferred techniques including the reallocation of space, the improvement of facilities, the hiring of new staff, and a modernization of revenue collection and spending were paramount to a successful institution. In this manner, the degraded state of the hospital and the types of abuses witnessed regularly in Jobim's capacity as a Santa Casa doctor served as an indictment of the Santa Casa's management structure. However, without solid evidence in the form of bookkeeping or other records, the commission could not substantiate a direct causal relationship between financial mismanagement and poor hospital conditions and nearly nonexistent therapeutic outcomes. Although the clean-slate approach was attractive to reformist politicians and doctors, limited access to revenue, and contested political and cultural fields, kept those ambitions in check. In order to both treat and manage the insane, doctors called for the construction of an asylum that eschewed not only physical punishment and total seclusion but also overt religion, which was quite radical in a city characterized formally by robust Catholicism and informally by ever-growing candomblé.

By the time the Medical Society leveled these criticisms at the Santa Casa during 1830, Emperor Dom Pedro I was already fighting a tide of Brazilian discontent. General anti-Portuguese hostility, mounting Brazilian concern over unpaid Napoleonic War debts, and an angry legislature representing scores of regional interests not aligned with the interests of the court were evidence of a regime under ever-increasing pressure. In April 1831, Emperor Dom Pedro I, like his father before him, departed from Brazil. The emperor left a son, Dom Pedro II (just five years old at the time) behind. Given the young monarch's age, Brazil was to be ruled by a Regency (1831–40). The Regency's main political concern was managing local and regional ambitions for power until Dom Pedro II turned eighteen years old.[35] This political opening emboldened doctors to become vocal advocates for the mentally ill. Building on their earlier critique of the Santa Casa, they initiated a campaign decrying what they felt was the barbaric care for—and immoral neglect of—the confined insane. Their critique was also more fundamental; they objected to the mental health regimes of the Santa Casa as inadequate and unscientific. Working in medical journals, they extended their critique to the quality of the imperial oversight that made such care possible. By the time Dom Pedro I departed in 1831, the Medical Society had enmeshed itself deeply in local politics, finding secular reformist and anti-imperial alliances within the city council of Rio. The council openly solicited the Medical Society to produce reports on various long-standing institutions in the city, some of which, many Society members believed, actually threatened the public's health. As Rio moved slowly toward republican rule, the city council was looking to consolidate its power. Specifically, council members hoped to transfer the traditional responsibilities of the Santa Casa from Catholic and imperial jurisdictions to municipal jurisdiction under a newly created bureaucracy, the Department of Public Health. By calling attention to the depth of the Santa Casa's problems, they hoped imperial authorities would back them in curtailing the role of the Santa Casa as the main provider of social services for the city.[36]

In its formal, commissioned reports, the Royal Society of Medicine expanded on its earlier positions alleging that the mad interned at the Santa Casa received "barbarous treatment." They argued persuasively that instead of "alleviating their disgraces, this institution aggravated their insanity."[37] Reports and articles written by members of the Medical Society stressed the significance of building an institution where madness could not only be medicalized but also managed humanely. Doctors decried the violent methods used to control the insane at the Santa Casa, positioning themselves firmly within Pinel's myth as a protector and liberator of the helpless. In place of Santa Casa violence, they argued that the insane needed an asylum where "they would receive physical and moral treatment that would restore them to reason." In order to do this, activities such as "labor, outdoor exercise, baths, and forms of leisure based on the principles espoused by Pinel and other medical philosophers who, for their reformist spirit, have improved the treatment of the mentally ill in almost all the cities of France, Italy, England, and the United States should be adopted in Brazil."[38] The invocation of Pinel and his therapeutic methods illustrates the extent to which doctors looked to him as a source of authority. In contrasting Brazil with France and other North Atlantic countries, the doctors were also making the case that the adoption of European-style Pinelist treatment of insanity should stand as part of the constellation of modern nationhood.

The documented problems of the Santa Casa cleared the way for members of the Medical Society to take further action. That they were documented primarily by the society itself meant that the society was learning to build structural depth into its critique; this was a strategy that would bring them and other budding scientific professionals results over the upcoming century. Using the imperial connections he had established while head surgeon of the navy, Soares de Meireles attempted to create a higher profile relationship with the imperial ministry to further advance the Medical Society's goals. After some negotiations, the imperial government agreed to elevate the status of the Society of Medicine from a local organization to a national one. In May 1835, the Imperial Academy of Medicine (Academia Imperial de Medicina) replaced its predecessor, thereby strengthening the relationship between imperial authorities and Rio's medical establishment. In an elegant move, the academy established the protocol of appointing the imperial minister honorary president of the organization. Soon the academy relocated from its headquarters in the city to an office in the imperial palace. In addition to Imperial Minister Antônio Paulino Limpo de Abreu, the ten-year-old emperor-in-waiting Dom Pedro II, members of the diplomatic corps, and other distinguished court guests were present at the official inauguration of the nation's foremost medical organization.[39] This group of reformers was growing in ambition and importance within the highest-ranking centers of imperial power.

After this elevation in professional status, the academy expanded the campaign for the creation of a modern asylum and began to lobby state officials on the overall benefits of Pinel's moral treatment. In so doing, they were entering into what would become a protracted contest of myths, ideas, and treatment regimes, with arguably both of the most popular belief structures in Brazil at the time: Catholicism and candomblé. They rejected the view that madness was either a spiritual disease or the result of demonic possession, as well as the traditional bleedings and other physical therapies associated with its cure. These Brazilian doctors, not yet psychiatrists, still applied Pinel's nosology of mental illness toward its cure. In much the same way that the pathogenic city and the Atlantic intellectual world's fear thereof had set the asylum conversation in motion, the moral treatment's approaches to the health of the mind would become the bedrock of Brazilian psychiatry. And the conflicts with Catholic—and later Kardecist spiritism and candomblé social structures would shape its scope of growth.

In 1837 Dr. Antônio L. da Silva Peixoto wrote the first medical thesis on the topic of mental health in Brazil. Titled *General Considerations About Mental Alienation,* the thesis examined madness and its treatments at length. Close scrutiny of this document shows the depth of Pinel's influence on Brazilian doctors interested in the new field of psychiatry. In the thesis, Peixoto explored Pinel's theories on insanity and the ways that a Brazilian moral treatment could improve the lot of the mentally ill. Peixoto's interpretation of the moral treatment proposed that there were four primary types of insanity, each with specific symptoms and manifestations. They consisted of:

melancholia (which exhibits depressive symptoms), mania without delirium (which exhibits overactivity and violence but only affects the mind), mania with delirium (which produces extreme passions and affects both body and mind), and dementia (which exhibits forgetfulness and lack of judgment). This interest in classifying types of madness was both the foundation for the eventual creation of a nuanced suite of treatments and a distinct departure from the Santa Casa's long-standing categories of "violent" and "peaceful."

The moral treatment put forth a four-part therapeutic regimen, which it stipulated would heal all (four) types of insanity if correctly and fully applied. First, physicians and hospital attendants were to be unfailingly kind to patients. Second, repressive methods such as straight jackets and chains were used only when absolutely necessary. Pinel asserted "the general government of the hospital, resembled the superintendence of a great family, consisting of turbulent individuals, whose fury it should be more the object to repress than to exasperate, to govern by wisdom rather than to subdue by terror."[40]

The third principle of moral treatment was labor. According to Pinel, an inactive life was one of the primary causes of insanity. Therefore, physical labor and exercise was one of the best methods by which to actively stimulate body and mind. He claimed that employment and exercise allowed the mind to focus its attention outward and not inward to the site of mental disorder. The fourth and final component called for compassionate management on the part of the head psychiatrist. Although this idea consisted of the aforementioned theories of kind treatment, limited restraint, and physical labor, it also placed emphasis on sound institutional governance. Pinel stressed that a psychiatrist who performs his duty should exhibit "great sagacity, ardent zeal, perpetual and indefatigable attention."[41] Functional management, therefore, meant a psychiatrist's ability to govern the asylum with absolute care and compassion along with fastidious attention to the details of patients' illnesses, treatments, and progress. The moral treatment functionally necessitated the creation of charismatic psychiatrist-managers and the maintenance of an attendant bureaucracy.

In advocating for the moral treatment, doctor-reformers were advocating for the building of the asylum. Although one could theoretically apply the moral treatment at any site, there were aspects of the treatment regime that better promoted patient recovery in a certain kind of dedicated space. In the *Revista Médica Fluminense* journal, Dr. De Simoni not only argued for the creation of an asylum but stressed that it needed to be in "a spacious and serene location with many trees so as to facilitate exercise and running water for baths necessary for the treatment of the mad."[42] Although amusements, recreation, exercise, and kindness were meant to support happiness and activity in the patients, there was one method that would dominate the institutional approach to moral treatment: patient employment. As a further extension of moral and humanitarian treatment, labor was believed to have natural healing powers. Patients could work at a variety of tasks, reinstating their sanity by simply preventing idleness, promoting mind distraction, relieving abnormal brain functions, alleviating symptoms of insanity by physically draining the patients: these tasks gave patients a sense of duty and responsibility while also preparing them for a life producing and consuming outside the asylum. In the words of future asylum medical director Dr. Barbosa, "Manual labor would be without doubt more necessary to the mad than to other men." Viewed as a "powerful curative measure" and "indicated in almost all types of madness, it should not tire the sick but merely provide one with the appropriate distraction, a tranquil dream, and a respite from intellectual functions." He went on to state, "In all of the countries observed where the mad in hospitals are employed in manual labor, the cures are more numerous than other establishments."[43]

It may have been convenient for the reformers, who were asking for support from plantation-based, slave-invested traditional Brazilian power networks to characterize their treatment as partly leading the mad out of their insanity and into a happily working state. It is worth noting here that Brazil's participation in the Atlantic slave trade (though not slavery itself in Brazil) was formally outlawed at approximately the same time (1850) as the actual groundbreaking of the asylum. The end of the slave trade undoubtedly generated multifaceted apprehensions about labor, productivity, and the nation's economic health. One can infer that these concerns, alongside discussions about the merits of a large-scale asylum project to aid the mentally ill, showed up in the same halls of imperial power that Simoni, Peixoto, and their cadre frequented. Whether they knew it or not, they were, among other things, positioning Brazilian psychiatry to be born as an adjunct utility to the institution of Brazilian slavery at a time when that institution may have been understanding its human chattel as less replaceable and therefore more worth repairing.

In their own worldview, Rio's not-yet-psychiatrists' faith in Pinel's labor therapy was greatly influenced by the discourse surrounding slavery. For reformist planners, the rise of industry in mid-nineteenth-century Rio in some ways sidelined the long-standing conversation about slavery and abolition in favor of a conversation about "functional labor." For the Medical Society, the existence of a rational and healthy nation depended on a populace with a work ethic compatible with the dictates of emerging industrial production; for them, the question of whether that population was enslaved or free did radically change their mission. Under these circumstances, the curing-cum-training of the mentally ill as laborers promised an opportunity to recoup economic loss caused by what amounted to a sort of mental breakage and resulting loss of productivity in the workforce. This perspective not only positioned doctors as managers of the mad but also as potential managers of the unruly and unpredictable within a largely African and Afro-Brazilian workforce. As the modernizing project in which psychiatry was born grew, slavery would be abolished, and with significant consequence, psychiatrists would find themselves attempting to manage a panoply of the needy, including those former slaves who offended the public order or the rules of the new economy in any way.

Although the tenets of moral therapy (and specifically labor therapy) found little criticism among state officials, the proposal to build an asylum caused serious controversy because it threatened the Santa Casa brotherhood's monopoly on philanthropic activities in the city. In a conciliatory manner, Pereira chose not to continue seeking the reduced role of the Santa Casa and elected instead to encourage the new emperor, Dom Pedro II, and members of the imperial court to construct an asylum under the Santa Casa's auspices. De Simoni noted that a "building constructed according to the outlook and precepts of medicine, could be capable of turning the alienated into useful persons."[44] The rationale for asylum construction that Pereira put forth to the emperor and other wealthy benefactors hinged on two premises: first, to remove patients deemed insane from the Santa Casa's general hospital as a means of reducing chaos and speeding the recovery of the other patients; and second, to develop an extensive rehabilitation program for the insane based on the tenets of moral treatment.[45]

An adept statesman and politician, Pereira recognized that the newly formed medical elite and its allied city politicians did not want the public health bureaucracy tasked to ensure the well-being of the mentally ill to be dominated by the lay brotherhood and, by association, the royal court. However, he also knew that the Santa Casa still enjoyed significant support among Brazilians and at the Portuguese court and that the lay brotherhood would not easily relinquish its primary charge. In finding a path forward, Pereira stressed that the management of an asylum was irrelevant and that those concerned about the mentally ill should be solely focused on the creation of the asylum. When this failed to fully convince some medical reformers, he promised doctors from the Medical Society some important-sounding posts in the newly built asylum. He also admitted that public health conditions in the city were indeed dire, and he assured the doctors and municipal authorities that the creation of a public health bureaucracy was at the forefront of the imperial government's agenda. This bureaucracy, the Central Board of Public Hygiene, was created in 1850, spurred on by a yellow fever outbreak. Pereira's combined strategy of concession and incentive proved politically effective and the new asylum was to be built with the support of the society but under the auspices of the Santa Casa.

On the day of his coronation on July 18, 1841, the first Brazilian-born emperor, Pedro II, marked the beginning of the Second Empire, the continuation of the monarchy, the unity of the nation, and the founding of the first public asylum in Brazil through Royal Decree 82. The decree authorized the purchase of land in the Praia Vermelha section of the city and the construction of the building. Santa Casa officials placed the symbolic first stone of the building in late 1842. After winning the support of the court and mollifying the Imperial Society of Medicine, Pereira now had to tackle the difficult task of constructing the asylum. A project on the scale of the asylum required large donations to complement the tax revenues generated by the Santa Casa. Furthermore, the asylum project necessitated the construction to be organized in stages so that funds could be raised consecutively. Pereira, who was head of fund-raising, concentrated on rich, single Portuguese men and women who had few (if any) heirs.

Pereira enlisted the rhetorical assistance of the medical community to encourage the rich to bequeath some portion of their estates to the asylum project. De Simoni, the academy's most respected man of letters, made a plea to the wealthy to donate out of a sense of self-interest. He reminded readers that unless a new, more humane insane asylum were built "rich and powerful men" regardless of their "high degree of social elevation and intelligence" might end up suffering the degradations of the old Misericórdia hospital asylum where the wards were so constricting that "even the sky [was] forbidden" from view.[46] Hinting at political pressures that might land persons of high-class standing in asylum wards, De Simoni pointed out that nothing, not even prison, presents "the individual to the risks of being victimized" like having to confront the Santa Casa asylum.[47] He went on to state that "your social position, your authority, your inviolability cannot guarantee you from this jail, from the poor treatment, Pitch in! Help the Santa Casa with your donations." By inference De Simoni suggested that donors would be protected from unnecessary humiliations in case they began to suffer from mental illness.[48]

With the support of De Simoni and the society, Pereira was able to push his tactics further, prevailing on the council to raise taxes on imported goods and on the Imperial Court to permit the Santa Casa to sell titles of nobility to status-obsessed members of Rio's rapidly growing class of nouveau riche. Reflecting upon his method of imposing a clever "luxury" tax, he observed in a private letter, "It was a meritorious project to build a hospital for poor people considered insane with the money of rich fools. The barons and commanders all [will die], but the hospital [for the insane will remain]."[49] He even groomed the young emperor to become the asylum's most important benefactor. In lieu of a customary statue, which other brotherhoods erected for the emperor upon his coronation, the Santa Casa proposed to dedicate the entire asylum in Pedro II's honor, and in turn, the emperor became the guardian of the Hospício Dom Pedro II. The emperor's support of the asylum ensured a constant flow of credit and donations.[50]

These efforts were met with success. On November 30, 1852, religious authorities blessed the asylum, and then on December 5 it opened to great fanfare.[51] The asylum was inaugurated with speeches made by José Clemente Pereira, Dr. José Martins da Cruz Jobim, and Dr. Francisco de P. Cândido in a ceremony in which faith, philanthropy, and science commingled to commemorate a compromise effort and a hybrid victory. The ceremony drew a large crowd including the archbishop of Rio and many members of the royal court.[52] By most accounts, those in attendance were greatly impressed with the building's architecture. It was politically appropriate that the building's large-scale design and stunning decorative details suited the grandeur of its greatest benefactor and namesake, the Emperor Dom Pedro II.

It was also only appropriate that the building's architecture be carefully planned to restore an irrational mind to reason. As scholar Christine Stevenson states, "Asylum appearances mattered in the same way their plans did; actively, instrumentally, in themselves therapies."[53] Pereira took great care to consult doctors regarding the optimum asylum design, since nineteenth-century psychiatrists considered the architecture and planning of their hospitals to be one of the most powerful tools for the treatment of the insane. The influence of Pinel and other French psychiatrists was visible in the layout and decorative details of the asylum. Planned by architects Domingos Monteiro, José Maria Jacinto Rebelo, and Joaquim Cândido Guillobel, the asylum was designed as one large rectangle with four large internal patios separated by one central bloc. The design was modeled after the famed Maison Nationale d'Aliénés. Created in 1796 in the Parisian suburb of Charenton, it was the flagship welfare institution for the mentally ill in France. Medical and state officials in Rio de Janeiro hoped that the Hospício Dom Pedro II would become a beacon of hope for the mentally disturbed inside and outside of Brazil. "Certainly in that moment, it was one of the best psychiatric hospitals in the world. Apart from clean cells, music, open spaces with gardens, and offices to perform clerical tasks were readily available so as to enhance therapy."[54]

Though architecturally austere, the asylum boasted seven statues made from coveted marble imported from Carrara, Italy:[55] two allegorical embodiments of Science and Charity, Emperor Dom Pedro II, José Clemente Pereira, Saint Peter of Alcântara, Philippe Pinel, and his notable student Jean-Étienne Dominique Esquirol. While Science and Charity guarded the entrance of the asylum, the statues of Dom Pedro II, Pereira, and Saint Peter of Alcântara were placed in different salon rooms. The statues of Pinel and Esquirol were placed outside the male and female wing, respectively. The powers that made the asylum clearly chose this pantheon of statues to represent the collaboration between medical, religious, and state authorities and to show respect to austere Catholic religious traditions and to French psychiatry. This grouping also shows a certain flexibility in the shuffling of myth, idea, and man in the leveling between Charity and Pinel, Dom Pedro II, and Science. This kind of cultural flexibility would both allow the newly minted psychiatrists room to build into the powerful force they would become, and in the end, it would also deeply frustrate their orderly and hierarchical city plans.

The building itself was one of the most impressive and largest buildings in the city (fig. 1.1). With its adjacent park and isolation spaces, it occupied an area of 140,000 square meters.[56] Referred to by city residents as the Palace of the Mad, it was commonplace for pedestrians to stop and look in awe at the majestic institution. The overall design and humanist medical vision greatly impressed national and international visitors. Foreign missionaries Daniel P. Kidder and Daniel Cooley Fletcher observed that "the Lunatic Asylum, or, as it is officially called, the Hospício de Pedro II, situated on the graceful Bay of Botafogo, is a splendid, palace-like structure inaugurated in 1852."[57] In a surprise visit to the facility, the notable Swiss-born American scientist Louis Agassiz and his wife, educator Elizabeth Agassiz, characterized the asylum as a "model of neatness and order." Moreover, they noted the serenity, which seemed apparent among patients that they saw during their short stay:

> As we went up the spacious staircase, the sound of music brought us to the door of the chapel, where the evening service was going on. Patients and nurses were kneeling together; a choir of female voices was singing sweetly a calm, peaceful kind of music; that somewhat monotonous chanting, so passionless in its regular movement, which one hears in the Catholic Church; the candles were burning before the altar, but the great window just outside the door was open to the setting sun, and, as I stood in the balcony looking out on the mountains and listening to the music, I thought that a mind which had gone astray might find its way back again in such scenes and under such influences. Certainly, if nature has any healing power, it must be felt here.[58]

It was in this optimistic environment that two of the doctors of the Imperial Society would be employed going forward, becoming Brazil's first experienced, secular, and scientific mental health professionals. The process of becoming experienced would coincide with the formal emergence of psychiatry, and with that, a clearer picture of what psychiatric care in its actual execution would entail. According to "Project of the Hospício Pedro II Statutes," the functioning of the asylum was divided into three parts: the administrative, the medical, and the religious. At its inauguration the asylum received 140 patients, of which Pereira listed 74 men and 66 women, of which 126 were classified as quiet, 10 as agitated and 4 as unclean. Most of the patients came from the city of Rio, with a smattering from around the country.[59] However, this number would grow to three hundred (150 men and 150 women) by 1854, when the building was completely finished. The

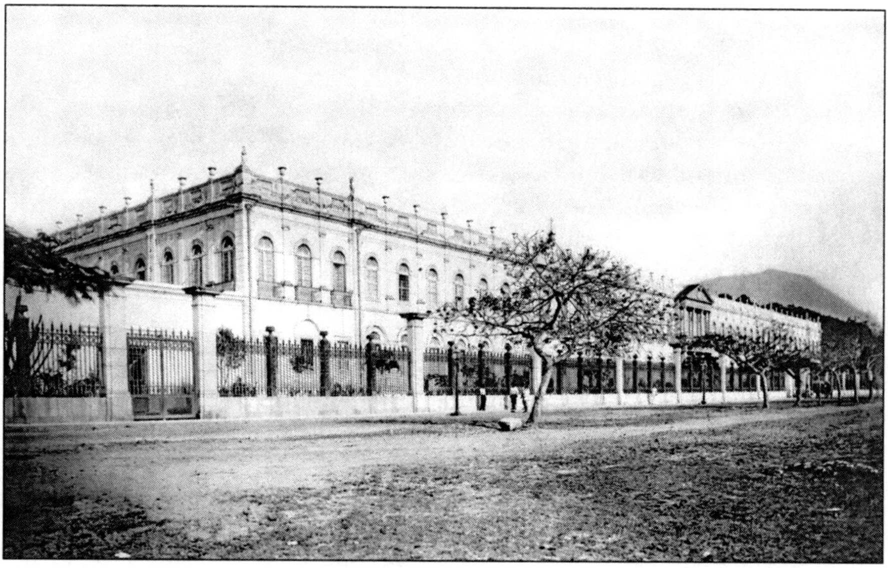

Figure 1.1. Hospício Dom Pedro II, built in 1852. *Hospicio de Pedro Segundo: Praia Vermelha* by Pieter Godfred Bertichem, 1856 lithograph, Biblioteca Nacional (National Library) of Rio de Janeiro.

doors to the asylum were open to "the mentally ill of both sexes throughout the empire, without distinction to condition, naturalization, or religion." Although all were presumably equal in their path toward institutionalization, stark differences separated patients once they entered the asylum. Apart from the division of sexes, residents were divided according to socioeconomic status: pensioners (patients for whom someone was paying), and those admitted "freely" (i.e., the indigent; slaves whose masters did not have the means to, or interest in, paying for their treatment; and sailors from merchant ships). First-class pensioners were entitled to a private room, second-class pensioners occupied a two-person room, while third-class pensioners, who consisted of free people of color and slaves, occupied the general wards. Patients were also segregated by comportment. The freely admitted indigents and third-class pensioners were divided along the following lines: (1) the tranquil clean, (2) the agitated, (3) the filthy, and (4) the affected by accidental diseases. First- and second-class pensioners would only be divided into the following: (1) tranquil and (2) agitated. Segregation based on social status and behavior was paramount since economic and social "promiscuity" among the mentally ill was thought to create "confusion, disorder, and anarchy [since] the idea of creating categories in the classification of mental illness . . . is an undeniable necessity in the moral, hygienic, and disciplinary running of the establishment."[60]

Conclusion

By the mid-nineteenth century, Rio's preeminence in Brazil was affirmed as the economy soared and the focus of export activity and real political power shifted from the northeast to the center-south regions. Rio's political leaders hoped that the city's dynamic development would lure foreign investors, while coffee and other exports would contribute to the city's reputation as an important trading center. As the country's capital, Rio was meant to be the showcase of Brazil's sociopolitical, economic, and cultural transformation from a backward monarchy—and a tropical backwater—to a modern capitalist state. In many ways, Brazilian modernists wanted to prove to themselves as well as an Atlantic community that Brazil could be a modern state and that they could create the necessary institutions from Brazil's existing culture, infrastructure, and populace. The struggles over where and how to manage the mentally ill were struggles between medical modernities and competing religious traditionalisms. On one hand, it was believed that the marriage of clinical austerity and the benevolent care of skilled medical psychiatrists in a secular site would be able to cure the mentally ill. On the other hand, it was commonly thought that the care of the infirm fell under the power and control of the royal court and its largely Catholic institutions. As doctors attempted to introduce new social policies to manage and improve the characteristics of city residents, traditional Catholic charity also became a symbolic field on which the emperor could display paternalistic and personal concern for the welfare of his subjects. The peculiarity of imperial modernity in the mid-empire period was this utterly improbable arena of political contest, compromise, and coexistence: the welfare of the population represented an end in itself for emerging medical bureaucracies, and at the same time it became a means for establishing both the legitimacy of all of the concerned parties and the power of the sovereign.

Furthermore, as the local chapter of the most prestigious lay brotherhood in the Portuguese world, the Misericórdia's careful selection of its members, based on lineage, wealth, and profession, provided many of the city's elite with an institutionalized measure of status. As historian Isabel dos Guimarães Sá asserts,

> Although the misericórdias played a leading role in local politics through their elite membership . . . , they were always allies of the king, to whom they answered directly. Their autonomy from Episcopal authority, together with their religious ideology in conformity with Catholic doctrine, made the misericórdias an institution that occupied an intermediate position between lay and ecclesiastical authorities, between central and local institutions, between the early modern state and local prerogatives.[61]

Fashioned after their counterparts in Lisbon, the Misericórdia signified the ability of the colonial order to reproduce not only metropolitan institutions but also metropolitan values such as piety, charity, propriety, and virtue. The Santa Casas had played an important role in Portuguese colonial societies by providing many of the social welfare services. A departure from this tradition represented a rupture in the sociocultural, political, and economic fabric of Brazilian society.

To critique the Santa Casa was to critique the imperial government, old networks of power and patronage, and the politics of care in the capital of the empire. Denunciations of the Santa Casa by a burgeoning urban elite influenced by Enlightenment ideals were an attempt to wrest power away from a colonial institution seen as too inept to handle the new challenges that came with urbanization, modernization, and the emergence of a post-colonial multiracial and multicultural society fraught with the real fears and extravagant rumors that prevailed. Pereira and others in the imperial government were able to directly confront the challenge of creating an institution for the mentally ill compatible with the modernizing goals of the new elite. The creation of the asylum—a political compromise built in stone—was touted as a political triumph, albeit briefly, for the imperial government. As a symbol, the asylum illustrated the political grandeur and the benevolent moral economy of the imperial state. For doctors the asylum was more complicated. It functioned as proof of bureaucratic and political prowess. Where once there had been only the Santa Casa, now there was a hybrid institution, one still largely under the control of religious authorities to be sure but dedicated to the scientific principles of the moral treatment. They had challenged the Santa Casa, and against generationally long odds, had gained some ground. This would inform Brazilian psychiatry's organizational structures and its sense of its own paths to empowerment moving forward.

The asylum would also, perhaps most critically for psychiatry, serve as a place in which to develop psychiatric knowledge and a place from which to both participate in Atlantic conversations with international psychiatry. Eventually, it would also launch further criticism of religious authorities. And at the intersection of all of these purposes, the asylum, in its physical work, was also meant to be a revolutionary healing technology. It was meant to be a new terrain for the reenactment of psychiatry's foundational myth, Pinel's gesture. Spurious though it was, doctors' dedication to the story illustrates the real, diagnostic, and curative optimism that marked the beginnings of a new approach to madness. Doctors approached the management of madness in Rio with the aspirational language of idealistic reformers; their time in the Hospício Dom Pedro II would season that language as they themselves took on more responsibility for the patients of the asylum. They placed the asylum building campaign and the modernizing movement in which it grew, in a public frame, using the mythic utopian zeal of Pinel and the ideals of the French Revolution as a means to galvanize their professional peers to provide order in the streets of the city and solace to the city's vulnerable mentally ill population.

Chapter Two

"Of Grand Intentions" and "Opaque Structures"

The Fight for Psychiatric Management of the Hospício Pedro II during Brazil's Second Empire, 1852–90

Born out of a political negotiation between religious officials from the Santa Casa de Misericórdia Catholic lay brotherhood, the imperial government, and the medical community in Rio de Janeiro, the Hospício Pedro II embodied the groups' often-conflicting hopes and plans. Each side envisioned a hybridization of medical and religious knowledge that might restore insane minds to reason and represent a new mode of therapeutics for insanity and a new sociopolitical experiment in collaborative governance; however, each envisioned it differently. Politically shaken by the crisis of legitimacy during the Regency period, the imperial government saw the asylum as an opportunity to project a magnanimous image of state power.[1] Experiencing multiple erosions of traditional religiosity, the Catholic lay brotherhood hoped to stake a new public claim to relevance by underscoring their roles as caregivers in a public partnership with doctors in which they intended to hold control. Doctors, in turn, viewed the very creation of the asylum, and its rhetorical commitment to the moral treatment, as a medical victory and hoped to use it to incubate and eventually launch the psychiatric profession and an array of attendant social reforms.

Compromise and power sharing between religious officials and asylum doctors inside the asylum inevitably failed, with each party diverting its energies to fighting the other and defending their respective domains rather than addressing the problems of the insane. Instead of serving as constructive checks and balances, rivals served as scapegoats for problems, and the asylum became a political battleground rather than a rational center for compassionate bureaucratic management. This chapter chronicles the complex contest over the governance of the Hospício Pedro II, which ultimately involved the French nun order, the Daughters of Charity, as well as the Brazilian Santa Casa Catholic lay brotherhood, emergent psychiatrists, and the state. It investigates how psychiatrists, as apostles of professional rationality, developed their ideas about reason and bureaucratic power in this contested site of religious charity between 1852 and 1890.[2]

Although these groups shared some ideological ground, agreeing for example that the insane needed to be secluded in the asylum, I argue that they brought divergent and entangled epistemologies about the constructions of madness, its treatment, and its bureaucratic governance. Chapter 1 closely examined the intellectual work of Brazilian doctors in which they charged that the imperial state had a responsibility to provide asylums to manage insanity as a problem within the urban population over which it claimed control. It demonstrated that Brazilian doctors increasingly sought to claim a medical and moral responsibility for the insane on behalf of the state, despite the incipient nature of medical infrastructure. This chapter looks at what doctors and others believed followed from that responsibility. By focusing on bureaucratic struggles and boundary work preservation between psychiatrists and their adversaries, it explores how psychiatrists used both their real works in the asylum and their articulated Pinelist intentions to ground their nascent but fast-growing profession. The governance frameworks they created in the asylum to care for, survey, and manage the insane inside the asylum were central, but their critiques of the Santa Casa employee management practices as techniques of power and as performances of both professional and moral commitment also became important in their rationale for being and growth. Psychiatrists' relentless activism and calls for asylum reform did garner them a degree of political clout, prompting state officials to grant them a series of professional concessions. As such, this narrative highlights how medicine and its institutional forms affected Brazilian state formation and, conversely, how practices of governance influenced bureaucratic cultures of Brazilian medicine and their relationship with religion.[3] Critically, this intra-elite conflict was the most important process work as it related to treating the mentally ill; this was different from treating the mentally ill themselves, given that it laid the groundwork from which doctors would be free not only to exercise therapeutic regimens but also to exercise the bureaucratic muscles to expand the reach of the psychiatric profession.

It cannot be taken for granted that the gendered values of psychiatrists aligned with those of patriarchy. As adherents of the moral treatment, early psychiatrists imagined themselves as father figures within the vast household of the asylum. The authority of the psychiatrist must be of prime importance so that patients would obey him and allow him to lead them to rationality. Deference, on the part of both staff and patients, to his rule was paramount. Although the position of psychiatric authority in the asylum (as in other medical contexts in the Atlantic world) sidelined women in positions of medical and managerial leadership, it did not preclude the exclusion of women as workers. Psychiatrists' self-presentations indicate a belief in gender complementarity wherein they performed expert labor related to the "curing" of mental illness and the direct management of patients while the Daughters of Charity provided the wraparound services, including most of the hands-on care, to facilitate and enhance the work of doctors.

Historians often portray Brazil as a unique outsider in nineteenth-century Latin American history. Events such as the transplantation of the Portuguese Court from Lisbon to Rio de Janeiro in 1808, the elevation of the colony to the status of co-kingdom with Portugal in 1822, and the near-bloodless final transition from monarchy to republic in 1889 have all led historians to picture the Brazilian state as remarkably successful in accomplishing important policy goals with little interference from antagonistic oligarchs or mass movements. Much of Latin America has lacked Brazil's stability. Mexico, with its turbulent periods of foreign military intervention, or Argentina, with its bloody conflicts between capital and hinterland, are prime examples. This does not mean that Brazilian development was without deep acrimonious conflict and precarious passages; on the ground sociopolitical and cultural conflicts among elites and between elites and nonelites affected both the micro- and macro-workings of state formation. Analyzing asylum bureaucracy alongside sociopolitical developments reveals oscillations in government policy and in the effective control that the government had over its institutions during the long nineteenth century, which complicates the narratives of stable governance and opens new approaches to bureaucratic battles and the cultures that they created.

Since psychiatry was an emergent profession in mid-nineteenth century Rio, proto-psychiatrists generated a plethora of material about the asylum as they wrote theses, journal articles, and asylum reports, among other texts. In constructing its own forms of legitimacy, psychiatry defined its initial audience and demonstrated its claims of expertise primarily for local and imperial state officials, foreign psychiatrists, other Brazilian doctors, and in rivalry, for Santa Casa religious officials. By molding their version of the profession's contours to negate the values of religious management of insanity, doctors used the body of knowledge they were creating to solidify their authority as expert men in the context of memo and journal. Religious figures, on the other hand, did not produce nuanced intellectual treatises on asylum management, effectively ceding an arena they thought was unimportant to the doctors. Santa Casa asylum managers' archival residues mainly consist of reports on the mundane operations of the asylum sprinkled with sporadic responses to the steady flow of medical denouncements that undermined their authority. While I examine these residual echoes in order to explore religious figures' articulations of insanity management and care, the doctors' foundational Pinelist belief in archive creation means that their writings necessarily provide my primary point of entry into an exploration of asylum governance, structure, and culture.

The Santa Casa de Misericórdia and the Care for the Mentally Ill, 1852–58

Created in Lisbon in 1498, the Santa Casa was a paradoxical institution. Although its foundation was credited to devout Catholics, both lay and ecclesiastical, from the beginning it was operating under royal patronage. By the early sixteenth century, it held responsibility for the management of virtually all of the charitable services throughout the Portuguese Empire.[4] An overview of its administrative structure illustrates the extent to which this institution reproduced a locale's status quo. Although the Santa Casa's membership included individuals from the gentry, the professional classes, ecclesiastics, and plebeians, its members had to be male, of good repute, God fearing, serve the brotherhood without question, and congregate when summoned by the order. The brotherhood barred individuals of black, indigenous, and Jewish ancestry. A *mesa*, or board of guardians, that consisted of thirteen brothers from the upper and lower classes, carried out the key duties of the brotherhood. The board consisted of a scribe, nine counselors, two stewards, and the *provedor*, or president, all of whom were elected for a yearly term.[5] Membership could be up to six hundred people in a given locale and covered a broad section of society, but the president was always chosen from the upper class. Even though the president was expected to defend the Misericórdia against the incursions of civil and ecclesiastical authorities, his position offered little autonomy. Only in minor decisions did he exert independence of action since he was obligated to convene the board on all matters of policy.[6] The prestige of the brotherhood was such that governors, viceroys, archbishops, and ministers of justice often coveted the role of Santa Casa president and frequently served in that capacity. The Santa Casa was, part and parcel, traditional Brazil.

During the period under examination, all the presidents of the Santa Casa were active or past politicians at the local or national level. For example, during his tenure as Santa Casa president, Pereira was deputy general (1838–41) and senator (1842–54) of Rio de Janeiro. Even though the Santa Casa was an independent institution, the decision of the brotherhood to annually elect politicians, and politicians' willingness to serve the lay brotherhood, reveals deep links between civil, state, and religious actors in the provision of social assistance to the needy. One of the key functions of the Santa Casa was the distribution of alms, or material aid and social services to the "deserving poor" and needy, which depended on the contributions of wealthy city residents. Charity in this context, as historian Miri Rubin posits, reflected the elite's perception of its social and religious obligations (to serve their own social standings and souls), rather than an effort to meet the actual needs of the poor.[7]

As a long-standing institution of imperial charity, prior to the construction of the asylum the Santa Casa offered a loose and attenuated system of care for the insane, housing the mad with other marginal populations, including the diseased, prostitutes, and vagrants. Doctors' denunciations of the "barbaric treatment" of the insane in this institution during the 1830s, as well as the fund-raising efforts of José Clemente Pereira, head of the lay brotherhood at the time (1838–54), ultimately convinced imperial authorities to construct an asylum. The simultaneous restructuring of the political system and creation of a national medical system greatly facilitated and impacted the eventual contours of the institutionalization of madness in Brazil. In the process, politics and medicine became the central arenas of contact between the asylum (and madness itself), on the one hand, and state and society, on the other.

State representatives decided to annex control and internal management of the asylum to the Santa Casa because the hospital and the imperial government enjoyed a mutually beneficial relationship in which each confirmed and legitimized the other.[8] Neither the barely nascent psychiatric profession nor the city council of Rio could offer equivalent bureaucratic and actual asylum-running man and womanpower, or the international goodwill that collaborations with the Catholic Church had traditionally given them. The subcontracting of assistance work to the Santa Casa also allowed the imperial government to assume fewer daily responsibilities, while taking credit when convenient for a welfare system highly visible to its subject-citizens. Imperial statesmen were also happy to entrust the asylum to the Santa Casa because it allowed some of the most powerful men in Luso-Brazilian politics to show their Christian charity without directly committing the state to costly social programs or the creation of an effective and resilient infrastructure of care. When imperial officials and Santa Casa president Pereira took on the construction and management of the asylum acquiesced to medical pressure to construct an asylum, inclusive promises made to medical establishment supporters were not forgotten, although as will become evident they were remembered primarily in name. Pereira dispatched Dr. Antônio José Pereira das Neves to France for two years so that he could study the "model psychiatric establishments" as a means to transplant the best psychiatric practices to Rio.[9] Beyond the importation of ideas, the Santa Casa director also recruited actual French professional nurses, bringing the Daughters of Charity nuns from Paris to Rio based on their reputation as premier hospital managers and nurses.[10] Historian Colin Jones's research on the Daughters as a Catholic order in seventeenth-century France depicts them as a centralized and tightly supervised organization where caring for the sick and poor took precedence over all of their other obligations, including religious devotions. It also shows that the nuns of the order were well-respected as hospital administrators in many poor-relief institutions and even as independent medical practitioners in their own right.[11]

The Santa Casa's decision to recruit French nuns to perform the work of charity in the Hospício Pedro II deviated from the brotherhood's traditions. The all-male Misericórdia adhered to a gendered notion of charity. Although their symbolic figurehead was Mary, the mother of Christ, men had traditionally performed the actual charity. This rupture in policy reflected the difficulty of an institutionally weak Brazilian Catholic Church in defining their proper public sphere of influence in competition from other religions. Moreover, it reflected the brotherhood's attempt to radically rejuvenate the Catholic Church. The Daughters of Charity had earned a transatlantic reputation as especially devoted and capable women who took on the role of nurses in the secular world while maintaining strong religious identities. Notably, their devotion to Catholicism was ostentatiously presented to communities through their wearing of the dark blue and white habits. This habit was both incongruous and conspicuous, an affirmation to the wearers and a dramatic "sign of consecration and a witness to poverty."[12] The Daughters of Charity were recognized as women who had decided to commit their whole life fully to God. Their partnership with Brazilian state and religious officials was part of, and significant to, the broader goals of the Catholic apostolic mission of ultramontanism, the belief that the papacy is and should be at the center of the church.[13] Since the Daughters represented the powerful combination of asceticism and pious service that often led them to be depicted as the physical embodiment of Mary, their work in the asylum can be understood as the Santa Casa's attempt to recenter the Brazilian Catholic Church on its strengths while the church was, for the first time, in collaboration, however slight, with the new scientific officials.[14]

Against the backdrop of Catholic revivalism and French cultural affinity,[15] the final agreement between Pereira and João Marques Lisboa, commander of the Imperial Brazilian Legation in Paris, gave the Daughters great authority in the Hospício Pedro II.[16] The nuns were subordinate only to the board of the Santa Casa, although they were technically obligated to follow the laws, decrees, and regulations of the brotherhood. While the Santa Casa board had responsibility for and control of the asylum, they endowed the Daughters of Charity full responsibility for the administration and religious divisions. They appointed a special three-brother board to in turn appoint a single medical doctor to the titular post of director overseeing the institution's medical and economic services, as well as two doctors to work under him, each of whom was titled to oversee one gender-segregated ward.[17] In the medical department, the Daughters of Charity served as nurses for the female population, nurse supervisors for the entire asylum and were tasked with providing support for the doctors as needed.[18] In the economic department, the Daughters would also supervise the pharmacy and occupational therapy rooms, in addition to all services related to the kitchen, dining hall, laundry room, and clothing closets.[19] In exchange for their services, the nuns received free room and board and a modest annual allowance to support their clothing budgets.[20] Doctors were a bit like the nobles promised titles by Pereira during the asylum campaign movement: the titles received held little substantial weight to influence meaningful processes. The asylum's medical director did not have control over the care being given because the Daughters of Charity neither believed in his goals nor were they answerable to him, and the administrative decisions were outside his purview. He was, thus, director in name only. He, along with the doctors under his direction, would be better understood primarily as psychiatric observers in the Catholic asylum. They would find their sources of power outside the asylum walls and use that power to increase their influence, but it would be almost thirty years before they saw any real change in status. During that time, it was abundantly clear that the Daughters of Charity were in control of the asylum.

Religious authorities understood the Hospício Dom Pedro II not as an asylum but as a general hospital. The idea of a hospital as a site where the sick were treated therapeutically and cured is a relatively late historical phenomenon. In the nineteenth-century Atlantic World, and anywhere where the Catholic Church was founding and running houses for the sick, the concept-goal of such places was something distinctly other. The word *hospital* has its etymological roots in the Latin *hospes*, meaning a kind of guest room. Until the seventeenth century, most of western Europe followed the ancient definition by allocating space more for the purpose of easing the sick into death rather than providing therapeutic intervention. Since the hospital remained subordinate to ecclesiastics and their associated lay interests, the logos of preparing the soul for its postmortem journey became one of its primary rationales—even though in the case of the mentally ill, some of the patients might live there for decades. This would take on great significance and urgency in the nineteenth century throughout the Atlantic World since, as historian Michael J. Steiner suggests, the rise of epidemics changed the meanings associated with death, in that the frequent possibilities of unexpected death during the sickly seasons led to a bifurcated understanding of death as either "good" or "bad."[21] The proliferation of diseased dead bodies led to a naturalization of death wherein bodies materialized in morgues, cemeteries, lecture rooms, and museums. In order to make death less profane, the hospital space then became imbued with sacred meaning so as to facilitate one's good death. When looking at the waves of epidemic disease that threatened nineteenth-century Rio, it becomes highly probable that the leadership of the Santa Casa and the Daughters of Charity themselves subscribed to this understanding of the asylum-hospital space as a passageway from life to death.

The Daughters were a strict and hardworking order, devoted to a life of chastity and service, and the women who came to Brazil were no exception; their reputation landed them the lion's share of the work that needed doing in the asylum. They were also an independent minded and capable group of women; in an environment of evident and public discord between psychiatrists and Santa Casa administrators, they embraced both nursing and management as their divinely ordained missions and parlayed their ubiquity in the asylum into significant control over the institution as a whole. What differentiated the Daughters of Charity from other kinds of nurses was their value-driven approach to sickness and healing; they pledged to use exceptional care to "reveal the healing presence of God" by acting "as God might act." They embraced their independent duties, skills, and responsibilities with a mix of deeply held values and religious devotion since they were part of "Christ's militia."[22] The Santa Casa board seemed content to stay out of the way of these pious, effective women-in-habits; the Daughters enjoyed deep international Catholic respect, and the Santa Casa did not want the work of directly caring for the mad. Doctors-cum-psychiatrists, with their budding professional desire for just that responsibility, would chafe under the Daughters' leadership.

Members of the Santa Casa Lay Brotherhood and the Daughters of Charity came to the asylum with long-established reputations as hospital managers, but the doctors chosen by the Santa Casa for the asylum posts brought very little professional expertise related to either bureaucratic governance or the treatment of insanity. While doctors with specific formal training in mental health were scarce in Brazil, doctors such as Simoni, who had extensive management experience and a high public profile, were either not offered or declined titular asylum positions. The doctors that did so typically had extensive training in clinical medicine and earned their medical degrees at the Rio de Janeiro College of Medicine, but in the first twenty-seven years of the asylum's existence, they did not have formal training in mental illness.[23] These novices closely followed developments in European psychiatric theories through books and journals and often traveled to Europe to study and to train with practicing psychiatrists. When Dr. Manoel José Barbosa assumed the position of first asylum medical director (1853–66),[24] he expressed great insecurity since he was not "qualified" to "talk about mental illness therapy, so difficult to cure."[25] Whether by Santa Casa design or not, the actual responsibilities of the post of director were commensurate with his confidence in the arena of mental health. It is no surprise then that until 1879, none of the "medical directors" within the asylum were part of the Imperial Academy of Medicine, the prestigious professional group that campaigned for the creation of the asylum during the 1830s. Doctors who served in the asylum were generally low-profile medical doctors who hoped to use the opportunity to not only learn about insanity and to experiment with different treatment models but to also network themselves into the nascent medico-state structure, for the albeit slim chance of long-term professional gain.

Dr. Barbosa was not mistaken when he said that he, and by extension the medical community, had much to learn about asylum management. Still, he and the men who would follow in his immediate professional footsteps would develop a method of advocacy from their postings-without-powers through steadfast observation. Treatment in the asylum under the Daughters was pragmatic and eclectic, reflecting both the belief in the manifold causes of insanity and the various and intertwined functions of a treatment. Therapy was divided into two categories, moral (psychological) and somatic (physical) treatments. While the moral treatment sought to control, manage, and make an impression on the mind, somatic, or "indirect methods" of treatment (e.g., blood purgings, the administration of emetics, purgatives, and blistering agents) acted on the mind indirectly through the body. As doctors tended to aspects of the moral treatment, the Daughters of Charity primarily supervised the somatic methods of treatment. This division of labor supposedly yielded separate spheres of influence whereby the labors of doctors and nuns would complement each other in a strangely gendered way, as the women cared for the bodies of the mad and the men cared for their minds. When Barbosa assumed medical directorship of the asylum in 1853, there were 136 patients, 10 nurses, and 10 Daughters of Charity nuns.[26] Thus, it can be inferred that the somatic treatments reached many more patients than the moral treatment did; it was, after all the Daughters' asylum, and the moral treatment was not their professed therapy of choice. The compromise cobbled together by the charismatic Pereira, one that worked so well as a culture of fund-raising, did not long remain functional while in actual contact with the asylum.

Contestations over Bureaucratic and Therapeutic Management, 1858–79

It took about six years for the doctors to become completely disenchanted with the asylum as administered by the Daughters and to find an arena that played to their strengths. Given the structures put in place by the Santa

Casa and cultures of care in play, the only real power position available to the doctors was outside the asylum walls. First and foremost, the doctors had the bureaucratic busywork of writing annual reports to the Santa Casa director. Ambitious and in the lower ranks of their own profession, the doctors began by denouncing their partners' methods and presenting a litany of problems in need of reform in their reports to the Santa Casa director. They followed that up with letters to state officials covering the same concerns. By classifying a series of practices as symptomatic of bad governance, they quickly established a relationship based on antagonism and suspicion with the lay brotherhood. They also used an aspirational process of public critique to project what the asylum might look like under their control. They criticized the admissions process that led to incomplete patient files and overcrowding. According to Dr. Barbosa, indiscriminate admissions of the "incurable indigent," the "turbulent and agitated," and the "paralytics, idiots, and epileptics" was the main cause of overcrowding and the asylum's high mortality rate.[27] He argued the asylum had admitted people who were incurable and burdensome:

> Without hope of recovering their reason, they live as automatons, or rather, they vegetate inoffensively. In this regard, after speaking to the director of the Santa Casa de Misericórdia more than once, I have taken the opportunity to remind him the necessity to remove the idiots and the epileptics among the alienated. They are indeed burdens to the asylum and certainly they should not be here.[28]

Dr. Barbosa's comment expressed a preoccupation of many psychiatrists during the latter half of the nineteenth century: the curability of madness. "Cured" patients validated the effectiveness of treatments and the primacy of the doctor in the hierarchy of asylum caretakers. Asylum doctors argued that the chronically mentally ill jeopardized others' progress by aggravating their already delicate states and diverting the attention of asylum staff. While the chronically insane consumed precious time and resources at the asylum, their presence, resistance, and immunity to the psychiatric therapeutic toolkit exposed the fallibility of a profession still fragile in its infancy. Meanwhile, in the Daughters' worldview, if a person needed care and support for decades as they moved toward death, then the Daughters would be rewarded in heaven for providing that care. It is worth noting as well that the Daughters, based on their Atlantic reputations, were consummate professionals and familiar with the mix of people that often found themselves inside a nineteenth-century asylum. The doctors, on the other hand, pointed their critiques at the Daughters of Charity, even when they were better understood as systemic complaints about the incompleteness of the infrastructure of care.

Doctors' objections to asylum procedures extended to the Daughters of Charity as well. They advocated for a new ethos of nursing and a new kind of nurse. Care was not an abstraction to be managed but an intimate relationship with medical, moral, and ethical components. From the perspective of doctors, nurses and other personnel were supposed to be subservient to the psychiatrist, conscientious, and scrupulous. Characterizing the preferred qualities of a nurse prior to the institution's opening, Dr. Luiz Vicente De Simoni, a key figure in the asylum movement campaign, advocated that "a nurse of an alienated [person] should wed severity with sweetness, bravery with prudence, discretion and charity and a certain intellectual sphere to understand the ill. [He] should be honest, active, industrious, intelligent, and with much experience."[29] Dr. Barbosa claimed that the actual nurses hired failed to meet this standard. His 1855 asylum report to the Santa Casa director emphasized that

> in the male division, there are twelve nurses under the immediate supervision of the Daughters of Charity. Generally, these employees serve poorly and they do not deserve any confidence. It is necessary to watch over them constantly, punish them often, fire them, etc. That is not, however, surprising: everyone knows the kind of men that among us would lend himself to a genre of service by the amount of 24 mil reis monthly.[30]

Dr. Barbosa also attacked the Daughters' competency as managers.[31] Such criticisms by doctors escalated after 1858, when the Santa Casa board formally gave the Daughters of Charity's mother superior authority over the nurses in addition to economic affairs. This contentious issue reached its zenith with the death of a patient, Sant'Anna, on January 18, 1874. Doctors Luis José da Silva, Custodio Nunes, and Ignácio Francisco Goulart, the medical director at the time, suspected that nurse Antonio de Oliveira had caused the patient's death, which occurred in isolation in a straitjacket after de Oliveira subdued and isolated him. According to Dr. Goulart, de Oliveira considered the insane as feral violent animals and had treated Sant' Anna accordingly. He argued that "it would be better to leave these abandoned unfortunates on city streets rather than to provide them with shelter here [asylum], under the cover of pseudo-charity" than subject them to "what the nurses do with their brutalities; only later to treat them like assassins and furious dogs, when they act in self-defense."[32] Goulart condemned the culture of impunity sanctioned by the Daughters of Charity. The doctors were learning about running an asylum, certainly, but at the same time (and perhaps to a much greater degree) they were enhancing their ability to manipulate the bureaucratic powers to their ends.

They quickly moved beyond formal complaints to the Santa Casa Board. Addressing imperial state administrators through letters, doctors depicted the asylum, within just a few years of its creation, as an ambiguous entity whose goals vacillated between perfunctory charity (i.e., to house and care for the incurable or chronically mentally ill) and rehabilitative therapeutic assistance (i.e., to treat the curable mentally ill so that they could return to society). They portrayed themselves as the sole defenders of the mentally ill against the nuns and their auxiliary nurses who provided inefficient and potentially perilous treatment as well as the Santa Casa brothers who mismanaged the asylum's infrastructure of governance. They staged performances of expertise and curative caring for state administrators. They also self-consciously performed psychiatry for other Brazilian doctors in articles and dispatches about asylum life in medical journals. In this they continued an existent narrative, building on Brazilian doctors' use of French psychiatrist Pinel's liberation of the insane from the Bicêtre and Salpêtrière mental hospitals as a grammar and a vocabulary from which to launch the asylum-building campaign in the 1830s and 1840s. Expanding upon psychiatry's origins story, asylum doctors corresponded with like-minded doctors about Hospício Pedro II but also broadcasted a message that reverberated long and loudly enough that it was eventually heard in the halls of Brazilian psychiatry's most exalted model, French psychiatry.[33]

The 1874 Sant'Anna incident followed by the landmark visit by a French psychiatrist in 1875 (and by another French psychiatrist later in 1880)[34] marked a dramatic turning point for asylum psychiatrists. Their indignation at the Daughters of Charity and the validation from an esteemed French professional combined provided them with a much-needed impetus to ceaselessly undermine the Santa Casa's governance of the asylum. While the institution operated as a patrimonial tourist site frequented by Brazilians and notable foreigners, it did not encounter the French psychiatric gaze until the visits of French psychiatrists Philippe-Marius Rey and François Jouin to the Hospício Dom Pedro II (1875 and 1880, respectively). The French doctors primarily concerned themselves with the asylum population as their main subject but also opined about Hospício Pedro II's operations and administrative shortcomings. Rey, a psychiatrist at the Parisian Saint-Anne Mental Hospital who stayed in Rio de Janeiro for a month, offered minor criticisms of the institution's built environment,[35] but he emphasized the paucity of medical authority within the asylum's administrative structure. After relaying that the senior staff consisted of an administrator, two doctors (one of whom was the medical chief), a medical assistant, a substitute for the doctor, a mother superior, and a chaplain, he declared, "There are no resident doctors. This absence is especially regrettable considering that no lay member of the senior staff resides in the asylum. Therefore, during the major part of the day and during the whole night, the management of the establishment is in the hands of the Mother Superior, to whom the regulation confers a high degree of authority."[36] Rey suggested an advanced medical student provide a permanent medical presence by residing in the asylum.[37] Although this recommendation echoed the Brazilian asylum doctors' critiques, his opinion about the structure of nurse accountability differed: "In the opinion of doctors, the nurses leave much to be desired, but their negligence and errors are severely punished, and the ill treatment of patients results in the immediate expulsion of the violator, and, if the case is severe, the courts can even try it. These measures, which are highly commendable, reflect the spirit of humanity that governs the management process."[38] Instead of reiterating the deficiencies of the nurses, Rey, a modernist's modernist, praised the administrative structures in place to address them. This may indicate that the asylum doctors' stated issues with the Daughters of Charity and the male Brazilian nurses under their control had more to do with cultural competition for power than it did with real deficiencies on the part of the nurses. Rey's favorable assessment of the asylum in his 1875 account generally credited the asylum doctors with its success. He remarked that, in comparison to other countries he visited, "Brazil has done a lot for its alienated. The capital has an asylum that, apart from its imperfections, could arouse the envy of more than one big city in Europe. Many asylums in Italy, to name only those we were able to visit, including the ones in Milan, Florence, and Rome, cannot even be compared to the Hospício Pedro II."[39] In contrast to the Santa Casa, which at the outset brought in a workforce of devout believers from and was ultimately responsible to the pope in Rome, this was the first substantive connection between Brazilian medical-psychiatric culture and the Atlantic World of psychiatry. This provided a much-needed boost to the doctors' dreams of running the asylum and taking some pride of place in their own modernist and scientific Atlantic World. Rey went further, describing the physical plant as both aesthetically pleasing and functional and taking the opportunity to endorse the asylum doctors' idea that a more scientific approach would complement the building:

> The buildings are beautiful. The granite, the marble, and precious woods of Brazil provide a truly sumptuous aspect. The rooms are tall, well ventilated through numerous large windows; the water is abundant for the needs of service. Everything is very clean; there are no bad smells. All these qualities make us regret further it is only charity and not science that led to the creation of the Hospício Pedro II.[40]

For all intents and purposes, the Daughters of Charity may have operated to the best of their abilities and, with the resources they were given, an efficient asylum. However, the execution of the moral treatment as an effective treatment for mental illness necessitated not only aesthetically pleasing and clean asylum structures but the actual workings of science and medicine. Rey suggested that the asylum had administrative problems but expressed confidence in doctors' expertise and ability to operate the institution. He described the facility as a model:

> The provinces, particularly in Bahia, Pernambuco, São Paulo, will soon be offering the same care that the Santa Casa da Misericórdia applies to their patients. If the establishment's internal administrative service continues to lag, we found through reports to the administration that the doctors possess a thorough knowledge of the necessary reforms and of the treatments applied to the alienated. With such elements in place, this interesting part of hospital care will develop a lot in Brazil, since it knows to protect itself from the spirit of routine and self-serving oppositions that are always encountered on the path to progress.[41]

Rey characterized the asylum doctors' eventual ascension and the resulting transformation of the asylum as inevitable, either as a gesture of solidarity or a measure of belief. He based this assessment on what he saw but also on the reports that the doctors had been filing to the Santa Casa board for more than twenty years. Pinel's blueprint for incorporating Catholic caregivers but using the tools of bureaucracy (e.g., annual reports, formal complaints, etc.) to wrest care for the insane from the hands of religious officials entirely was starting to bear fruit. Rey's report was the first external confirmation that this strategy would bear success.

Jouin's report conveyed a more somber tone as he notes the overrepresentation of chronic patients and the lack of a special facility for them. Reiterating the criticism of Dr. Gustavo Balduíno de Moura e Câmera, director of the asylum's medical service (1878–81), Jouin noted that

> the hospital organization in Rio de Janeiro has nothing in common with what we observe in Paris and cannot be compared with a Sainte-Anne, for example. This fact is bitterly criticized by Dr. Moura e Câmera in his last annual report, because there is not, apart from this house . . . No Bicêtre, No Salpêtrière, no Vaucluse, no Ville-Evrard, etc., to which they could send their chronics, that can also not be compared with the organization of Salpêtrière, that we know so well.[42]

He likewise restated concerns raised by Dr. Moura e Câmera that the asylum did not provide clinical training to students of medicine in Rio de Janeiro.[43] Like Rey, Jouin parted company with asylum doctors in praising the asylum's administrative structure as sensible. However, this was based on the presumed hegemonic power and authority of asylum doctors, which was in turn more based on their titular power than on their actual authority within the still-religious institution. After mapping out the institution's administrative structure, he stressed that "all of these officials, we repeat, are under the immediate supervision of the medical chief. Thus, do we need to emphasize how perfect the functioning of the asylum is? With what care the details of administration are taken into consideration?"[44] The visits of Rey and Jouin to the Hospício Pedro II proved a turning point in Brazilian psychiatry, legitimizing the management, therapeutic, and bureaucratic work of Brazilian asylum doctors within the context of Atlantic medical cultures and lending moral support to their Brazilian colleagues in their activist struggle to become the managers of the asylum. Professional missions to assess asylums in Europe and the Americas were common at the time, and the arena of the professional medical journal had emerged as a place where medical competencies were grown and measured. By publishing their findings, Rey and Jouin made Brazilian asylum doctors and the Hospício Pedro II discernible members of an Atlantic psychiatric constellation. Foreign science and medical experts who traveled to Rio after Rey and Jouin consistently lauded the architecture of the asylum and the great care provided to the insane within its walls.[45]

Rio de Janeiro asylum doctors received the enthusiastic professional legitimacy and support from the French psychiatric standard-bearers during a period of political crisis alongside tremendous economic and intellectual growth in Brazil. By 1870 the increasing momentum of the Industrial Revolution in Europe and the United States had swept Brazil up into the vortex of the international economy, stimulating the thriving export market in raw materials. As Brazil constructed various modernization schemes in the areas of communications and transportation, the political threads of the imperial government began to unravel.[46] Disaffected Emperor Dom Pedro II's sporadic intervention in political disputes and infighting has led many historians to argue that he bears "prime, perhaps sole, responsibility" for the dissolution of the monarchy.[47] The emperor's weariness and his heir's lack of interest in ruling led to a political vacuum that statesmen hoping to modernize Brazil would fill. Asylum doctors, among others, joined this movement for the dissolution of the monarchy and what they believed were its atavistic institutions and practices.[48]

Comtean positivism provided asylum doctors with a lexicon and an ideological framework with which to attack the Daughters of Charity and the Santa Casa as representatives of an old order that hindered national progress.[49] As one intellectual of the time succinctly explained, "Previously Brazilian philosophy . . . went its way in isolation from the progress achieved in the old world. It seemed to us that Positivism was the best system to rescue our thought from this depression, because only Positivism contained a strong and coherent structure to pose against the Catholic structure that was dissolving."[50] Positivism appealed to psychiatrists who wanted economic and professional development without social mobilization that would alter existing class and race structures. Since they regarded the mass of their patient population as ill-prepared for the rigors of modern society due to, among other factors, illiteracy and "inferior" African racial background, positivism appealed as a model of modernization that rationalized the continued concentration of power in the hands of modernizing experts and technocrats.[51] As a good complement to the rise of a robust professional class in Rio de Janeiro, positivism flattered the organized professions' assertion of specialized expertise and offered secure recognition for the importance of their skills.[52] Sectors such as commerce and manufacturing grew during the period, but the knowledge-based professional classes saw the most notable growth. In this "professional society," members of collective organizations superseded occupational groups and laid claim to specific skills to declare themselves a profession. The concretization of psychiatry as a legitimate field came to hinge upon asylum doctors' ability to wrestle power and control away from the Daughters of Charity. Asylum doctors had the respect of foreign colleagues, recognition for their work in medical journals, and a close affiliation with legal medicine at the Rio de Janeiro College of Medicine, but the Daughters' presence prevented asylum doctors from possessing fully the object, the asylum, that reified psychiatry. However, in the face of republicanism's growing popularity and abolition's looming presence and social turmoil that threatened to dissolve the cohesion of the empire,[53] psychiatrists staunchly advocated for greater professional power and autonomy. In turn, modernizing state officials who surveyed a riotous public appealed to asylum doctors and other professional groups as a means to garner political support; lessen resentment; and in the case of psychiatry, manage supposed problem people and populations. As markers of the beginning of the end of Brazilian psychiatry's time as observers in the religious asylum, the passing of education decrees that paved the way for the institutionalization of psychiatry as a professional field are important.

The End of an "Exceptional" Governance Model, 1879–90

Legislative Decree 7.247, passed in 1879, authorized the creation of psychiatry as an autonomous and specialized unit in the nation's two medical schools: the Rio de Janeiro College of Medicine and the Medical School of Bahia.[54] The decree effectively granted psychiatry its first autonomous academic and professional space within Brazilian civil society, and opened the door to the creation of homegrown Brazilian psychiatrists. Two years later, Decree 8.024 authorized the Rio de Janeiro College of Medicine to hold a public contest for the first Chair in Psychiatry. Referring to this decree, the psychiatrist Manoel Joaquim Fernandes Eiras asserted that "this creation, already long claimed, is one of the largest benefits provided to science and to the country . . . nothing is more important, that demands study . . . and thorough observation, than the mental afflictions."[55] These decrees marked a pivotal moment in the tenor of contestations over asylum governance. They made it possible for psychiatrists to promise a future workforce equal to the task of managing Rio's mentally ill, altering the balance of power between asylum doctors and religious authorities. It is no coincidence that it was just following the passage of 7.247 and 8.024 that the asylum attracted its first socially and professionally prominent psychiatrists to serve as asylum doctors, who were in turn able to more effectively lobby to displace the Daughters as administrators and unlink the asylum from the Santa Casa.

The decrees had immediate effects on the asylum. Unlike their predecessors, the new doctors at the asylum used new outlets (such as the press) and new rhetorical strategies (the framing of institutional problems within the context of welfare reform at the moment of abolition) to assume administrative control of the asylum. Specifically, Dr. Nuno Ferreira de Andrade, the interim Chair of Psychiatry at the College of Medicine and the asylum medical director, solicited the head of the Santa Casa to remove the nuns from the asylum. He came to the institution as an impassioned doctor and academic but also as an untested administrator. Soon after earning his medical degree from the Rio de Janeiro College of Medicine in 1875, he occasionally taught as a substitute in the medical sciences (1877). He would formally become a professor after his "Physiology of Epithelios" won him the 1877 professorship in Clinical Medicine over the works of notable doctors. His role as a provocateur could most readily be observed with his unpublished "Memória Histórica da Faculdade de Medicina do Rio de Janeiro" (1879). Fastidiously detailing the history of the educational curriculum, this polemical document stressed the ineffectiveness of the measures taken by the imperial government in relation to medical education even after the April 19, 1879, Leôncio de Carvalho reform decree. Although the decree sought to radically alter education requirements at the primary and secondary levels along with the faculties of law and medicine, Andrade found them ineffectual and inadequate within the context of medical training.[56] Underestimating his resiliency, state officials responded to his impassioned critiques with silence and perfunctory promotions. He was named general health inspector of the port in 1881,[57] and in 1882, director of sanitary service of the Hospício Dom Pedro II.

Andrade engaged in a tense yet revealing exchange in a series of letters with the then-director of the lay brotherhood, Senator José Ildefonso de Souza Ramos, the Viscount of Jaguary (1878–83) over a two-month period in 1882. In the doctor's first letter, he cited a series of flaws and inconsistencies in the asylum statutes of 1852 that failed to protect the interests of effective staff personnel against the supposed whims and pettiness of the Daughters of Charity. He described the overall governance of the asylum as an "opaque structure" and its internal regimen as "the most radical negation of applicable legislation to an asylum."[58] He posited that even though the statutes of 1852 dictated that the Daughters of Charity perform auxiliary roles in the medical service, the internal order of the institution confirmed that they operated as the "discretionary government of the asylum."[59] Directly attacking Santa Casa and the nuns as the embodiment of a moral framework of religious care counter to the therapeutic ethos central to the moral treatment, he argued that the nuns sought "spiritual joy" by seeking "to redeem venial sins with the money of wretches" rather than acting in the best interests of the poor insane.[60] The power and authority granted by his position as Chair of Psychiatry at the College of Medicine and as the director of asylum medical services, as well as his own professional standing, enabled Dr. de Andrade to press for more autonomy. He bristled at the possibility that the Daughters might obstruct his instruction of medical students: "Should I consider my teaching secured against the unforeseen stumbles of others' bad will?. . . If today, before I open my course, I see my authority as doctor dwarfed by the authority granted to the Daughters of Charity . . . what will tomorrow be, when the necessity to teach creates for me new impositions and more serious obstacles?"[61] Dr. de Andrade proposed that the brotherhood cede the administration of the establishment to state regulation. Appealing to the humanitarianism of the Viscount of Jaguary, he inquired, "Why not place Your Excellency in front of the movement, and with the prestige of your name, recalling your past, brightest one, for the love of 500 unfortunates. . . . [Why] not promote the alluded separation?"[62] Sidestepping the leaded jargon of institutional management, he assumed a position of deference and employed flattery to establish an affective terrain whereby the Santa Casa director would be compelled to sever the asylum from the Santa Casa as a means to protect the mentally ill as well as the Santa Casa's reputation as an institution of care.

Approximately a month later, Santa Casa's president wrote a letter that would defend the asylum's internal regulations and the works of the Daughters of Charity. He first affirmed that the privileges granted to the order were in keeping with the statutes of 1852, given that a provisional article in the statutes allowed for the order to assume more administrative control as the Santa Casa saw fit. He claimed that "the regulations of the asylum are not, as you think, an 'opaque structure' but they are complex judicious dispositions perfectly appropriate for the grand intentions of this institution. And furthermore, the internal regulations were not the inventions of the director in his office; it is a consecration of intelligent practices developed through long and thorough experience, in perfect accordance with the statutes."[63] Moreover, the Viscount of Jaguary suggested that the combination of functions performed by both nuns and doctors would make the medical service more effective. Specifically, occupational therapy could make use of the talents of both. He proposed the following: "The doctor is, without the slightest question, the only person competent to determine the type of work appropriate for the alienated . . . but the doctor does not know the . . . aptitude of each patient, nor is this knowledge of the profession, while the Mother Superior, who has the responsibility for the inspection of work spaces, would be useful to him." Praising the Daughters' "bravery," "enthusiasm," "evangelical patience," and "disposition to religiously complete their duties," he contended that the order fastidiously contributed to the good treatment of the insane.[64] Within the world of Catholic Charity the devoted and tireless Daughters were still regarded as the functional earthly embodiments of Mary, the brotherhood's symbolic icon.

Indignant about the proposal to separate the asylum from the Santa Casa, the viscount noted that the idea was extremely unjust, given that the asylum was "a charity position" within the Santa Casa that was "carried out in a manner that the state could not do better."[65] He denied that the institution was "an anomaly of a hospital," as de Andrade had labeled it. He lauded the asylum's exceptionalism by asserting that it was not only a national model but also an exemplar in South America since it emerged in a constitutional monarchy and not a republican regime. He referenced the opinion Dr. Barbosa expressed upon assuming the post of asylum medical services director in 1853 by declaring that

> it is not only the city and province of Rio de Janeiro who reap the benefits and enjoy the advantages that one has in mind with foundations [the asylum] of this order: of all the provinces of the Empire the insane are sent, and even neighboring countries, recognizing the excellence of our hospital, they turn to Brazil for treatment and relief of the unfortunate insane of these countries, and with reason they do, because if the asylum of Pedro II is not superior, it is also not inferior to any of the best establishments of the same kind that exist in Europe, that in the magnificence and grandeur of the building and its well ordered proportions. . . . The Hospício Pedro II is a unique and model establishment in South America; and a little glory to Brazil and not the neighboring republics, extolling its institutions, they see the prosperity that has given us peace and recognize the happiness of a country, that establish such large establishments under the constitutional monarchical regime.[66]

Ultimately, the Viscount of Jaguary judged the intentions of the psychiatrist to be "unfair and unworkable" and proclaimed that "it would be a poignant injury to his administration . . . to dismiss himself a charge of charity, [of] their own institution, that has performed in a manner that the state could not do better."[67] Dr. Nuno de Andrade's reply insisted that he was not criticizing the Santa Casa but proposing remedies the Santa Casa could make to improve the asylum. He emphasized that his ultimate goal was to improve the lives of the unfortunates interned in the asylum.[68] On May 4, 1882, the Santa Casa director, "fully aware that Dr. Nuno de Andrade only wanted the best for the unfortunates, but piously believing that this was not the intention of the Santa Casa," fired de Andrade.[69] In this, de Andrade can be seen as a medical director like many of those who would follow him. He had the standing and the desire to make the case for psychiatric control of the asylum, but much like the directors he succeeded, he did not have the standing to confront the director of the Santa Casa.

However, Dr. de Andrade advanced the conversation in his time in office. His focus on the state as a critical actor in safeguarding the welfare of the mentally ill upset the tenor of formulaic discourse about urban assistance. The Santa Casa had possessed a monopoly on meting out aid to vulnerable populations; by pulling the state out of the proverbial shadows, he instigated a critical discussion on the state's ability to fulfill the rights of its subjects-citizens. Dr. João Carlos Teixeira Brandão, his successor as Chair of Psychiatry in 1883, expanded upon the critical foundation Dr. de Andrade built by proposing that republicanism, and not constitutional monarchism, was the political formation suitable to address the varied needs of the insane. This position also undermined the Santa Casa's use of the monarchy as a justification for its authority. Brandão embodied the vital reformist spirit characteristic of his psychiatric-minded colleagues.[70] Born in in the parish of Arraial de São Sebastião, in São João Marcos, a former municipality of Rio de Janeiro state, Brandão attended the Colégio Pedro II in Rio de Janeiro city before attending medical school. After defending an 1877 thesis on the urinary tract and graduating from the Rio de Janeiro College of Medicine, he commenced a clinical practice in Barra Mansa city, another municipality in the state. He practiced medicine there from 1878 to 1880 before going to Europe, and specifically to France, Germany, and Italy to study psychiatry. Returning to Rio de Janeiro in 1882, he would be one of the founders of the Policlínica Geral do Rio de Janeiro (General Polyclinic of Rio de Janeiro) and one of its doctors specializing in mental illness. In 1883 he delivered a pessimistic report on the institutions for the insane in Brazil to the Sociedade Médico-Psicológica de Paris, of which he was the only Brazilian member at the time. Instead of being reprimanded or chided by Brazilian colleagues, Brandão's career quickly took off upon his return to Rio.

Upon earning the nomination of Clinical Chair in Psychiatry at the medical school in April 1883, he joined the clinical faculty (as a professor) of the Hospício Pedro II in 1884. Two years later, his professional accolades were recognized by the Imperial Academy of Medicine when he was formally elected a member, and soon after, the administrative director of the asylum.

During the course of 1886, he published a series of articles in the popular newspaper *Diário Oficial* titled "The Alienated in Brazil" and popularized criticisms of the institution. The republican and secular psychiatrist voiced the most virulent criticisms against the Daughters of Charity. He asserted, "Entrusted to the Daughters . . . [the asylum], resembled a convent more than a hospital. . . . From morning to night, the religious chants mingled with the din of the mad entrusted to uncultured nurses while the Daughters of Charity carry out the tax precepts in the statutes of the congregation."[71] He characterized the government of the Daughters as an exercise in arbitrary power that displaced the doctor in the center of decisions: "Arranging the keys of the establishment, they did what they wanted, giving ingress and exit to whom they pleased."[72] Brandão believed it was nearly impossible to affect change, since "the directors and the doctors were restricted to the information that the nuns distributed. And if one of them would dare to inquire about some fact that did not appear normal, he heard unrelenting insults."[73] In contesting the right of the Daughters of Charity to intervene in the asylum's medical service, Brandão claimed to fulfill "the humanitarian and civic duty to call the attention of the government to the dangers that can arise from power of reactionary ultramontanism, of which they are mere passive instruments."[74] By associating the nuns' supposedly poor administration of the institution to a foreign influence, Brandão acquitted the imperial government of culpability and repositioned it as a victim.

According to Brandão, only a psychiatrist could rescue the asylum from foreign deleterious forces. Here, he was commenting on the appropriate role of the doctor:

> The director of an asylum should have the right to interfere in all the determinations that relate to the occupation, employment and distribution of the ill. His influence should be exercised constantly above all the service and the personnel charged with guarding or surveillance of the alienated. . . . Thus, all the other reforms should be subordinate to that which is supreme: give autonomy to the director of the medical service, turning him directly responsible for all that occurs in the asylum.[75]

The demand for the doctor to be accorded absolute authority is explicit. Further, Brandão proposed the dissolution of already existing institutions that purportedly served the mentally ill and the creation of a comprehensive network of asylums in all regions of the empire.[76] As Rio de Janeiro's economic growth in the latter half of the nineteenth century led to a precipitous increase in its population, the poor and working classes who were unable to keep pace with modernization suffered from a series of socioeconomic ills that a number of aid institutions sought to address, such as the Shelter for Beggars. Created in 1854, it provided shelter for the indigent encountered on city streets, public plazas, and the forecourts of churches.[77] During the 1860s, if the "tamed mad" (or "gentle mad," as psychiatrists referred to them) were found roaming the streets, the police would lead them to the asylum. If denied admission due to overcrowding, they were then sent to the Shelter for Beggars. On the other hand, their more "agitated" counterparts were sent to the House of Detention.[78] Similarly, the Refuge for Begging, created in 1879, also served the needs of the indigent and homeless poor.

In accordance with its statutes approved in 1884, individuals requesting entrance who could prove their absolute indigence, as well as those who were of advanced age or whose physical state was extremely weak could be granted admission. Admission was also granted to minors up to fourteen years of age who wandered the streets along with "idiots, imbeciles, and the mad," who were not admitted to the asylum.[79] He noted that institutions such as the Shelter for Beggars, the Refuge for Begging, and the House of Corrections all housed the insane in Brazil. Brandão estimated that 350 out of the 400 individuals housed at the Refuge were mentally ill while the remainder of the population consisted of "vagabonds, the old and children," making it a "deposit for the indigent insane."[80] For Brandão the reclusion of "the insane without homes" in the Refuge, with its lack of sufficient water and boards for beds was "a monstrosity in our social environment"; it was where the "mad, the old, men, women, children, and vagabonds lived in revolting promiscuity" that promoted idleness since it failed to follow the precepts of sound psychiatric treatments, such as occupational therapy.[81]

Public institutions were not the only targets of Brandão's vitriol. He also criticized the practice of interning the insane in small private health centers, known as "houses of health."[82] An article published in the *Diario do Rio de Janeiro* in 1871, by an author with the suggestive pseudonym Lucidus, asserted that during lucid intervals, many of the insane would be removed from the asylum and placed in a house of health, where they would be held for observation for a limited time. If they took a turn for the worse, they could be placed back in the asylum with the permission of their families or a guardian.[83] Brandão believed allowing doctors who did not have any psychiatric training to operate (and often own) these establishments made them viciously circular. He pointed out the lack of evidence to support their use, as well as the lack of regulatory standards for treatment and suitable accommodations in these establishments. While he conveyed that he did not plan to "bother any of the owners of the existing houses of health in the Empire," because they were not "capable of entering in an indecent conspiracy," the doctor's admonishments made tensions between psychiatrists and general medical practitioners over the therapeutic management of insanity clear. Brandão made the case that, in the face of unrelenting foreign religious movements mismanaging the asylum, a weak imperial government, decrepit public institutions, and unspecialized private establishments, legislators should generate comprehensive laws concerning diagnosis and treatment of the mentally ill, thereby ending an era in which the "state does not assist the insane as he is but as a vagabond, a beggar, or a criminal that he appears to be."[84] Furthermore, he adopted an alarmist rhetorical strategy by suggesting that the onset of modernization and civilization would lead to a rise of mental maladies and that it behooved the state, in order to avoid an epic crisis of public health and order, to heavily invest in providing systematic assistance to the mentally ill.[85]

The multiple criticisms Brandão leveled at various authorities and institutions resonated with the President of the Senate (1882–85) and Prime Minister (1885–88) João Maurício Wanderley. Wanderley, also known as the Baron of Cotegipe, was to be the director of the Santa Casa from 1883 to 1889. Wanderley came to the position already seasoned by dealing with criticisms leveled at Santa Casa de Misericórdias. Prior to his arrival in Rio, he served as the president of the province of Bahia (1852–55) and witnessed firsthand the problems that plagued the Santa Casa de Misericórdia Hospital of Salvador. He had overseen the amelioration of problems such as overcrowding, unhygienic conditions, and economic deficits through the sale of Santa Casa properties and the purchase of a building to house the insane (as opposed to treating them in the hospital), in a move that officials and doctors alike acknowledged had succeeded.[86] Cotegipe appointed Brandão as asylum medical director in 1887 and supported him in creating a series of reforms to dramatically reduce the administrative authority of the Daughters of Charity and expand the responsibilities of medical officials in the asylum bureaucracy. Importantly, after a restructuring of personnel and their duties, the medical director took full control of operating the economic service (in addition to taking on the appointment and dismissal of both nurses and their assistants), thereby leaving the Mother Superior with the sole responsibility of supervising the domestic staff (i.e., servants and slaves). These processes make apparent Brandão's adept skills as a seasoned professional able to harness his experiences as a student, doctor, and institution builder in Rio and abroad toward productive bureaucratic ends. Although Nuno de Andrade's and Brandão's goals were similar, the former managed only to advance the debate and get himself fired by asking too much, too publicly, and too quickly. In contrast, Brandão got the better part of the control for which de Andrade was asking, but by bringing the leadership of the Santa Casa onside rather than antagonizing it, and by couching his moves against the Daughters as a "restructuring" rather than as their removal from power, or from the institution. His conciliatory and yet insistent approach got further bureaucratic concessions in that the medical director, going forward, was given full control of generating medical information about the asylum. He had final authority on the diagnoses of those allowed to enter the asylum, archived critical documents related to their medical history, and created annual reports sent to the Santa Casa that thoroughly discussed therapeutics used and results obtained.[87]

These measures set the stage for Brandão to make further initiatives. During his tenure as medical director, Brandão brought the asylum and psychiatry into a congruency, one that moved both closer to the long-standing goals of public and mental health modernism. He transformed the institution into a productive laboratory of psychiatric experimentation and ushered in a new era of psychiatric optimism. Brazilian psychiatrists would, at long last, be in a position to achieve and fail as apostles of Atlantic modernity on a national stage. With the declaration of the republic in 1889, the balance of power would even shift away from the Santa Casa, tipping the balance of power in psychiatrists' favor as they formally became the institution's new administrators. The old power alliance between the crown and the Santa Casa was giving away to a new axis held by the city council and the powers of secular public health, including psychiatry. By 1890 the republican administration separated the asylum from the Santa Casa, designated it the National Insane Asylum, and made it a state entity.

Under full republican-backed psychiatric leadership, the asylum saw the departure of the Daughters of Charity. The August 15, 1890, edition of the weekly medical magazine *O Brazil-Médico*, to which Brandão contributed frequently, stated that the Daughters of Charity had "abandoned the institution" on August 11, 1890, and emphasized how powerful the nuns' motives must have been for them to have left so quickly even though the unfortunate mad people were entrusted their care.[88] While casting aspersions on the nuns by suggesting irresponsibility and betrayal on their part for the abandonment of the insane, the news announcement subtly also acknowledged that, to the delight of psychiatrists, the experiment in the supposed harmonious hybrid governance and therapeutics between religion and medicine had finally come to an end.[89]

Conclusion

A close examination of the Hospício Dom Pedro II as a microhistory of bureaucracy reveals a small yet significant process of state formation that has been generally overlooked. Instead of looking at asylum managerial struggles as one long political impasse until the creation of the republic, a focus on specific episodes reveals a connectivity within a field of conflict critical in establishing the qualities of the social contract associated with the emergence of republican rule. Though seemingly disparate, the efforts by asylum doctors to carve out professional space at the expense of religious officials, the consequences of the imperium's episodically waning involvement in Brazilian affairs, and the espousal of a positivist modernity by the burgeoning professional class, all taken together would become remarkably constitutive of the contours of modern Brazil. Specifically, the rivalry between religious officials and doctors over the asylum's bureaucracy as an indicator of state-formation process during the years 1852 to 1879 illustrates the extent to which the imperial government began abdicating authority by allowing new actors (i.e., emergent psychiatrists) and old ones (i.e., Santa Casa directors) to assume positions and pursue their rivalry within state institutions, such as the Hospício Pedro II. The pervasive inaction of Santa Casa directors in the face of asylum doctors' early complaints suggests the staunch approval that state actors, in addition to the city's urban elite (many of whom were members of the lay brotherhood), conferred upon the Daughters of Charity's bureaucratic management of the asylum. By 1879, however, the impulse of Brazilian government officials to quell dissent among a clamorous psychiatric class by initiating a series of modernizing reforms in higher education gave asylum doctors decisive victories. Although the proclamation of the republic signaled not only the effective separation of the asylum from the Santa Casa as well as the expansion of psychiatry's potential for professional growth, what Scull calls "the capture of the asylum" occurred because psychiatrists such as Brandão projected onto the asylum during the 1880s not only the notion of insanity as a form of mental illness but new forms social assistance and citizenship. By linking these terms in a causal chain to project a sense that they act together as natural, or rather naturalized forces in the domain of the asylum, psychiatrists espoused a compelling rhetoric of state welfare and responsibility for the insane and rode that rhetorical wave to a series of reforms inside of the asylum, and in the following years, outside its walls. This was the most notable consequence of the formalization of psychiatric control of the asylum. Psychiatrists and state officials crafted a host of legislative measures that formed the basis of a medico-juridical public welfare system that singled out mental illness as a state category with sociopolitical and economic implications. The first critical organ within the welfare system was the Medical-Legal Care for the Mentally Ill (Assistência Médico-Legal a Alienados), created in 1903. Under this body, treatment of the insane became centralized and differentiated as the National Asylum was the only institution to receive pensioner patients, offering practical therapy in nonagricultural activities and serving as a point of admission into the care system for mentally ill individuals to be referred to other services and institutions.

Another significant consequence of psychiatric control of the asylum was the reorientation of psychiatry. As the state formally recognized madness as a psychiatric domain and with the asylum firmly under their control, psychiatrists almost immediately began to cast their gaze on the public sphere as they entered more deeply into the new republican struggle to define the normative rational ideal of the Brazilian citizen. Since the declaration of the republic followed on the heels of emancipation, a recently emancipated Afro-descent or African-born citizen, to the dismay of many elite Brazilians, was the normative Brazilian citizen. Influenced by antiblack racism and the rise of scientific racism, Brazilian psychiatrists designated the nation's largely mixed-race population on the outskirts of rationality. As they strove to foster and preserve a social and moral order that supported existing class, gender, and racial hierarchies, they depended upon the alignment of psychiatry with a public health epidemiological model in which institutions of assistance (whether they served the mentally ill or not) were subjected to psychiatric regulation. Historian Heitor Resende observes that during the early twentieth century, "Public health *and* psychiatry give their hands in the common task of sanitizing the city, removing the filth [from] . . . the centers of infection which are the slums, the sources of disorder which are the unemployed ragamuffins, infesting the outskirts of the port and the streets in the center of the city"[90] (emphasis added). Versed in the argots of criminology, eugenics, and degeneration theory, psychiatrists heralded science, expertise, and efficiency to address not only mental illness but also a range of issues such as poverty, crime, and delinquency. Fashioning themselves as architects of Brazil's modernity, psychiatrists worked closely with state actors in order to underscore psychiatry's vital use as a public health utility. However, an immediate consequence of psychiatric ownership of the asylum was the institution's remaking. With the aspirational phase of their professional development behind them, asylum psychiatrists were poised to enter a managerial era full of optimism as they devised a series of measures to remake the institution into a paragon of moral treatment. While the extent to which new institutional measures would transform the asylum into a monument of therapeutic cure would be quite limited, an examination of these initiatives provides glimpses into the discursive interiors of psychiatry.

Chapter Three

The Government of Psychiatry

The National Insane Asylum's Interior Lives, 1890–94

After the declaration of the republic and the subsequent official sanction of the complete psychiatric control of the Hospício Dom Pedro II, Brazilian psychiatrists were poised to enter a halcyon period. Under the Santa Casa's management, the belief that patients needed to choose rationality over insanity led to techniques centered on intimidation. Purging, bloodletting, blistering, physical restraints, threats, and straitjackets were employed to achieve this end. Moreover, sedatives, as any other treatment, could and would be applied with force, if necessary for punitive purpose and to improve behavior on the wards, thereby alleviating nursing strain. Morphine, hyoscyamine and hyoscine (often combined with atropine) could be turned into very powerful sleeping draughts for severely disturbed patients whose noisy behavior disturbed the ward routine.

Psychiatrists assumed the leadership of an institution riddled with accusations of torture, abuse, and neglect. Patients were known to be chained to walls, left unattended for many hours, and mistreated by staff members. Doctors who worked in the Hospício alleged that conditions were unsanitary, inhumane, and dangerous and that the asylum used painful and uncommon punishment. They noted that conditions were not only dangerous but also inadequate for the care and habilitation for the mentally ill. Some even concluded that the physical, mental, and intellectual skills of most patients had deteriorated while in the asylum. Similar to other asylums, abnormal patient behavior resulted in staff applying therapeutic interventions "to react to inmate initiative rather than the other way around."[1] As psychiatrists shunned the Santa Casa's system of restraint and corporal treatment, they hoped to follow a regimen of conciliatory and gentle management free from coercion and corporal punishment.

The severance of the asylum from the Santa Casa and the departure of the Daughters of Charity represented palpable markers of success for psychiatrists after a decades-long trek of professional emergence through rugged and shifting terrain. With disputes over the creation of the asylum itself behind them and struggles with religious authorities seemingly won, they embarked on an ambitious program to rehabilitate and rejuvenate the asylum into a paragon of regenerative therapy. Psychiatrists were ready to prove that they could restore the mad to sanity and fix the broken. Attuned to the latest Atlantic intellectual and psychiatric currents, Brazilian psychiatrists embraced the republican and positivist government that came to power vowing an end to the cultural stagnancy within the asylum and other imperial institutions. As theorist Henri Lefebvre might have suggested, the republican asylum produced the actions of the political and social superstructure as surely as those forces had created the asylum.[2] Whereas many historians have addressed the sociocultural and economic implications of the republican revolution, few explore the emergence of legislative decrees that sought to expand the rights of the mentally ill through the implementation of social assistance initiatives. By instigating the passage of Decree 206 (the establishment of Medical-Legal Assistance to the Alienated), Decree 791 (the authorization of the Professional School of Nurses, EPEE), and Decree 1559 (the establishment of the Observation Pavilion), psychiatrists hoped to finally have the space with which to revolutionize the asylum, creating a monumental engine of therapeutic care. The reorganization of people and space by these decrees offers insights into how psychiatrists understood the mentally ill, their medical collaborators, and most importantly for my purposes (and for the shaping of the social fabric of the new republic), themselves. By adding and removing bodies deemed appropriate or inappropriate and manipulating the asylum's space, these measures sought to remedy problems such as unscientific nurses, overcrowding, and the pervasive presence of the chronically incurable. Psychiatrists invented and shaped complex relations between the inner and outer dimensions of asylum space that ultimately constituted the core of their professionalization. Since the asylum did not reflect the ideal institution psychiatrists had envisaged, material and discursive reform continued to seek an ideal that the asylum could only fleetingly meet. Similar to the house in philosopher of science and phenomenologist Gaston Bachelard's *The Poetics of Space*, the asylum functioned as a shelter that reflected the inner workings of psychiatrists' ambitious projects.[3]

In this context, the reforms and assistance decrees that continued to change the asylum had little bearing on the daily care of the mentally ill. Rather, they reveal much about the inner workings of early Brazilian psychiatry. A focus on psychiatrists' actions and initiatives that sought to improve and expand care for the mentally ill reveal the sometimes overlapping ways in which class, race, and gender biases undergirded the profession, as its practitioners actively sought to make it integral to Brazil's republican project of national order and progress. Considerable intellectual growth and institutional consolidation characterized psychiatry during 1890–94 as doctors initiated a flurry of initiatives that reflected key ideals of the modernization ethos they shared with the republican government, one based on the solemnization of race-cultural segregation and the socioeconomic uplift of the sectors of the citizenry they felt were deserving. This chapter focuses on not only the form and function of the asylum reforms but also on both their apparent and latent meanings. It predominantly traces the evolution of Brazilian psychiatry, as evidenced by the transformation of the asylum, through the prolific writings and speeches of Dr. João Carlos Teixeira Brandão, the first psychiatrist-administrative director (1890–97). As the fully empowered director of the asylum, the chair of psychiatry at Rio College of Medicine, and the key architect of the Medical-Legal Assistance to the Alienated Act (1890),[4] Brandão became the institution's (and by extension the psychiatric profession's) mouthpiece. He was a formidable advocate and both reflected and structured the views of his profession. As such, a concentrated study of his acts and words reveals the intellectual development of psychiatry during a volatile socioeconomic and political period.

In 1888 the nearly one million Brazilians of African descent still held in bondage were freed. A year later, militant republican elements in Rio's military academy and local republican political parties staged a bloodless coup that resulted in the emperor's exile to Europe and initiated the era now known as the First Republic in 1890. Bitter political conflict among factions of the agrarian oligarchy, the army, and the navy marked the political transition from monarchy to republic as civil wars continued intermittently throughout the country. Rio's role as the national capital and port city crucial to Brazil's export economy protected it from the worst of the violence, as the nation became more deeply involved in international trade as a supplier of raw materials such as coffee. During 1890 the new republic plunged headlong into a speculative financial fever that included a currency expansion that would cause economic turbulence well into the twentieth century. One side effect of the inflation that this economic upheaval brought about was industrial and commercial expansion, as well as increased protection for domestic production. Growth in agriculture and an enormous wave of foreign immigrants also stimulated industry by providing both the capital and the labor. Distinguished Brazilian jurist Evaristo de Morais captured the feeling of the 1889–91 surge in the Rio de Janeiro's stock market (Bolsa de Valores): "The Republic came and with the Republic, the Encilhamento. There was a profound transformation in this country. There was a fever, a madness. Money spread itself around here in a real flood. One was given the impression that everyone had gone insane."[5] This frenzy made and broke fortunes, but it had an across-the-board negative effect on the majority of the urban poor. The cost of living, already inflated by the demands of immigration, shot up quickly; the increased demand for consumer goods by the newly rich grew aspects of the economy that had little to do with the needs of the poor and newly emancipated; and the new government's tendency to look to the sinking export economy as an all-purpose solution led them away from investing in meeting the needs of the city's wage earners.

Against this backdrop of uncertainty, the new republican structures and ideologies promised a new exaltation of the individual and his or her rights as more traditional, imperial institutions shrank or dissolved. For the racial majority of Rio, the language of rights and freedoms that the republic brought in with it functioned primarily as a mirage, while in law and in police practice, their citizenship and freedom of movement were significantly curtailed. The passage from slave to free labor and constitutional monarchy to republic (in 1888 and 1890, respectively) brought about new public order concerns regarding security, political stability, vice, and morality. As officials undertook political policing of, for example, anarchists or participants in the several revolts that threatened to topple the new republican government, they also expressed a great intolerance and antipathy toward a broad spectrum of previously tolerated vernacular practices of city's Afro-descent majority.

An official obsession with the unruliness of Rio's masses generated such an extreme demophobia among national political elites that a movement to relocate the capital to a peaceful inland location began to gain some momentum. Professing the viewpoints of a new republican elite class leery of Rio, Prudente de Morais noted in an opening session of Congress on January 27, 1891, that they wanted to relocate the government to keep it from the "evil influence of this terrible city, so saturated with elements harmful to the moral life of the nation, that it has become accustomed to their continuous absorption, to the intellectual endosmosis that itself expands to the ancient capital of the Empire." Politicians such as Virgílio Damásio, head of the Republican Party of Bahia, were more strident. On December 15, 1890, Damásio argued that the federal government's location in Rio de Janeiro threatened the new Brazilian federation:

> The conditions of the population clustered in this city are very contrary to the existence of a large capital and a large federation such as ours. Moreover, in a crowded city where the social sediment consisting of the masses lives, in which, unfortunately, instruction has not yet penetrated, nor the minimum of civic education; where we find many people, let's speak the truth, who, entirely outside the community of the industrious and honest, live between idleness and manipulation and small crimes; this great mass of men is a weapon, a very powerful lever in the hands of agitators.

Although the change in capital did not occur until many decades later, the fact that politicians in the new republic seriously considered the idea clearly illustrates the concerted elite apprehension about the city's residents. In spite of their disagreements on many issues, a growing consensus was fashioning itself, almost involuntarily, among the different elements of the nation's and the city's elites concerning the state of the working poor, of which Afro-Brazilians became a special population given their newfound status as citizens. In a city where the majority of households had slaves, making slavery an endemic part of the city's rhythms, the abolition of slavery, for the slaveowning classes, was not solely about the loss of slaves whose labor generated income. Abolition represented the disquieting erosion of personal paternal authority and augmented already popular racist constructions of Afro-Brazilians as unreliable, licentious, violent, newly out of control, and therefore suspect. Against this background of disparaging perceptions of Africans, Afro-Brazilians, former slaves, and the poor, the moral panic proposed by social scientists seemed congruent with somewhat more broad-based preoccupations about public safety and public order, although likely out of balance with the actual threat posed by Rio's disenfranchised. Cultural theorist Stuart Hall described sociocultural moments like this one, noting that

> when the official reaction to a person, groups of persons or series of events is out of all proportion to the actual threat offered, when 'experts,' in the form of police chiefs, the judiciary, politicians and editors perceive the threat in all but identical terms, and appear to talk 'with one voice' of rates, diagnoses, prognoses and solutions, when the media representations universally stress 'sudden and dramatic' increases (in numbers involved or events) and 'novelty' above and beyond that which a sober, realistic appraisal could sustain, then we believe it is appropriate to speak of . . . a moral panic.[6]

The antivagrancy campaign that emerged as a result of an 1890 antivagrancy statute is a good example of such a panic. The statute, as many historians of Brazil have noted, was the legal expression of an ideology relative to vagrancy that had begun its evolution with the arrival of the first slaves in the new Portuguese colony of Brazil as it linked dark skin and poverty to backwardness. The most prominent postabolition version was based in "a firm and unshakable belief in the innate laziness and irresponsibility of the black and racially mixed Brazilian masses."[7] Thus, moral panic over the disorderly masses was also exacerbated by the pauperization of the working classes, and of Afro-Brazilians in particular.

By the late 1880s, the city's free people of color earned varying degrees of prosperity and stability as some achieved modest wealth organizing small shops and even purchasing their own slaves. However, a great many more etched out a fragile existence working as day laborers, street vendors, and domestic servants. Historian Mary Karasch stresses that "what awaited so many freedpersons was not the golden dream of freedom but rather the nightmare of poverty."[8] Free black poverty was exacerbated by the coming of full abolition. Rio's population ballooned from 275,000 in 1872 to more than 1 million in 1920 as migrants from across Brazil and abroad came into Rio.[9]

As authorities sought to stamp out vice and divide licit from illicit forms of work, they instituted a series of brutal campaigns to "civilize" and "sanitize" the city center, pushing out low-income, mixed-race, and black populations to try and make the city center safe for bourgeois culture. It was in the poor parishes of the city that industry thrived, along with construction, informal commerce, and day labor, and these parishes swelled with Rio's internally displaced. Even before the 1890s, when the population and industry grew dramatically, the pattern of overcrowding had intensified steadily. Between 1872 and 1890, the Old City's population grew 52 percent, and the three poorest parishes, São José, Sant'Ana, and Santa Rinta, grew 100 percent, 75 percent, and 42 percent, respectively. Historian Jaime Benchimol references figures illustrating that an average of 14.7 persons per building in 1872 had increased to between 32 and 35 persons in 1890, with the greater proportion of this crowding occurring in the Old City center. Indeed, by the 1870s, the poor began to construct their own shelters on the hills separating most of the city from the dock. The most famous, known as Favela, was founded in the late 1890s and would give its name to what has become an enduring practice in Rio of unauthorized (though often organized) informal city expansion by the poor, in which tents give way to informal houses that eventually give way to more formal structures. For those who lived in these districts, conditions were difficult. In addition to the construction of informal settlements from the ground up, late colonial- and imperial-period townhouses and mansions were transformed by subdividing and redividing every room into several, making dense rooming houses using wooden boards, fabric, or other materials as walls. These buildings became known popularly as *cortiços* ("beehives" of small, irregular dwellings, usually overcrowded and without plumbing); their presence, like hyperdense poverty housing structures in many moments of moral panic, haunted city planners and their "civilized" dreams for Rio. The fusing of this poverty combined with under- and unemployment only fed the popular construction of the masses as a deviant class. As poverty deepened, elites blamed the city's underclass for its own poverty and for the visible manifestations of that poverty including *cortiços* and *favelas*, while generally not engaging with structural or institutional causes of disenfranchisement.

These developments gave the Hospício Nacional de Alienados a renewed significance in maintaining emerging disciplinary routines and structures as police officials, followed in frequency by family members, brought an extraordinary population to the doors of the asylum. As the classic work on Rio's police by historian Thomas Holloway documented, the republican state and the elite classes used the police as a tool against the lower classes through an enforcement focus on petty crime.[10] In addition to crimes against persons and property, the police repressed popular practices and habits deemed incompatible with Europhilic notions of Rio's progress toward becoming a true cosmopolitan showcase of an Atlantic capital. According to Holloway, "The establishment and development of the urban police system were a necessary precondition for the transition from slavery to the free labor regime." The police were instrumental in coercively resolving the paradox of slavery and liberalism in the deeply incomplete modernity that followed abolition.[11] Within this imagining of the cityscape, it became quite commonplace for police officers to bring individuals who displayed unusual characteristics, features, and behaviors to the asylum in the name of public order and normalcy. This chapter follows the path of studies concentrating on particular municipal institutions and the compromise bureaucratic incorporations of different social sectors that sought to maintain sociopolitical stability and order against both real and phantom threats. It focuses on the role of psychiatrists in imposing, through their work, the rules of the "state"—rules whose creation psychiatrists had themselves influenced. These medical professionals, employed or contracted by the government, were the agents of regenerating and reinforcing entrenched practices imposed differently on different social layers. Between the formal state and the informal population at large, they sought to bring the government's sociopolitical projects of "order and progress" into reality through the management of the asylum.

Before delving into the underpinnings and implementations of each of the three key asylum reforms in this chapter's time period, it becomes critical to explore the workings of the institution Brandão and other psychiatrists actually inherited. Asylums are, by their nature, less perfect than the ideas of their making. In this, the Hospício Dom Pedro II was no exception. The psychiatrists were bequeathed an asylum that was chronically overcrowded with patients who were predominantly indigent and hailed from the city (table 3.1). During the institution's formal imperial thirty-eight-year life span (1852–90), it prominently featured people of African descent of varied statuses that included free, emancipated, and enslaved. Notable, the majority of foreign admissions to the asylum from December 1852 to December 1856 came from Africa (tables 3.2–3.3). From 1852 to the 1870s, mania and dementia were the predominant ailments attributed to this population of color. By the 1880s (and into the early twentieth century), the majority of people of color (i.e., blacks and mestizos) in the asylum would suffer from epilepsy (51 percent), followed by hysteria (48 percent), alcoholism (45 percent), and dementia (42 percent). From the 1880s onward, the majority of the white population there would suffer from paranoia (73 percent), followed by mania (65 percent), dementia (58 percent), and alcoholism (55 percent). Concurrently, the majority of men were diagnosed as alcoholics whereas most women were diagnosed as hysterics, followed by alcoholics. While the military brought the majority of white patients (men in particular) to the asylum, the police brought people of color.[12] Closely reading the work of historians Daniele Ribeiro and Lourence Cristine Alves, it can be presumed that the asylum, between 1888 and its closure in 1944, was increasingly occupied by white indigent men. Among the various reasons put forth to account for this racial demographic shift, the most compelling are the multicausal ones that examine how the gradual process of abolition alongside the influx of European immigration displaced many Afro-Brazilians from the urban public marketplace. While the pauperization of Afro-Brazilians and others generated anxieties about the breakdown of public order, Afro-Brazilians were frequently criminalized while whites were medicalized. As police authorities placed the former in carceral institutions such as the House of Detention, their white counterparts were placed in the National Insane Asylum.

In 1890, however, the asylum under Brandão's leadership had a patient population of approximately three hundred, the majority of whom were people of color and indigent. It was an asylum whose nurses cared for the mentally ill with methods from traditional religion, not of science. By most measures, those methods were ineffective, and in the eyes of psychiatrists like Brandão, the nurses' pervasive reliance on methods such as somatic remedies like sedatives or hypnotic agents and straightjackets led to deeper insanity on the part of many patients. Prior to the asylum's passage into full psychiatric control, the psychiatrists had diligently advocated for the moral therapy from their position of relative powerlessness with the idea that a commitment to therapeutics over palliative care and a change in tactics, management, and staff, would solve the asylum's problems. Up until the Daughters of Charity left the institution, they had laid the blame for the asylums faults on inept religious staff who did not follow their directions or on the Daughters of Charity's management.

The Pinelist rhetoric of these early psychiatrists notwithstanding, the archival record reveals that, upon taking control of the asylum, they did heavily rely on a wide variety of restraint methods believing them, at best, to be necessary parts of the asylum's therapeutic regimen. Use of coercive methods, according to Dr. Ludovino da Silva, could not be abolished in a Hospício "whose population consists of individuals of various conditions and of diverse [manners] educations, of habits, and of varied customs."[13] Even though psychiatrists came into power on the strength of a purely curative regime, in practice the distinction between curative and punitive therapies is often difficult to ascertain as doctors sometimes presented what appear to

Table 3.1. Estimated population of the city of Rio de Janeiro (urban districts)

	1799* (%)	1849** (%)	1872** (%)
Free people of color	8,812 (20)	13,361 (5)	73,311 (27)
Slaves	14,986 (35)	110,622 (41)	48,939 (18)
Whites	19,578 (45)	144,403 (54)	151,799 (55)
Total	43,376 (100)	268,386 (100)	274,049 (100)

* Urban districts.

** Urban and rural districts.

Sources: Manolo Florentino, "Alforrias e Ethnicidade No Rio de Janeiro Oitocentista: Notas de Pesquisa," *Topoi* 3, no. 5 (2002): 10–11; Herbert S. Klein and Francisco Vidal Luna, *Slavery in Brazil* (New York: Cambridge University Press, 2010), 183.

Table 3.2. Geographic distribution of patients from December 9, 1852, to December 31, 1856

Region	Admissions	Discharged	Died	Remained
Court municipality	232	91	54	87
Province of Rio de Janeiro	147	60	57	30
Minas Gerais	23	7	11	5
São Paulo	28	10	13	5
Paraná	3	—	—	3
Goiás	1	—	1	—
Santa Catarina	18	6	6	6
São Pedro do Sul	23	4	10	9
Bahia	80	21	31	28
Pernambuco	33	14	10	9
Espírito Santo	6	1	1	4
Sergipe	4	2	—	2
Maranhão	8	4	1	3
Piauí	2	—	—	2
Alagoas	6	1	2	3
Rio Grande do Norte	2	—	—	2

Source: Arquivo Nacional, Série Saúde / Ministério do Império, Maço IS3, 1854–57.

Table 3.3. Movement of foreign patients from December 9, 1852, to December 31, 1856

Nationality	Admissions	Discharged	Died	Remained
Portugal	158	79	44	35
Spain	5	4	1	—
France	23	17	4	2
Germany	27	13	7	7
England	12	10	2	—
Italy	4	2	—	2
Prussia	5	4	—	1
Switzerland	3	2	—	1
United States	4	2	1	1
Chile	1	1	—	—
Buenos Aires	1	1	—	—
China	2	—	1	1
Africa	249	152	72	25

Source: Arquivo Nacional, Série Saúde / Ministério do Império, Maço IS3 5, 1854–57.

be punitive measures as the best cures. For example, the use of leeches on the anus, referred to by Dr. Barbosa as of great benefit in the treatment of maniacs, was undoubtedly uncomfortable and humiliating.[14]

In practice the doctors used a variety of remedies that closely resembled the punitive religious traditions of care, including bloodletting (through leeches or mechanical suctions), blistering agents, purgatives, and a variety of pharmacological substances. Among the drugs used during his tenure as asylum director, Barbosa mentioned ammonium acetate, opium, purgatives, and digitalis-laurel water,[15] while in 1974 Dr. Rey observed that potassium bromide (anticonvulsant and a sedative in the late nineteenth and early twentieth centuries), potassium iodine, chloral hydrate, morphine hydrochloride, and espelina leaves (cayaponia espelina had been known to aid in the treatment of syphilis) were the most commonly used drugs at the time.[16] Hydrotherapy, a ubiquitous Hospício treatment method, was another therapeutic measure often used to deleterious ends. Water was long thought to be an effective treatment in asylum settings because it could be heated or cooled to different temperatures, which when applied to the skin could produce various immediate reactions throughout the rest of the body. The framing of treatment and punishment as a distinction without a difference could most clearly be seen when cold water was poured over unknowing and surprised patients. This popular hydrotherapy method was used to lessen the "heat of madness" or to rouse the melancholic. Still, having the staff jump out and pour cold water on those of fragile mind when they least expected it may have had its actual roots deeper in the whips and chains of the Santa Casa than the language of Pinel. Although the reputation of physical and other types of restraint was sullied by an emerging psychiatric profession, they were widely used in the asylum during its imperial history. The imperial asylum was an asylum chronically overcrowded with indigent people of color, an asylum in which violently inhumane methods were expected by staff and patients alike. It was the imperial asylum in which psychiatry was born, the imperial asylum that psychiatrists inherited, and the imperial asylum that would serve as the bedrock on which a greater psychiatric modernism would be forged.

By 1890 the republican state was operational, however fragile, and the idea, however abstract, of the consensual free and rational citizen, more widespread. The madman presented an iconic problem, and for the first time, the sanity of all citizens became an ideological imperative and a political concern, not merely a matter of convenience. Flushed with long-sought-after triumph, newfound professional power, and buoyed up by the republican political culture that exalted "order" and "progress," psychiatrists sought to finally construct the empirical and discursive framework from which to make the asylum a vital curative center. Central to the remaking of the institution was the operationalization of the moral treatment. This process involved the regimentation of patients' lives in the asylum setting, where they would be convinced to regain their rationality through prolonged and intense interactions with a medically trained psychiatrist. This was not "talk therapy" but rather an individualized and routinized method of care designed to bring patients back into the community of productive citizens through a series of interactions meant to convince them of their madness and subsequently inspire them to reject it.

Combining close surveillance and paternal concern, rapport was established and cooperation engendered between doctor and patient. Such therapeutic strategies often depended upon the charisma of the doctor and in turn had the effect of increasing his prestige and authority. Since the psychiatrist's use of the moral treatment "actively sought," as the historian Andrew Scull suggests, "to *transform* the lunatic, to remodel him into something approximating the bourgeois ideal of the rational individual,"[17] the psychiatrist served a vital political function in the context of the new republican era in addition to a medical one.

Since the asylum's 1852–90 period represented a thwarted attempt at fully exercising the tenets of moral therapy, the creation of the nursing school, the agricultural colony, and the observation pavilion in the immediate aftermath of psychiatric takeover of the asylum serviced its implantation. The logic of an asylum that sought to treat the mentally ill with moral therapy does not suffice, however, to account for the internal transformations of the asylum. Alongside the asylum-as-instrument, developed as a psychiatrist's primary tool in aiding the mentally ill, there was a more covert model, but perhaps an even more influential one—that of the asylum as a republic in and of itself. According to this model, the asylum functioned as a closed system, something akin to a small self-sufficient state with, as Pinel predicted, its own "little government."[18] From the choice of nurses, the construction of new facilities and management decisions, to the trends in psychiatric practice itself, this image of a self-governed entity weighed continually on the fate of the psychiatric institution.

Recruiting Nuns "Without Habits"

Having banished the Daughters of Charity, psychiatrists at the asylum welcomed the opportunity to staff the institution according to their ends by working closely with Minister of Justice and Interior Affairs José Cesário de Faria Alvim. Together, and in a testament to the breadth of Francophilia among elite Cariocas, they recruited secular nurses from France and established a nursing school linked to the asylum. These measures cemented a new, post–Daughters of Charity tradition of gender relations between doctors and nurses that validated the paternal and epistemic authority of psychiatrists, who unlike the previous nurse-managers and very much like most of their modernist cohort, were all men. Seeking to no longer be ideological voices in the wilderness, Brazilian psychiatrists desired nurses trained at the Salpêtrière School of Neurology since, by the close of the nineteenth century, Salpêtrière was famous worldwide as a psychiatric center and as the place where psychiatrist Jean-Martin Charcot and his students had laid the foundations of modern neurology.[19] One of his students, Désiré-Magloire Bourneville, would succeed Charcot as director of the Salpêtrière. While Bourneville is most popularly associated with the mental diseases of children, he was also renowned for being militantly anticlerical during his tenure as school director. As a staunch promoter of nursing education, his *Manuel de la Garde-Malade et de L'Infirmière* (1888–89) served as the foundational text for the Brazilian nursing school. Apart from detailing knowledge about anatomy, physiology, and pharmacology, the text stressed linkages between learned knowledge in school and its practical application for asylum patients based on their specialized needs. Ideally, the Salpêtrière nurse would know principles of medicine and diverse treatments for the insane and be capable managers obedient to the needs of their psychiatric superiors. Thus, the recruitment of French female nurses trained according to the dictates of an eclectic therapeutic pedagogy that rendered the asylum a secular space dovetailed well with the goals of psychiatrists hoping to inculcate a new mode of labor and gender relations in the asylum. Their ideal relationship, as a group of male psychiatrists with women in their workplace, seems uncomplicated (if regressive) in terms of women's power. Instead of subscribing to the voguish Atlantic Nightingale nursing pedagogy that framed nursing as separate from "doctoring" and exalted the nurse as a seminal figure in the therapeutic process (e.g., the Daughters of Charity), Brazilian psychiatrists coveted Bourneville nurses, often known as "nuns without habits," due to their promotion of a professional identity based on devoted care and control of their charges and deferential compliance to their medical superiors. But the recruitment of secular nurses was not sufficient to meet the revolutionary goals of Brazilian psychiatrists. They encouraged state officials to emulate the desired qualities of the Salpêtrière asylum nurse through the creation of Brazil's first nursing school. The Professional School of Nurses opened in 1890. Although the school was formally open to both men and women, its intended and actual use for the majority of its history was the education of female nurses. An article in the *Jornal do Commercio* noted that "if the creation of such a school was an advantage for men, it was even greater for women, where the activity widens their horizons and provides them a future in which they may provide important services."[20] Upon successful completion of courses and clinical work in the asylum over the course of two years, women would earn a nursing degree and have their choice of hospital and state facilities to work in.

Apart from serving the needs of both the mentally ill and psychiatrists, the school also purported to uplift women since it would serve as a "vast field of women's activity, where, due to their delicacy of feelings and refinement of affections, there will be no competitors, whether at the hospital bedside of the sick or in private homes, where they would complement the doctor."[21] It is clear that the identity of the nurses coming out of the school was to exist entirely within and under the identity of the doctors they were to serve. The medical journal *O Brazil-Médico*, bestowing praise upon Brandão for creating the school, observed that the school was a magnificent project in that it provided psychiatrists with "true assistants" while engendering a productive moral economy by creating a labor market for women that constituted "an honest and highly humanitarian means to acquire subsistence."[22] Moreover, state officials argued that the school could also transform the lives of wayward young women. A few months after the authorization of Decree 791, Faria Alvim inquired about the possibility of the Santa Casa director sending underprivileged women over the age of eighteen, who resided at the brotherhood, to the nursing school. Such a collaboration between the Santa Casa and the school would "support, direct and educate underprivileged girls," making them "creatures useful to themselves and their homeland."

He emphasized the need to "broaden the horizon of aspirations" for girls who "do not find immediate and remunerative application" in the absence of professional education other establishments offered to boys.[23]

While statesmen and psychiatrists alike saw the school as a social, public, and medical good, its admission requirements privileged the socioeconomic and cultural mobility of certain Brazilian women. Psychiatrists conjured a specific profile of the desired nurse in developing criteria for the nursing school. Eligibility guidelines stipulated that women had to be at least eighteen years old, know how to read and write correctly, understand basic arithmetic, and submit a certificate of good conduct. The devisers of the criteria knew that elite women rarely sought out employment; they remained cloistered at home or in convents in order to maintain class and caste privilege.[24] Yet women had minimal access to formal education during the nineteenth century, so the education admission requirements posed a barrier to nonelite women as well. Many women in Rio had poor to nonexistent rudimentary reading, writing, and math skills.

The requirement of a certificate of good conduct barred many women from the school as well. Professional men of every stripe provided such attestations of professional comportment, respectability, and moral character as a right and duty of position in the nineteenth and early twentieth centuries.[25] The Daughters of Charity had needed no such certificate; membership in their esteemed order was sufficient. Few women had the dense and complex ties within the embedded patronage network to conjure up such a certificate. As a document that purported to represent and standardize an official set of relations, the certificate operated as a congenial trope of sociality that linked ideologies of gender, class, and race. Good conduct was not simply a mode of relations but one that indexed past behavior with an expectation of its continuance.[26] In this manner, the procurement of a certificate of good conduct demonstrated one's ability to maintain a stable and mutually reinforcing patron-client relationship. As historian Kim D. Butler put forward, in the aftermath of abolition in 1888, few Brazilians of African descent would have access to such certificates since state-subsidized immigration for Europe pushed many Afro-Brazilians out of the best remunerated posts in the agricultural and industrial economies (particularly in the southeast). By 1850 many plantation owners had stopped buying slaves and were refusing to employ freed persons by arguing that they were inherently indolent, preferring immigrant (read as European) workers instead.[27] Thus, even though no legal barriers prevented black laborers from obtaining jobs in the postabolition period, Brazilians of African descent encountered a hostile labor market where employers had a de facto preference for white labor and a legal mechanism that allowed them to invest in white labor *and* the well-established network of patronage.[28] Formal and unstated elite concerns about the nation's fundamental demographic and cultural Africanness provided both the rationale for subsidized white immigration and for the marginalization and pathologization of black workers in postabolition Rio.

Based on the demographic and sociological profile of late nineteenth-century Rio de Janeiro, the majority of women who met the admissions criteria for the nursing school came from the European immigrant population. Likely to possess rudimentary skills in reading and math, these women did not have to contend with antiblack racism and discrimination that would keep Afro-Brazilian women and most women of color from getting a certificate of good conduct. The figure of the asylum nurse, then, served as a meeting ground for the cultural politics of whitening.[29] By directly influencing the process of nursing recruitment from France and the training of nurses in Rio, psychiatrists manufactured their ideal subordinates within the asylum domain. Presumably unlikely to challenge the authority of the psychiatrist yet drawn to the prospect of respectable work that could facilitate social mobility, the ideal asylum nurse could adhere to the new gender regime where the psychiatrist served as the paternal professional and the nurse, his obedient and maternal feminine subordinate.

Constructing Medico-Legal Citizenship and the Virtues of Agricultural Labor

Psychiatrists also asserted their professional authority through Decree 206 (The Medical and Legal Assistance to the Alienated), which not only cemented the professional authority of psychiatrists over the medical care of the insane but expanded the asylum's terrain of confinement. The first article of the measure designated the asylum as the central entry point into the care system for the mentally ill and authorized the construction of two agricultural colonies on the Ilha do Governador, known as the São Bento and Conde de Mesquita colonies. Instead of continuing the practice of haphazardly placing the presumed mentally ill in the city's social assistance institutions, they would be taken to the asylum first, where they would be referred to other institutions if necessary per psychiatric reference. Prior to the declaration of the republic, the Santa Casa director and the Daughters of Charity's Mother Superior had almost uniformly guaranteed entrance to the asylum after police authorities or family members brought the presumed to the asylum. No medical screenings or psychiatric exams such as anthropometric tests preceded admission to the asylum. Psychiatrists had been the last members of the administrative staff to enter the patients' therapeutic regimen. Decree 206 positioned psychiatrists as the first, and the primary, professionals to oversee the care and management of the mentally ill.

This landmark decree also articulated a new form of medico-legal citizenship for the presumed mentally ill both inside and outside of the asylum.

Similar to legislative statutes in France, England, and Belgium, the reform measure included language about safeguarding the interests of the mentally ill through a series of guarantees and rights that included legal representation, due process, and access to expeditious medical treatment. While Decree 206 seemed to mandate the "protection" of the insane, the only structures of defense for their rights came from an illiberal framework of differential medical citizenship. In his study of the construction of "inclusively inegalitarian citizenship" and the historical uses of citizenship in Brazil since 1881, political anthropologist James Holston argues "citizenship is a measure of difference and a means of distancing people from one another. It reminds people of what they are not—even though paradoxically, they are themselves citizens—and defines citizens as others."[30] According to Holston, the Brazilian state created "differentiated citizenship" based on a "gradation of rights" that shaped and regulated political, social, and civil spheres and legitimized different treatment for different types of citizens. This hegemonic process qualified and normalized personal and collective notions of citizenship based on social differences, such as education, property, income, family name, race, gender, and occupation. Hence, the popular use of the term "*cidadão qualquer*" to mean "a nobody," or an anonymous "citizen" with no formal identity rooted in family, labor, or community relations—yet still an individual and still a citizen. Holston's argument of "differentiated citizenship" provides a useful theoretical context for what historians Olívia Gomes da Cunha and Flávio dos Santos Gomes have recently defined as the "almost-citizen" (*quase-cidadão*), which from the perspective of historical anthropology, describes the status of the postabolition working poor in Brazil and the problems the social structure had generated.[31] If the working poor occupied a position of "almost-citizen," the working poor and indigent who were presumed insane and admitted to the asylum resided in a state of "bare life."[32] Even within that bareness of life, they experienced citizenship according to socioeconomic categories that differentiated them according to psychiatry's discursive construction of citizenship.

Within the asylum domain, psychiatrists bestowed varying degrees of citizenship rights to patients based on economic standing. When the asylum first opened, it quickly became a coveted site occupied by rich, poor, black, and white alike; but over time, the indigent, with the pressure of the police and popular public order concerns pressing for their institutionalization, became its main clientele.[33] While the majority of occupants at this early juncture in the asylum's history came from the municipality of the court, this trend would ebb and flow as numerous petitions to house the insane in the imperial capital's flagship asylum poured in from province presidents and Santa Casas from throughout Brazil and neighboring countries. For example, an 1853 letter by Santa Casa director José Clemente Pereira documents that Isabel Dorrego, daughter of General Dorrego from Buenos Aires, who had resided in Rio since April 1852, was anxiously waiting for the asylum to open.[34] Reminiscent of Foucault's mad on the Ship of Fools in seventeenth-century Europe, ships bound for Rio de Janeiro brought the mentally ill from all over Brazil and Latin America; upon disembarkment, they would wander the streets until, in a best-case scenario, police authorities brought them to the asylum, where they were classified as indigents. Although statistical records are not available for every year, a sampling of the asylum population during its formative years (1852 to 1856) shows that the majority of patients' country of origin was identified as Africa (some classified as "freed," meaning that they had been enslaved), followed by Portugal.[35] Echoing the assertions of historian Magali Engel, slave owners readily freed those slaves they suspected were insane before sending them to the asylum, or they left them to wander the streets so that the slaveholders, as property owners, would bear no financial or legal responsibility for those that had once served them. Of the 1,746 admission records from 1850 to 1888 that contained the social status of patients, there were 207 slaves, 153 freed people (*libertos*), and 1386 free persons (*livres*).[36] While the racially indeterminate category of "free" could include those marked as black, white, or mixed race, the statistical record shows that a majority of the free were brought in as indigent and were classified as black or mixed. The records state that between 1883 and 1900, 85 percent of the indigent class were black or mixed,[37] and the asylum population was 40 percent white, 35 percent black or mixed, and 24 percent without racial designations.[38] In 1870, a rare year where the patient population fell below 300, the records categorize 209 patients out of 297 as "indigent."[39] Thus, these statistics indicate a mutually reinforcing relationship between poverty, insanity, and blackness. The early preponderance and continuing significant presence of indigent patients as a permanent defining fixture of the asylum not only reflected the extent to which the police and others would use the institution; it also reflected the ways in which the elite classes and a succession of republican administrations spawned a series of urbanization and economic plans that disproportionately left out the city's heterogeneous poor (composed of former slaves, freed persons, rural migrants, Spanish and Portuguese immigrants, and Rio natives). In the immediate aftermath of the messy transition to republican rule, anxieties about lawlessness, disorder, and danger, whether well-founded or not, were commonly projected upon those of African descent as the tide of antiblack scientific racism spurred on apocalyptic fears of national chaos and ruin. Within this schema, the presumed indigent insane, of which those of African descent presumably constituted a large segment, became a vulnerable surplus problem population. As writer and asylum patient Afonso Henriques de Lima Barreto observed of the asylum in *Cemetery of the Living* (1922), "All is black," referencing the "dark pigment of most of the ill. . . . Black is the most trenchant, most arresting color."[40]

Psychiatrists were united in their belief that the Afro-descent people and the indigent population would hinder the asylum's modernist becoming and looked to the agricultural colony as a therapeutic management tool. The emergence of agricultural colonies in Rio was part of a wave of agricultural colonies that spread throughout the Atlantic World. Agricultural colonies were built concurrently in France, England, and the United States, among other countries, in the late nineteenth and early twentieth centuries.[41] The establishment of these agricultural colonies (often small farms attached to psychiatric hospitals) first emerged in Europe as a response to broader calls for psychiatric reform dating from the mid-nineteenth century. With mounting concerns over asylum overcrowding and accusations of patient negligence, psychiatrists began to experiment with alternative forms of patient care that relied on new uses of space and the environment; instead of chaining or isolation cells, psychiatric reformers argued that putting people to work in the fields in the open air would be more humane and therapeutically effective. Discussions about the uses of labor as therapy actually centered on a much older idea rooted in antiurban discourses and a vogue for experimental farms dating from the early nineteenth century. The first colonies were introduced in France as rural outlets for a revolutionary urban underclass and as penal colonies for orphans and juvenile delinquents, including the famous colony of Mettray.[42] A condemnation of urban industrial society marked early discussions about the colonies and a countervailing valorization of the countryside as a site for the restoration of authority, order, and social discipline. Reformers embraced these agrarian utopias, but for reasons that went beyond an appreciation of their aesthetic or romantic qualities. As the French historian Ceri Crossley writes, "Rurality was not so much emblematic of an earlier, simpler world as constitutive of a passive citizenry. This was not the countryside as escapism: agricultural work—with religion in support—was understood as a process of socialization."[43] For psychiatrists in republican Brazil, fresh from victory after four decades of conflict with religious authorities and struggling with the disconnect between the reality of the indigent population within the asylum on one hand and their therapeutic ideals on the other, the intended focus of the agricultural colonies was on the socialization or resocialization of the largely Afro-descent indigent and the freeing of the asylum.

While Brandão advocated moral treatment and isolation for melancholics and maniacs within the confines of the asylum, he stressed that chronic patients needed to "exercise outdoors, [so that] the distractions [of] manual work [can] produce the complete integration of the primitive mental personality."[44] In this manner, the agricultural colonies were constructed around the notion of dual function of providing patients with both work and rest, characterized as a great comfort to the insane who "in moments of calm" could move outdoors, "outside the heavy and gloomy atmosphere of the asylum, that for them is a prison."[45] According to Brandão, the agricultural colonies were suitable for the treatment of the insane from both therapeutic and economic perspectives.

Brandão claimed that by working the cultivation of crops and livestock, the mentally ill could convert their work into profit.[46] And he stressed that the government should prefer these institutions since they would cost little.[47] Once established, individuals from both the National Insane Asylum and the Almshouse could be transferred there. Sidestepping the rhetoric that privileges the interests and well-being of the insane in the construction of agricultural colonies, it becomes apparent that these sites also benefited psychiatrists since they allowed psychiatrists to focus away from Afro descent, indigent "problem" populations. Founded a few months after the proclamation of the republic, the agricultural colonies were built in two preexisting buildings on the Ilha do Governador (Governador's Island). While the first was situated on the farms of São Bento and belonged to the Benedictine Brotherhood, the second was the property of the Conde de Mesquita (Earl of Mesquita). Separated by approximately 1.5 miles (2,500 meters), the Colonies of the Alienated of Governador's Island (Colonias de Alienados da Ilha do Governador) were initially intended for men with strong physical abilities. However, they quickly became open to both men and women. At the end of 1890, there were 142 people in the colonies, and official documents described them as employed "in the tilling of the land, cultivation of cereals, beans, and the raising of animals and domestic birds."[48] While those at the São Bento Colony focused on the cultivation of crops, those at the Conde de Mesquita Colony tended to livestock. In addition, those with knowledge of mechanics were employed in the construction of houses and stables, while insane women were responsible for washing clothes and sewing work.[49] In this manner, it was possible to organize the insane according to their aptitude and dispositions for labor according to the state of their diseases. Transatlantic psychiatric writings had long held assertions about the healing power of nature and, specifically, agricultural work in the open air, citing the rhythms of the seasons as contributing to the restoration of the mind.[50] Foucault himself explored similar ideas in eighteenth-century French discussions of treatments for insanity, where the return of the patient to the "immediacy" of nature through agricultural labor had the ability "of liberating man from his liberty."[51]

Scholars of colonialism have focused on the proliferation of the agricultural colony model as penal colonies for political prisoners, reformatories for paupers and juvenile delinquents, and as sites for the occupational training of poor white settlers in many countries; however, the use of labor and, specifically, agricultural labor, as a psychiatric intervention, has been largely overlooked.[52] Academic focus on the natural and built environment as hindrances to the agricultural colonies' success too benignly portray Brazilian psychiatrists, and namely Brandão, as well-intentioned but ill-informed professionals. Even though some works have taken this rendering of psychiatrists to task by focusing on the colonies as sites of total exclusion that effectively segregated and excised the chronic indigent insane, they too have been limited in their analyses.[53] Class, rather than mental disposition, was the shared material condition of those sent to the agricultural colonies. Presumed maniacs, imbeciles, idiots, and alcoholics, among others who were poor or indigent, overwhelmingly resided under the large conceptual umbrella of incurable. The placement of indigent peoples in agricultural colonies in a postslave colony so quickly after abolition should immediately spark suspicion on the psychiatric elision of presumed deficient minds and forced labor within a space eerily reminiscent of the colonial plantation. The absence of overt racial references in the agricultural colonies' archival record should not be understood to preclude, much less excuse, the latent operationalization of class and race of psychiatric measures in postemancipation Rio de Janeiro.[54] A contemporary reader might regard the use of the agricultural colony as a reflection of progressive, innovative ideas, since agriculture provided a wide range of possible activities for the presumed insane, ranging from the cultivation and harvesting of the fields to working with livestock and maintaining the estate. In theory there was a job to suit every possible temperament and aptitude, and placing the insane to work on a farm meant reinserting them into an uncanny hierarchy with the asylum director filling the role of landowner, or master, the staff of skilled farm managers serving as overseers, and the patients that of worker, or slave, providing the labor according to directions and supervision from above.[55]

When tracing the contemporary uncanny to its late eighteenth-century European foundations,[56] historian and architect Anthony Vidler notes that the malaise of a newly formed bourgeois sector uneasy with its social position often projects a fear "carefully bounded by the limits of real material security and the pleasure principle afforded by a terror that was, artistically at least, kept well under control."[57] Brazilian psychiatrists were fearful of failing, keenly aware of their precarious professional roles in an asylum inundated with chronic and indigent patients. This population forced psychiatrists to probe the limits of their professional security, all the while discovering the failed recourses of a pleasure principle grounded in therapeutic tools such as the moral treatment. In a way, the agricultural colonies were the expression of psychiatrists' professional insecurities projected on the indigent and institutionalized. Thus, Brandão's rendering of the agricultural colony as an ideal site for primitive minds can itself be read as a "primitive" response in the context of a postemancipation Brazil hoping to exorcise slavery in the republican imagination but yet turning to it as a referent. The settlement of the agricultural colonies with the indigent insane removed from the mainstream asylum patient population a subgroup that reflected "attitudes and practices of the system of repression [that] were transferred smoothly to the non-slave lower classes and persisted."[58] Apart from symbolic or hyperbolic academic value, the elusive slippage between madness, indigence, and blackness is important because it motivated psychiatrists to remove this "problem" population from the asylum and place them in a zone of bare life, represented by the agricultural colony.

Observing the Mad City: The Observation Pavilion

Altering the asylum's built environment as a means to maximize reform measures was a central component to the psychiatric revitalization of the institution. The creation of the pavilion was motivated, in part, by concern about the health of hospitals and related institutions in the city that were, themselves, considered unhealthy spaces.[59] As an international standard during the late nineteenth and early twentieth century, the pavilion-plan hospital, with its open wards separated by long corridors, was hailed as an ideal architectural form since, according to miasmatists, it allowed for cross ventilation.[60] The Observation Pavilion in Rio was a sprawling structure that was supposed to maximize ventilation, minimize the crowding of wards, and reduce the risk of infection. Even though this functionalist building was supposed to contribute positively to healing, it was not devoid of (ideological) form much less ideology. The notion that architecture is invested with meaning and is a means of conveying meaning is not a new one. Architects and writers in the architectural field have discussed how the built environment occupies and shapes the physical social context as well as influencing the perceptual nature of human behavior.[61] More than utilitarian, architecture stands in evidence of social life, conveying social and intellectual meanings through form.[62] Since architecture can be understood as a self-contained sign system with its own grammar and syntax, the importation of structuralist methodology to understand the built environment can facilitate the reading of the pavilion as a "text."[63]

In Rio de Janeiro, the exercise of professional authority over insanity and marginality, followed by medical imperatives, anchored the construction rationale of the pavilion. In reports sent to the Ministry of Justice and Interior Affairs soon after the declaration of the republic, Brandão critiqued police authorities for the convoluted and inefficient process of sending the presumed insane to the asylum. Often, the police took them to the Almshouse, where they would be observed for eight days before being transferred to the National Hospice. In the asylum, the majority of individuals would languish in bureaucratic and therapeutic limbo as they lacked proof of identity or documentation attesting to their mental ailments. In order to address this issue, Brandão suggested the construction of a structure on the asylum grounds where individuals could be carefully observed before they were processed and admitted into the institution, an investment in infrastructure to support the distribution and categorization roles that psychiatrists now commanded in the wake of Decree 206 (the establishment of Medical-Legal Assistance to the Alienated). Moreover, since many individuals brought to the asylum suffered from infectious diseases, he argued that psychiatrists needed a triage site where they could address somatic diseases, an argument that resounded profoundly in a city where residents were keenly familiar with the ravages of epidemic diseases. Thus, the creation of the Observation Pavilion hinged upon its functioning as a type of waiting zone or space that imposed a spatial-temporal control over the presumed insane and, therefore, authority over the actors who brought them to the asylum.[64] Convinced by Brandão's arguments, state officials authorized the construction of an observation pavilion on October 23, 1891 (Decree 1559).

Contracted in 1892, it was finally finished in 1894 under the management of a professor of clinical psychiatry and nervous diseases from the Medical School of Rio de Janeiro rather than the asylum director. Inaugurated in March 1894, the Observation Pavilion consisted of an amphitheater for classes, a place of residence for student-psychiatrists, and two sections for patients (Magnan for women and Meynert for men). When the presumed insane were brought to the asylum, they would be placed in the pavilion for fifteen days and subjected to a battery of anthropometric tests and disease screenings. After thorough surveillance by the medical gaze, they would be diagnosed and sent to the appropriate facility, be it the asylum, an agricultural colony, or prison. Upon arriving at the Observation Pavilion, patient Vicente Mascarenhas reflected on his degradation and debasement: "All of us were naked and I was full of bashfulness. I remembered the steam bath of Dostoyevsky in House of the Dead. I cried, but I remembered Cervantes and Dostoyevsky, who must have suffered worse."[65] Built along the ideological schema of the panopticon model, the Observation Pavilion also functioned as a laboratory, where the practice of psychiatry became a reiterative process.[66] The creation of both living and learning spaces within the pavilion offered medical students a full experiential immersion, thereby facilitating their emergent abilities to marry theory and praxis.[67]

Instead of turning strictly to European, and predominantly French, psychiatric theories, burgeoning Brazilian psychiatrists were able to craft a national psychiatric tradition responsive to Brazilian realities. The pavilion may be understood as what sociologist Zygmunt Bauman defines as an emic space and a phagic space.[68] While emic spaces are employed to segregate, phagic space engulfs and consumes otherness, recruiting and incorporating into its own logic rather than physically excluding. As an emic spatial technology that separated the indigent insane, the pavilion was also a site of consumption and transformation. As the indigent insane became the focus of constant surveillance, remaining under close scrutiny by psychiatrists for how they lived and died, they also fed and satiated psychiatric appetites.

Conclusion

To what extent were the initiatives described in this chapter successful? Did they realize the asylum's potentiality as a curative technology? While these measures did not serve as panaceas, they had varied degrees of success and failure. For example, an 1899 asylum report presented to the minister of justice and interior affairs claimed that it was difficult to operate a nursing school due to the absolute lack of candidates who could adhere to the school's requirements. According to this report, it was also "impossible" to train the orphans from the institutions of social assistance within the city's municipalities since they were "illiterate, with little love for work, and ill will towards the mentally ill."[69] As a result, more secular nurses from France were recruited to work in the asylum and to train Brazilian nurses.[70] Despite the nursing school's slow start, its establishment, along with the recruitment of French nurses, did ultimately provide psychiatrists with complementary assistants who conferred upon them deference and authority. Like the asylum and the nursing school, the agricultural colonies experienced a tenuous beginning due to overcrowding. For example, in December 1892, the colonies' population had risen to 211 patients,[71] and it surpassed 250 by the end of 1894.[72] In addition, the efficacy of the agricultural colonies was compromised for agricultural reasons, including small plots of unproductive land ravaged by endemic drought during hot months. The psychiatrists were poor farm planners. This combination of factors produced decreasing income and increasing expenses.[73] Apart from these issues, the accommodations for patients were in poor condition, in need of expansions and renovations, and the patients suffered the numerous epidemics that hit the colonies and also "suffered in the winter, as they were also attacked by worms in their feet." Furthermore, their location presented difficulties, as it was hard to transport food and medication from the National Hospice to them.[74] The litany of problems plaguing the colonies was not lost on the colonies' directors, who consistently documented them in their reports to the Ministry of Justice and Interior Affairs. When Brandão's successor, Juliano Moreira, the director of the asylum and of the Assistance to the Alienated welfare program (1903–30), extolled the virtues of agricultural colonies as excellent means for caring for the mentally ill, he proposed the creation of a colony on the mainland based on family care in lieu of reforming the colonies on the Ilha do Governador.[75] In 1924 the federal office of Ministry of Internal Affairs implemented his proposal, transferring the Ilha do Governador patients to the newly created Jacarepaguá colony in the city in 1924. It remains hard to argue for the therapeutic success of the agricultural colonies; however, it is true that the colonies served to remove a percentage of the largely Afro-Brazilian indigent from the asylum population, leaving psychiatry to therapeutically succeed or fail with the remaining, more insane, wealthier, and whiter asylum population.

The Observation Pavilion, on the other hand, represented, in many ways, the pinnacle of psychiatric success. Apart from offering psychiatrists considerable discretion in the admission of patients into the social welfare net, it offered them a captive subject base. In turn, this population functioned as the means to facilitate psychiatrists' end, their professional becoming. The Observation Pavilion paved the way for the creation of more specialized pavilions like the Bourneville Pavilion for Children and consequently more specialized psychiatric knowledge production.

An examination of the first asylum reforms initiated by psychiatrists in the aftermath of the republic's declaration allows for a sociopolitical and cultural understanding of early Brazilian psychiatry's interiorities. Early republican reforms that sought to modernize the asylum illustrate the extent to which gender, class, and racial thinking were constitutive of psychiatric mechanisms for treating the mentally ill. Indirectly and to varying degrees, these psychiatrists were inspired by the sociological positivism that dominated military thinking and technical training in late nineteenth-century Brazil. Many expressed variations of Comte's laws of human progress and his belief that society could be examined and "perfected" through the "rational" application of scientific principles. They shared a commitment to scientific method and a belief in inherent differences among individuals and between categories of individuals. They generated a phenomenal array of psychological, sociological, and physiological criteria for classifying types of insane peoples in the interest of treating them and in the interest of the defense of Brazilian society. In their attempts to remake the asylum into an ideal site, they created a constellation of at least putatively therapeutic institutions, but they still could not abate the series of problems that plagued the institution. Indeed, problems such as overcrowding, among others, garnered the attention of state and civil authorities during the late nineteenth century and catapulted the asylum and its psychiatrists into the public sphere.

The asylum, previously praised as the aspirational site of moral therapy and cure, was not able to cope with an increasing number of admissions, under psychiatrists much like it had been under the Daughters of Charity. Over time, a pessimism replaced the curative optimism typical of early nineteenth-century psychiatrists. In the second half of the nineteenth century, asylum psychiatrists noticed that while some patients recovered from some mental disorders, most patients did not recover, and some even worsened while in the asylum. Many patients suffered severe and persistent forms of illness and only left in coffins. Individualized attention was virtually impossible; most patients suffered from conditions that were barely amenable to treatment. The most realistic hope of relief for many patients was spontaneous recovery as asylum psychiatry, increasingly, consisted of curating the chronically incapacitated. There were no known effective treatments, much less cures, for any psychotic disorder.

The optimism associated with the asylum and the belief in its inherent therapeutic benefits had begun to wane, and its custodial character was harder to ignore. Thus, the late nineteenth-century period that witnessed the flowering of psychodynamic psychiatry, in the form of the moral treatment, was followed by a deep onset of therapeutic pessimism in asylum psychiatry. Brazil was not unique in this matter. The number of institutionally confined in the first half of the twentieth century doubled in England and Wales and more than trebled in the United States, where patient numbers in state and county asylums surpassed half a million by 1950. The majority of hospitals housed well over a thousand patients each. After, in many ways, unsuccessfully pitting rationality against madness, psychiatrists, and the people to whom they had promised a new, morally therapeutic world, reapproached insanity as more mature modernists but with a large measure of resignation.

This psychiatric pessimism was, in part, the result of the kinds of persons populating the asylum and its adjunct institutions of care: patients with intractable and irreversible organic diseases (e.g., tertiary syphilis) were flooding into the asylum. Not surprisingly, psychiatrists in Rio increasingly posited that most mental disorders were hereditary and particularly starting in the 1870s, degeneration theory became a dominant framework through which to explain insanity. While this term has implied a hereditary and biological model of insanity wherein psychopathic traits could be transmitted from parents to their children, its understandings took on varied meanings and textures in various contexts. Brazilian and other Latin American medical professionals did not understand degeneration theory through a racially deterministic model. Given the region's extensive history of racial, ethnic, and cultural miscegenation, they understood degeneration theory not through genes but through sociocultural structures. According to this logic, any Brazilian could become degenerate if they treaded too close to the presumed inferior cultural terrain of Afro-Brazilians and thereby denigrating the cultural integrity of the nation.

While the internal structures of psychiatry's self-image were undergoing dramatic transformations with the significant failure of the moral treatment and the rise of degeneration theory, the field had to contend with pressing public scrutiny about psychiatrists' professional competencies. The loss of hope around the asylum's potential and the consequent decline in profile of the asylum led to popular denigration of its medical superintendents and to a public reappraisal of the role of the psychiatrist. In place of self-confident declarations about growth, prosperity, and improvement, commentators characteristically discussed psychiatrists' inability to grapple with mental illness, which had been their central claim to relevance.

Chapter Four

"The Service of Disinterested Men"

Psychiatrists under State and Civil Scrutiny, 1894–1903

After four years as the full governing authority of the National Asylum for the Insane, psychiatrists encountered a barrage of criticism from state and civil actors who charged that psychiatrists' institutional remedies had failed. Many state officials defended the asylum from these attacks, but they also sought to intervene in asylum functioning. For these officials, the asylum's modernization served as an example of state power. It operated as a physical and symbolic object that enabled the state, through the provision of health care as a public good, to showcase its functions and duties. Wresting the offices of charity from colonial Leviathan institutions such as the Santa Casa de Misericórdia was fundamental to the republican administration; it had come into power with promises to federalize social assistance. While this process elevated the importance of assistance to all the nation's poor and "unfortunates," the insane held a special place in a hierarchy of the needy. Unlike young, able-bodied vagrant men or criminals, they constituted one of the populations that, in the republican modernist mindset, deserved aid and rehabilitation.

Republican spokesmen who sought to increase the infrastructural power of the state through the secularization of key colonial institutions seized upon the asylum and the insane as sites on which to graft a political program of liberalism. Infrastructural power refers to the capacity of the state to coordinate society by diffusing law and administration into areas of social life that, before the nineteenth century, had remained outside the scope of state concern.[1] In the case of early republican Brazil, the administration that came into power focused on the insane because the imperial government had marked this vulnerable population as one of its significant clients for state patronage. Just as imperial statesmen used advances in the treatment of the insane and the asylum itself as a political tool to garner public favor during a period of crisis, republican officials used the conversion to psychiatric control and functionality to validate their legitimacy. Imperial public institutions and ways of life had to be rejected, fully appropriated, or possibly even eradicated in order to create new political forms and new social mores in their stead. The infrastructural power of the republican state, after declaring the asylum to be under new psychiatric management, could be measured in part by the success of its management of the asylum.

This chapter explores how denunciations of the asylum and its administration and psychiatric rebuttals revealed the juxtaposition of, on the one hand, a strong antistatist tradition rooted in imperial nostalgia, and on the other, secular bureaucracies of expertise. Scholar Svetlana Boym's reminder that "while the longing is universal, nostalgia can be divisive" applies here.[2] Nostalgia, in late nineteenth- and early twentieth-century Rio, both for the imperium as an abstract, and for the specific profile previously enjoyed by imperial institutions of social assistance such as the Santa Casa, arose from the contested political significance afforded to the provision of welfare assistance to society's marginalized during the transition from empire to republic. While this chapter examines official state records to understand how psychiatrists and state representatives alike discussed the management of the mentally ill, it also uses newspapers as a critical forum for public debate. As elsewhere in Latin America during the last decades of the nineteenth century, journalists in Rio found themselves in a position that seemed both vulnerable and promising. Throughout the monarchic period, journalists did not constitute a distinct professional class, and their role could not be clearly dissociated from the parliament and party politics. However, with the significant technical and cultural transformations of the press that coincided with the proclamation of the republic, educated men saw reporting, editing, and owning newspapers as a chance for upward social mobility and access to political positions. Professionals who employed journalism as a secondary occupation saw in it a possibility of attaining intellectual and literary prestige and advancing causes often connected to their primary professions. Struggling to affirm their social status, journalists claimed the position of masters of the letter as well as shapers of public opinion who, at the same time, were shaped by it. As they struggled to construct and defend their public image and to become the new and authorized doctors of culture, they championed transparency, accountability, probity, courage, freedom, and equality among peers.

The editors saw themselves as educators. They believed their profession made them responsible for educating the populace in theories of self-government and cultivating in policymakers the ability to rule effectively. In creating this role for themselves, the editors very consciously followed the philosophy of Enlightenment. The element of Enlightenment philosophy most central to the role of the journalist was educating the people by involving them in discussions of the state. By publishing their ideas, the editors believed they were preventing the government from taking undue liberties with the direction of the state. While the editors believed they wrote to and for the "people," it is not immediately clear exactly who those people were. In many ways, the "people" was a rhetorical construction to lend weight to the analysis of the editors. If an editor could say that "a great number of people" felt a certain way, then his arguments gained a sense of authority. In other ways, the people were very much present and played an important role in the development of the political philosophies present in the newspapers. To borrow a term from Marco Morel, the newspapers cultivated an "active public" and competed for a "passive public."[3] Public opinion, as an expression, became increasingly associated with the power of the press and its audiences.

In late nineteenth-century Rio, as in historian Jeremy Popkin's description of the French Revolution, newspapers operated as both "purveyors of information and ideology" and as significant zones for the creation of sociopolitical and cultural identities.[4] As in Popkin's formulation, this chapter will address newspapers as an interactive literature of reform. The publications that captivated Rio's reading and listening publics both informed readers and provided them with the means to become active participants in state matters. While historians posit that the widespread availability of newspapers led to an increase in the number of prospective readers, less than 20 percent of the free population of Rio could read.[5] Therefore, late nineteenth- and early twentieth-century Rio was an oral culture. However, the power of newspapers came in part from the fact that reading newspapers aloud provided the crucial means for the transference of ideas and ideology between the literate and illiterate urban populations.[6] Visitors to Brazil at the time such as the Reverend Robert Walsh observed the oral delivery of newspapers; he reported that after the newspapers were distributed, he "constantly saw groups of neighbors assembled in some shop, and one of them sitting on the counter, reading a sheet of correspondence to the rest."[7] Other scholars have noted how common it was to find ideas being discussed in the street that were originally printed in the newspapers. In 1871 historian J. M. Pereira da Silva reported "the curious population read [newspapers] from sunrise to sunset, repeating the subject of the paper from mouth to mouth and the most extravagant calumnies [passed] as truth."[8] Editors frequently adopted writing styles that reflected the patterns of oral communication."[9] As newspapers began to characterize the new asylum with many of the same criticisms that psychiatrists had brought to bear against the Daughters of Charity, the new psychiatric authorities felt compelled to leave the comforting confines of the asylum, the medical school, and the halls of government in order to critically engage with the Brazilian public. Brandão, the charismatic asylum director, responded vociferously to critics. Indeed, as I will explore below, his responses can be read as exegeses of a profession coming of age as a modernist project inside the wide littoral of postimperial Rio.

The Asylum under Scrutiny

In 1894 Senator Francisco de Paula Leite e Oiticica from the state of Alagoas instigated a debate about the national budget and the use of public coffers for social assistance programs. It placed the shortcomings of the asylum and the managerial and medical pitfalls of psychiatry in sharp relief. Through various diatribes citing the asylum's numerous defects and attributing them to Brandão, the senator hoped to return the asylum to Santa Casa's management. While religious officials began to discuss whether Santa Casa was the proper organ to oversee the institutional and therapeutic treatment of the insane in 1890, the federal Senate did not comprehensively debate issues of state welfare, in addition to the moral and political economies of state responsibility for the insane, until November 9, 1894, during the Senate's 130th session. Taking a position squarely within the bounds of laissez-faire liberalism, the senator asserted repeatedly that the state should not bear complete responsibility for the insane. He advocated for tight conceptual limits on the state's role in social welfare wherein public assistance should be complementary or cooperative with private/religious efforts, freeing up the state to focus its primarily concern on its basic functions such as the defense of national territory.

Senator Leite e Oiticica reconciled laissez-faire with interventionist liberalism in public welfare by linking limited public assistance to the encouragement of religious entrepreneurship in charity. Since the meeting's topic of discussion was the budget of the Ministry of Justice and Interior Affairs for 1895, Senator Leite e Oiticica denounced irregularities in the relationship between legislative and executive powers surrounding the production of laws and budgets to regulate and allocate public spending. He condemned the executive for spending more than the legislative branch mandated, which ultimately made it necessary for the president to open lines of credit annually. According to the senator, this viciously circular process warranted immediate attention;[10] it was bad economic policy that undermined the constitutional power of the legislative branch to regulate spending and to determine the scale of programs by limiting their budgets. Moreover, he argued that the new republic was misguided, and falling victim to the fascination of wealth, suffering from "the mania of grandeur" and having "profligacy" as "one of its consequences."[11] In order to avoid imperiling the nation's economic future, it must cut unnecessary expenditures. Clutching the 1893 assistance report Brandão sent to the minister of justice and interior affairs office, the senator identified the Assistance to the Alienated as one of the seminal sources of excess, calling it "a drain on public funds and a slaughterhouse of the needy." He charged that "stripping the Assistance of its formal dress of affection, of dedication, of love for another," the asylum was nothing more than a prime example of "mercenary charity, perhaps with scenes of horror, unimaginable scenes, except with terror and indignation."[12] His lengthy monologue attributed such horrors and terrors to Brandão's and other psychiatrists' failures as administrators.

While Brandão's report argued that the constant pressure of police drop-offs created problems segregating the insane according to apt diagnoses, the senator focused on the "promiscuity" of classes in the asylum. Although the asylum's admissions based on class divisions was supposed to institute a de jure segregationist order, chronic overcrowding led to a de facto higgledy-piggledy space where the wealthy were "clustered [with the poor] and exposed to a common life."[13] He also lambasted Brandão directly for subjecting children to the "lust and violence of insane adults":[14]

> As sad as it is heartbreaking that, in the middle of all this dire lack of love, these reprobates of fortune do not encounter in the least a compassionate look and gentle authority dedicated to the relief of suffering, and the cold stare without expression of the Director of Assistance, to reject the innocent that will not compete! Yes! It was not for this they paid him; sheltering children was not the purpose behind the establishment's foundation, to pay for all the staff, to spend rivers of money, and the director is unwilling to be bothered by the dissonant wailing in that house of madpeople of all types.[15]

Further, the senator offered a litany of vital statistics based on mortality and costs. Again citing the 1893 annual report, he noted that by December 31, 1893, the asylum had housed 672 patients, 510 of whom had entered that year, 270 of whom had died. Finding the 30 percent mortality rate of those admitted as alarmingly high, he found it unacceptable that the federal government would financially support such an institution. Presenting the balance sheet of the asylum for the year 1888–89, when it was under the direction of the Daughters of Charity, he asserted that the asylum possessed sufficient finances to cover its costs according to that budget and did not need the financial support of the federal government. He inquired, "By what right, in the name of principles, did this service, which did not previously cost the public coffers a dime, pass from the Santa Casa to the federal government from private patrimony to the federal budget?"[16]

While Senator Leite Oiticica had voted against the restitution of the asylum to the Santa Casa the year before, in 1893, he called his change of position the result of serious study. He called the government's appropriation of the asylum as "a violence of the most unjustifiable, an attack on the right of property of others."[17] He put a heavy spin on the narrative of the asylum's origins, effectively crediting the Santa Casa and the Santa Casa alone with its creation. Citing the wording in the original decree that affirmed the creation of the asylum, its "incorporation with the Santa Casa," whose board accepted the task of ruling the institution's administration, the senator argued that the decree legitimized the retroactive annexation of the institution to the lay brotherhood. Strangely, given the asylum's name and imperial namesake, this alternative history of the asylum stripped it of any ties to the imperial government as well as to the medical community. It hid the efforts of doctors such as Xavier Sigaud and Luís Vicente de Simoni in the asylum-building campaign of the 1830s and diminished Emperor Dom Pedro II's role to perfunctory echo. The senator bestowed mild praise on the emperor for donating funds to the asylum's founding but gave the Santa Casa's director, José Clemente Pereira, full credit for the asylum's creation. In support of this argument, he referenced the 1853 financial report of the asylum to demonstrate that the Santa Casa, not the state, paid the deficit incurred by its creation.[18]

According to the senator, Pereira's tireless mobilization of benefactors was indispensable to the construction of the asylum. Calling Pereira "a great citizen," and "a great friend of suffering humanity," he nostalgically invoked benevolent pious institutional care. Neither the senator nor his hearers had any memory of the kind of benevolent care he figured Pereira as exemplifying. Scholar Douglas Coupland described this kind of nostalgia divorced from lived experience as "legislated nostalgia," that is, forcing "a body of people to have memories they do not actually possess."[19] The power of the senator's proclamations stemmed from a yearning for an actual or imaginary imperial Brazilian patrician world of pious and functional care that sanctified the insane, the lay brotherhood, and the state that oversaw but did not intervene in the curative endeavors of religious orders. This idea lived in the popular imaginary in ways that it never had lived in the reality of an overstrained institution inundated with the mentally ill like the Hospício Dom Pedro II.

In an interesting further revision of history, the senator marked 1882 as a watershed moment when the care of the insane took a turn for the worse as a result of the simple emergence of the *idea* of state responsibility for the care of the asylum's insane. Revisiting the tense exchange between Dr. Goulart and the then Santa Casa director, Viscount of Jaguary, the senator described the doctor's failed attempts to oust the Daughters of Charity as a medico-state victory.[20] According to the senator's formulations, the doctor's arguments planted a deleterious seed that bore fruit. According to him, the worsening of services for the mentally ill rested on the transition, however slow, to state governance. The statesman described a medieval cosmological vision where charity should be the unique domain of private religious institutions, since only religious charity was "disinterested," "dedicated," and "passionate"—capable of providing its services with dedication for its "love to suffering humanity," having in its reserve a "legion of goodwill men." Public charity, "mercenary" in nature, critically lacked such qualities or people, since its political and economic interests converted "asylums into budget nurseries, where money, meant to support unfortunates, was absorbed."[21] Hoping to convince fellow politicians of the virtues of private charity, he went on to cite various institutions that were models of "order, respect, and dignity." For example, the asylum for orphans, which the Society for Lovers of Instruction (Sociedade Amante de Instrução) maintained, "breathed the love for another, virtue, and dedication to humanity," and the School of Arts and Crafts (Lyceu de Artes e Oficios), an institution that received little state subsidy, was "beautiful . . . with lovely results!"[22]

Others, ranging from state officials to newspaper writers, would echo the senator's concerns. Brandão crafted a series of pointed responses to his accusations even before the speech was published. The psychiatrist attacked the senator's rendering of history, accusing him of bringing before the senate "slanderous talk," without the care "to turn to legislation or to the asylum archive for an inquiry/investigation into the truth."[23] Obligated to expose "facts that would be better buried in oblivion," Brandão offered another historical vision that forever linked the asylum to the state. To counter the senator's arguments, he stressed that the asylum was built on grounds owned by the emperor and that the asylum was not only constructed in territory reserved for public deeds but that the Santa Casa usurped property bought for the asylum, ceding it to other institutions such as the asylum for orphans.[24] Further condemning the Santa Casa, he claimed that the lay brotherhood borrowed from the asylum's coffers when necessary during times of "financial embarrassment."[25] Describing criticisms directed at himself as the "excessive frenzy of the Senator's imagination," Brandão deflected them point by point with reference to key passages from reports and memos sent to state officials regarding asylum deficiencies. Referencing an official record of identifying asylum problems, their causes, and possible remedies to state officials, he established a pattern of institutional transparency. For example, tackling the issue of "promiscuity" among patients, he referred to specific passages in a report sent to the minister of justice and interior affairs in which he urged the need to better isolate patients according to education and social position. He emphasized this task was not possible without the direct financial intervention of the government in order to create pavilions able to support the appropriate segregation of patients. As he asserted, "I asked for a special section for minors and I justified its necessity. If the Assistance cannot be exempt from receiving them, it is intuitive that it attempts to accommodate them."[26] With a hint of sarcasm, he addressed the issue of children living among adults: "The Assistance was created to help and to treat all the insane. When the police encounter an insane pregnant woman, they do not ask her to postpone the delivery in order to provide her aid."[27] Labeling the Santa Casa's practice of sending children of insane women to the House of Abandoned Children (Casa dos Expostos) as "inhumane and criminal," he defended his practice of allowing children to reside with their mothers.[28]

Responding to the senator's critique of the asylum's high mortality rate, the psychiatrist asserted that when patients arrived at the asylum, they were already in poor health since the police and families used the institution as a last resort and not a preventative recourse. He argued he could only improve the quality of care for asylum patients through increased government funding. Countering the senator's statistics, Brandão noted that from December 9, 1842, to December 31, 1889 (or forty-seven years and twenty-two days), 6,040 patients entered the asylum while 2,454 died. From January 1, 1890, to November 9, 1894 (or three years, ten months, and nine days), 3,043 patients entered and 1,089 died.[29] Here he argued that the asylum had higher mortality rates under Santa Casa than under the federal government and that the senator failed to take into account a proportioned approach to statistical mortality analysis. Moreover, he intimated that rising admission rates would guarantee an increase in deaths if government funding failed to keep pace with patient costs.

The high rates of admission and the staggering high rates of patient deaths were undoubtedly attributed to the ways in which the asylum operated as a multifunctional site of last resort. The patient population consisted of a motley group that included people with varying grades of learning disability: those addicted to drugs and alcohol, either acutely or chronically disturbed; those with personality disorders of protean varieties; vagrants; the aged who had become an embarrassment to their kin; pregnant single women who had been cast out by their relatives; and anyone who by hook, and not infrequently by crook, could feign whatever the law and medical standards required to be "certified." When these people entered the asylum, they were greatly stressed by the vestiges of poverty, dire living conditions, and poor bodily health. No sooner than they had entered the asylum, many died from diseases and ailments years already in the making. Demonstrating an awareness of the economic and social vulnerability of their patients, psychiatrists situated the pressures the asylum faced in the broader context of economic downturns alongside the consequent increase of poverty and costs of care.

In a dramatic attempt to prove that the senator's criticisms were groundless and to garner political support, Brandão submitted his resignation on November 10, 1894, a day after senator's speech before the assembly. His notice to the minister of justice and interior affairs specifically referenced the senator's statements, "Needing to respond to the tirades of Senator Leite e Oiticica who . . . misrepresenting the excerpts from the report I had the honor to present to you, violently attacked the Medical-Legal Assistance organization and my administration, I implore you, beseech you, after defending myself to the fullest extent, to concede to my resignation."[30] In this manner, Brandão portrayed himself as a selfless administrator without ego who was willing to martyr himself by assuming full responsibility for any problems related to the asylum and the welfare system for the mentally ill, however groundless. Marechal Floriano Peixoto, the vice president of Brazil, rejected his request, asserting that the psychiatrist performed his job with "such dignity" and should "continue to give this branch of public service the valuable resource of his proficiency and well known dedication." Playing into the feelings of the new republic and of President Prudente de Morais's progressive administration, the psychiatrist justified renewing his request, calling it an act of love for the republic and stating, essentially, that he would rather resign than countenance continued debate about returning the asylum to the Santa Casa. He asserted that

> I feel that the reason, for the political attitude assumed, either in republican propaganda, either in the events that followed the advent of the republic, of the reactionary attacks against the institution I manage. In this case, I prefer the sacrifice of my own love, exonerating me, to the realization of a fact that would constitute, in the republic, a medieval anachronism, a monstrous retrograde: the deliverance of the service to the insane to a confraternity.[31]

The vice president rejected this request and Brandão sent a personal appeal to the president, which was also denied. While the true intentions behind Brandão's numerous requests may never be known, it is notable that he framed the senator's criticisms, along with campaign to have the asylum be returned to the lay brotherhood, as an attack on the republic. He further constructed his own professional self as an expendable social soldier for the republic. When the senate resumed session on the November 19, Senator Ubaldino do Amaral from Paraná opened the meeting by accusing Senator Leite e Oiticica of attempting to convert the senate into the judiciary branch by returning the asylum to the Santa Casa. He stressed that the asylum was not a house of charity and that its management was an obligation of government, as it rendered a "service that dealt with public peace . . . with the very important rights of families," and as such, could not be trusted to a private institution.[32] Casting aspersions on the emotional fragility of Senator Leite e Oiticica for having been "excessively moved by the Santa Casa director's report and the depiction of children among adults," Senator Ubaldino do

Amaral claimed that other institutions, such as the Shelter for Beggars, were also in dire straits and that Senator Leite e Oiticica's concerns necessitated a larger and more comprehensive discussion of the national budget in relation to needy institutions, not just the asylum. Nevertheless, Senator Leite e Oiticica proposed a repeal amendment that would authorize the return of the asylum to the Santa Casa. The amendment was tabled for lack of a quorum in the 1894 session, but the issue resurfaced during the May 20, 1895, senate assembly. Perhaps sensing resistance from his colleagues in the previous senate session, Senator Leite e Oiticica refocused the rhetorical weight of his argument on the virtues of charity as opposed vices of state-funded public assistance. He stated that

> the service performed by the state is more expensive than the one offered by disinterested men, from institutions of charity such as the Santa Casa de Misericórdia do Rio de Janeiro: an institution that honors Brazil. . . . If we understand charity, in its most sublime, the most delicate, to not enter into these houses where there are those who are not responsible for their miserable state, who have lost what man holds most noble, what constitutes superiority over animals; if we remove compassion, the sentiments of charity would be lost because this service is solely made by the desire to earn money.[33]

In putting forth the idea that labors performed in the asylum should not yield monetary gain, the senator renders the ideal psychiatrist as a devoted practitioner motivated by his "love to humanity" and not by professional affirmations, except for the ones bestowed upon him by the unfortunate insane. The senator exposed, in subtle ways, the protectionism and the system of camaraderie in public activity, affirming that many doctors benefited from public services through a system of patronage (and nepotism).[34] While the senator's discussion of government patronage seemed to be a potentially volatile issue from which to rally his colleagues, it ultimately fell flat when the majority of the senate rejected Senator Leite e Oiticica's amendment and confirmed the management of the asylum and the provision of service to the mentally ill to public administration. Psychiatry had developed, in Brandão, the ability to defend itself as a provider in the intricate landscape of social assistance. This marked its growth beyond its identity as a pressure group for modernist thought or a profession of ombudsmen to state and church actors. Still, psychiatrists had to articulate a captivating narrative of their usefulness so as to avert potential professional death, since it was not yet able to rely on its works or its stature as a profession. The rejection of the senator's proposals signaled a temporary victory for psychiatrists in the realm of state legitimacy; however, a series of asylum patient escapes in 1896 would reignite discussions about the relative virtues of private charity versus public welfare.

Escaping the Asylum

Within a two-day period in 1896, Paradeda Junior, Jayme Paradeda Junior, and murderer Custódio Alves Serrão, among the other criminally insane, escaped from the asylum. Although patients had been escaping from the asylum ever since its founding, these three escapes received much attention in the city's leading newspapers. They reverberated profoundly in the popular imagination and gave rise to questions about the state's and the psychiatrists' ability to manage the mentally ill and to protect the public. In the public discourse, asylum psychiatrists' inability to protect the public from the danger posed by its patients created a rift connecting the placid liberal surface of society and the charged and violent substructure populated by the various margins of the presumed mentally ill. The public saw the escapes as evidence that the republic's circumscribed liberalism concealed and accompanied incompetent social administrations such as the asylum. Newspaper outlets' attacks on the asylum's administration and the welfare service for the insane demonstrate a genuine nostalgia for the particular reassurances of the paternalism of imperial times and a malaise surrounding the symbols of republican modernism, including the prominent, formerly imperial, republican asylum. Newspapers such as *O Jornal do Brasil* and *O Jornal do Commercio,* historically antirepublican, attacked the asylum's administration and Brandão in particular with renewed vigor.[35]

The antirepublican editorial board of the *Jornal do Brasil,* which had attempted a monarchical revival during the occasion of Dom Pedro II's death in Paris in 1891, proved to be among the most determined critics of the asylum and its psychiatrist-director.[36] Many members of the journal's editorial staff had once held prestigious titles conferred upon them by imperial authorities. In the first part of a series of articles titled, "The Abandonment of the Alienated," published on the May 29, 1896, the journal depicted the asylum, under government administration, as a site where "disorder" and "disorganization" reigned.[37] In the new modernist republic founded upon "order and progress," these were serious charges. The article highlighted the slow and steady "decadence" that had befallen patients at the asylum, describing the insane as "hungry, barefoot, brutally beaten, without even a mattress to rest [on], to sleep on the floor like dogs." It proclaimed, "And this is called the consolidation of institutions. And it is this they call order, they call progress. Miserable homeland!"[38] The newspaper further condemned what it called the active silencing of scandals and a culture of impunity sanctioned by Brandão and the minister of the interior. This criticism echoed the words doctors had used approximately forty-five years earlier in their eventually successful bid to take over directorship of the asylum. Although psychiatrists relinquished their roles as critics and became managers, the asylum was still haunted by the same deficiencies of the late imperial period.

The *Gazeta de Noticias* expanded on these basic criticisms in responding to the escapes: "The conditions that amaze us and everyone is the escape of three insane people in consecutive nights, without the asylum's administration being aware of them, or being cognizant of them, and since then, not taking the necessary precautions given the gravity of the case."[39] It called the flights "shameful evidence of the unfortunate situation of the establishment, that while it was managed by the praiseworthy Sisters of Charity did not drain actual funds and satisfied with integrity the necessities of guard and curative treatment of the insane."[40] Brandão's defense of his administration to the Ministry of the Interior received both state and public attention. A few days after he submitted it, the *Diário Official* published the defense, which repeated a number of rebuttals he had used against Senator Leite e Oiticica. He claimed that the escapes occurred because the asylum was an establishment "destined for the common mad" and as such, "it did not offer the necessary security nor does it have sufficient personnel to confine the dangerous, criminal, and condemned mad." After a detailed exposition of asylum conditions, he requested the minister take the necessary "measures against the sending of such mentally ill individuals to the asylum."[41]

The *Jornal do Brasil* countered, "Under the administration of the Santa Casa da Misericórdia there was all the security and they did not spend as much as now."[42] The *Gazeta de Tarde* called the placement of the "furious" insane in strong cells "incredible, cruel, hideous, infernal."[43] Vehemently denying that the asylum practiced corporal punishment on patients, Brandão stressed that the "morbid malevolence of some madpeople" necessitated the "energetic action" of nurses.[44] As the editorials increasingly attacked the integrity of the asylum by raising the Santa Casa as a perfect establishment of care, Brandão directly took the lay brotherhood's management of the mentally ill to task. Labeling the newspapers that praised the asylum's administration under the Santa Casa as "despiteful," "clerical," and "false friends of republican institutions," he found it remarkable that they would support an institution that hindered the development of psychiatry in Brazil.[45] He decried, "For five years I supported the silly impertinences of sacristan rats without saying a word. The present moment is not the same." Brandão's derisive characterization of care exercised by religious authorities toward the mentally ill ultimately rendered these caregivers as obstacles to psychiatric progress. "Breaking the silence" on what occurred in the asylum under the Santa Casa, which was "often buried with the strictest confidence," he asserted that "when, perhaps, the doctor, by chance not surprised by the offenses, the unfortunate insane leave their cell into the ditch of cemeteries, as if they were victims of an attack."[46] According to him, "murders were committed by nurses with the acquiescence of the sisters who affectionately defended them when the fact came to the knowledge of a doctor or the [then Santa Casa] director."[47]

To support his claims, the psychiatrist sent a series of documents concerning the death and cover-up of patient Sant'Anna that Dr. Ignacio Francisco Goulart had compiled in 1874 to the *O Paiz* newspaper. The *Jornal do Brasil* jeered, "Turning a deaf ear to direct positive accusations, [Brandão] intends to lead the public's and the government's attention astray with unjust rebukes against the Sisters of Charity."[48] The *Jornal do Brasil* defended the nuns, describing them as dedicated women who were a "seraphic example of Christian charity and love of others." Their sanctioned use of force by the asylum staff, the *Jornal* claimed, prevented patient escapes.[49] The *Jornal*'s assassination of Brandão's character continued; they accused him of removing objects from the asylum and placing them in his private estate. They inquired, "Is this what is intended to still be called an administration?" Calling on the government to act, it lamented, "Wretched Country, that supports the ignominy of an administration so defective! And is the government not shamed by so many setbacks?"[50]

On June 9 the *Jornal* presented an open letter from a reader, Joaquim Pedro dos Santos Silva, to the president of the republic, Prudente de Morais, and "to the honest public." Silva had a family member confined at the institution for many years under both the administration of the lay brotherhood and the state. His letter took umbrage with the facility in which Brandão employed political labels (i.e., republican) as a means to obfuscate the "suspicious business" of the institution receiving remuneration from the state. He stated that

> nowadays, anyone can point out the mistakes and faults in whatever establishment without being later labeled as a monarchist, Sebastianist, etc. . . . as if those that label and the very own Sr. Dr. Teixeira Brandão were true republicans. . . . If [Brandão] is today a republican it is because he is employed in a state establishment and for (whose) his services receives their fees and because of this says he is a republican. . . . [So he] should not lose suspicious business, he writes in papers saying that he is a republican.[51]

The *Jornal do Brasil*'s relentless attack on the asylum continued on June 16. Joaquim Ferreira de Mesquita narrated a sensationalist tale of sadness and death. His daughter Eva Ferreira de Mesquita had been a patient in the asylum since May 21, 1894. He claimed he had requested her release and been told it was not possible because his daughter was a murderer.[52] Ferreira de Mesquita alleged this was false. Without investigating the veracity of the case, the *Jornal do Brasil* spun a web of intrigue, implying asylum officials might have any number of motives for keeping Eva imprisoned. When, in a move that reflected growth in the institution's public truth making, the *O Paiz* newspaper conducted an investigation and revealed that Eva was indeed a criminal, the *Jornal* justified its conduct by claiming that it had been "on the side of the people" in reporting the misleading story and that it would never leave off "giving shelter to everyone who is judged oppressed and lacks protection."[53] Reaffirming its role as an organ of communication always in service of the public, the *Jornal* asserted, "Maybe this is a defect we cannot fix. We have become accustomed to hearing complaints of the people, to tend to them and to give them publicity because we understand that, however exaggerated they are, something of truth always comes out in them."[54] The jockeying for truth-teller position concerning the asylum among psychiatrists, journalists, and lay people alike illustrates how one's positioning "on the side of the [marginalized] people" had become a positive value on both sides of the private charity versus public assistance debate.

The debate in the press exposed the public to the messy operations of a state institution. Newspapers critical of the asylum acted as a political lever to obtain accountability and transparency. In an unprecedented move, the barrage of criticisms led Brandão to invite the president and the press to the asylum. Although the visit from the president failed to materialize, an editor from the *O Paiz* went to the asylum and observed, using familiar words like "moral," and "scientific progress," that "the mad deserve all the affection of society; and the society that has an establishment such as the one we visited, should feel proud and satisfied. . . . The National Asylum is an eloquent note of our moral advancement; its conservation testifies to the refinement of our affective qualities; and its development will attest to our scientific progress. . . . The Asylum is already a monument of great veneration."[55]

The visit also compelled the senate to revisit Senator Leite e Oiticica's previous rejected amendment to conjoin the asylum to the Santa Casa. On the July 28, 1896, senate meeting, Firmin Pires Ferreira (Piauí), Justo Leite Chermont (Pará), Antonio Nicolau Monteiro Baena (Pará), Barão do Lavradio (Rio de Janeiro state), and F. Machado and Domingos Vicente Gonçalves de Sousa (both Espírito Santo) supported the senator's amendment. To skirt discussions about the rightful proprietor of the asylum, Senator Thomaz Delfino (representative of Rio de Janeiro), a fervent defender of the republic, affirmed that the asylum was doing the best it could since it provided a service that other institutions (e.g., Beggars' Shelter) no longer fulfilled or were meant to ever fulfill. Resurrecting past arguments about the asylum's inefficiencies, Senator Leite e Oiticica, in turn, took great care to underscore the asylum's inefficiencies by speaking at length about the various escapes, as newspapers such as the *Jornal do Brasil* had chronicled. Delfino, quick to defend the institution, asserted, "Nothing more common throughout, in places intended for the reclusion of the mad, one observes attempts at evasion and evasions."[56] To which, Quintino Bocaiuva, former senator turned journalist, affirmed, "If this happens in a public establishment, one can imagine what should not happen in a private establishment, where the action of authority does not have to interfere!"[57] Defending the asylum under psychiatric rule, Bocaiuva also stated, "The

National Asylum, is today for us, a standard of Glory" and added that "the Medical Assistance to the Alienated in the city of Rio de Janeiro is today much more well done and complete than in ancient times."[58] He declared that "the State does not do charity nor philanthropy, but governs, namely, it guarantees order and distributes justice. Between their normal duties is the assistance to the alienated, relief to the community and the provision of public safety."[59] Thus, some senators held the view that insanity not only impacted the presumed mentally ill and their immediate communities but also society at large, placing it firmly within the purview of the republican government. In a statement that called madness an ailment that can affect anyone, Senator Delfino pronounced the state's ability to cure the indigent mentally ill if they were caught in the bureaucratic safety net of poor relief through public establishments, as opposed to private ones. He claimed that

> no one can ignore that the suggestions and actions of certain substances can disturb the psychic functions. . . . The section of public power avoids bad practices by preventing the admission of persons, such as the alienated, without public intervention in private establishments. . . . If madness attacks the indigent . . . they can be cured if at the beginning of the illness they are supported by free public assistance.[60]

Although the senate still voted to maintain the asylum under state auspices, the statesmen's discussion is noteworthy for its ability to show how defenders of the asylum exalted the state's capacity to administer vital duties for the public's good. Thus, while the debate changed nothing in actual institutional policies, it did advance a discourse of social assistance that framed both the asylum and psychiatrists as vital republican fixtures in state and civil spheres.

Redeeming an Ailing Institution (1898–1903)

The state's commitment to the asylum and to psychiatry's professional mission would strengthen during the transition from the administration of President Manuel Ferraz de Campos Sales (1898–1902) to the administration of President Francisco de Paula Rodrigues Alves (1902–6). Brandão's departure from the asylum in 1898 to pursue a political career, in addition to the national financial crisis, wreaked havoc on the asylum's operations and created a leadership vacuum that ushered in a wave of institutional inertia characterized by infighting among asylum psychiatrists. While Brandão's governance of the asylum was far from ideal, his fastidious rendering of the institution as a national treasure, and of himself and by extension other psychiatrists as dutiful patriots of the republic, framed psychiatry itself as a vital state discipline. Indeed, he left an indelible impression on the asylum;

when he left the office in 1897 to pursue a career in politics, the institution had a series of relatively ineffective directors that added up to approximately sixteen years of institutional instability.[61] The psychiatric asylum, like many newly hatched institutions, depended on the charisma of its first director for its public defense and internal stability.

The relationship between state officials and psychiatrists became strained in Brandão's wake as the Sales administration instituted a program of fiscal austerity over the asylum and other large state institutions during the outset of his administration in order to curtail national inflation and devalorization.[62] A dramatic increase in the numbers of impoverished persons entering the asylum as a place of last resort was ostensibly brought on by the nation's dire financial straits and deepening urban poverty. Despite cost-saving measures (such as an increase in pensioner fees),[63] overcrowding persisted to such a large extent that in 1898, the director general of public assistance sent a notice to the mayor of Rio asking him to act against the process the police had adopted of sending to the asylum "all the insane or those pretending to be insane encountered roaming the streets or removed from poor houses." He claimed this practice generated great costs to the city given the extent to which it taxed the institution's resources.[64] Budgetary problems plagued the asylum, as did internal conflicts between the psychiatrists who oversaw the administration of the Observation Pavilion and those responsible for the rest of the asylum. As an institution, it was extant but fractured. By 1901 renewed attention by the press revealed the microworkings of an ailing institution.[65]

On January 22, 1901, the *O Paiz* journal, once a supporter of the asylum, published "National Hospice of the Alienated: A Visit," offering a scathing depiction of the institution: "When God administratively regulates hell, creating in it a series of small bureaucratic formalities, of divisions and subdivisions . . . as Dante fantasized . . . the hell would [not] be less horrible. It is what happens in the mental hospitals."[66] The exposé noted that problems abounded even in the admissions process, since the Observation Pavilion was filled to capacity with people suffering from contagious diseases. Echoing the concerns of Senator Leite e Oiticica, the newspaper abhorred the categorical "promiscuity," a euphemism for the unification of classes and races, among patients: "What confusion! Everything is combined, mingled, fused! It is a delirious salad of all the known mental illnesses!"[67] Focusing on the plight of a young black girl of seven or eight years of age with sporadic attacks of epilepsy with long intervals of lucidity, the article claimed, "She is alive, she is cheerful, she has a malicious and intelligent look. What will happen to this poor unfortunate? If there was a school for degenerates, such as the one Bourneville created in France, she could perhaps educate herself, learn a trade, be useful. This one however, is doomed to a miserable life, cloistered between madpeople and idiots. . . . Poor child!"[68] It is noteworthy that while *O Paiz* was extremely critical of the asylum, it still called for yet another institution (a Bourneville-esque school for troubled youth) as part of an expanding modernist republican safety net.

Newspaper criticisms and administrative discord led to two government-initiated visits to the institution and, ultimately, direct state intervention in asylum affairs. The first visit, on February 7, 1902, consisted of an initial inquiry by Minister of Justice and Interior Affairs Sabino Barroso in order to evaluate the veracity of the accusations made against the institution. After three and a half hours of scrupulous examination, the minister noted that the organization of the asylum was not "entirely in accordance with the progress made in similar establishments in other advanced countries."[69] Singling out the poor management of actual patients, the government official stressed the lack of division among patients as a result of the apparent lack of segregation or distinction of age, sex, social status, and mental condition. In particular, he lamented the equal treatment of first-class and indigent pensioners, lamenting first-class pensioners' inability to receive treatment according to the price they paid.[70] Observing that the nurses were attentive to the patients, "treating them with tireless patience," the minister ascribed the asylum's problems to asylum director Pedro Dias Carneiro's bad leadership. Describing him as "a man obviously tired and who does not even have the energy, nor the vitality that the position requires," the minister called him "a weak man" and one "who is not well aware of what is happening in the establishment which has been entrusted to him and who does not have the precise conditions to direct it."[71] Newspaper sources unabashedly called for a change of director, calling for a man of recognizable competence and recognized energy and severity."[72] Minister of Justice and Interior Affairs José Joaquim Seabra launched a federal commission in December 1902 to formally review the asylum. Drs. Carlos Fernandes Eiras, Egydio de Salles Guerra, and Antonio Maria Teixeira, in addition to pharmacist F. M. da Silva Araújo, conducted a thorough examination of the asylum.

This commission represented the first serious government attempt to reform the institution, harnessing the knowledge of medical experts from outside the asylum to guide the hand of the state. The commission itself made a concerted effort to be comprehensive by using a "scientific" methodology that included close observation of the institution and accounting for the perspectives of its workers through a brief "survey" at the outset of the investigation and informal interviews during its duration.[73] Ultimately, the commission concluded that social assistance for the mentally ill did not exist in Brazil because the National Insane Asylum was functioning as a house of detention only. They described the patients at the asylum as "kidnapped from society" denied "the charity that they deserve as sick people."[74] Calling for effective social assistance based on rigorous scientific-medical standards in Brazil, as in European countries, the commission declared that "a people with venues of civilization cannot tolerate in their midst the embarrassing spectacle of 1200 unfortunates, deprived of reason, caged, as irrational, in an era where science boasts of resources, many times to cure them, always to soften their sufferings and sorrows. . . . These poor insane do not require large luxurious palaces; modest hygienic constructions would suffice, little cost, but where they can turn free of cares, classified and separated according to forms of alienation, and their social conditions."[75] The push toward medical classification and segregation by diagnosis and the medicalization of the overt class prejudice and barely covert race prejudice encoded in the phrase "social condition" was a central ordering principle of the asylum, and indeed, other turn-of-the-twentieth-century institutions of social assistance.

Conclusion

When psychiatrists assumed control of the asylum after the proclamation of the republic, they became public functionaries, subject to the critical gaze of the state and of civil societies in new ways. Criticism of the asylum caused many state officials to rally around the institution and to defend its bureaucracy of expertise. In defending the asylum, statesmen articulated a political outlook in which social assistance was largely the prerogative of the state and not private charity. Policymakers' consistent framing of social assistance as a matter of public security, medical-scientific expertise, and the citizen-in-need as a dependent, projected an image of a potent republican state. Indeed, the provision of care served as a marker of efficient governance. Moreover, the great extent to which republican statesmen defended psychiatrists and the asylum against their more critical colleagues illustrates the institution's significance to the infrastructural power of the central state. In early republican Rio de Janeiro, successive administrations sought to use infrastructural power (i.e., the power to rule society through the administrative coordination of social life), in contrast to the state's despotic power (i.e., the power to rule over society via monopolization of the means of physical coercion), as a means of exercising their authority. Attempts to rehabilitate the standing institutions of the state during the transition from colony to republic in Brazil sat at the nexus of the political project of building the administrative infrastructure and authority of a modern state, the cultural project of constructing bonds of loyalty to the modern nation, and the medico-scientific project of generating knowledge about the populations in whose name the roles of doctors were legitimated.

Criticisms against the asylum were not unwarranted. Within the walls of the institution, psychiatrists were coming to the understanding that madness could not be cured. To a large degree they would let go of the environmental determinism that understood the built environment as the touchstone of care, no longer believing that kind words and the asylum environs would bring most of their admitted back to reason. Insanity, the enemy they had been hoping to finally meet in the arena of a fully psychiatric asylum, remained a real social problem in spite of the implementation of the moral therapy and, in the main, the good intentions of the psychiatrists in question. Therapeutic pessimism replaced curative optimism as psychiatrists, influenced by transatlantic currents surrounding Darwinian theories of evolution, believed that the laws of selection and survival operated as strongly in the mental medical field as they did in the social world. The confluence of newspaper criticisms of the asylum and the cogent official defense put forward by asylum director Brandão represented a coming-of-age moment for psychiatry. Public scrutiny functioned as a formative experience for an embryonic profession that had yet to confront scrutiny about its use value. Indeed, psychiatrists adeptly countered the morass of countless criticisms leveled at them with a narrative of evolutionary progress in which they asserted their roles as the humble, tireless servants of both state and nation. Less audacious (yet no less determined) than their embattled pre-republican Pinelian selves, psychiatrists, when facing the glare of the public spotlight, reconstituted the profession in light of their asylum experiences. What emerged was a more mature profession less cloaked in the symbolic heroism of Pinel's gesture and more attuned to material institutional realities and the limits of therapeutic success.

Chapter Five

Breaking Out of the Asylum

Rio de Janeiro's Mental Hygiene Movement, 1903–37

Antônio Dias Barros replaced Dias Carneiro as the National Insane Asylum director on July 12, 1902, following a litany of complaints and criticisms from the press and state officials about the institution's functioning. Instead of expressing pleasure at the prestige of this appointment, Dias Barros lamented that "any person to assume this position would already be doomed to failure, and publicly dismissed for incompetence, but [he would] be charged in error, when it should be the asylum itself, in this situation [as it is] due to internal excesses of every kind, [perpetrated] after the declaration of the Republic under the authority of those who more worthily should have defended and solidified, in the spirit of [the] public, their claims and spirits."[1] In many ways, his assessment was accurate, and his tenure lasted only a year. When Dr. Juliano Moreira succeeded Barros in 1903, he brought an unprecedented series of political and medical techniques to the asylum, which ushered in an era of institutional optimism despite the asylum's reputation as a failure under republican rule. No longer a site devoted to the passive stewardship of the mad, the asylum began to carry out the dual, and perhaps somewhat contradictory, goals of containment and treatment. Treatment techniques included hydrotherapy, light therapy, and suggestive therapies. Although evidence does not suggest that these methods were particularly effective in curing mental illness, they reflected a paradigm shift within Brazilian psychiatry. Historians have discussed the evolution of scientific medicine over the course of the nineteenth century and analyzed the institutional, social, and cultural changes that followed the well-known epistemological shift in medicine most commonly associated with post-revolutionary Paris.[2] Beginning in the second half of the century, the asylum, in addition to the general hospital, underwent a fundamental transformation from a place of respite for the poor or the sick to a site defined by science. Historians have also demonstrated that in the world of early twentieth-century medicine, research, education, and the making of careers all became bound to the hospital. Laboratory training and bedside instruction at a university-affiliated hospital largely displaced the medical apprenticeship, and the identity of Brazilian physicians rested increasingly not on traditional therapeutics but on shared educational experiences and a claim to specialized scientific knowledge.[3] By the end of the nineteenth century, medical researchers in both Europe and the Americas increasingly studied physiological functioning rather than static anatomical structures.[4] The new generation of psychiatrists investigated the biological functions of the nervous system using many different approaches. In Germany, psychiatrist Emil Kraepelin used psychological experiments and statistical analysis; French neurologists experimented with the effects of hypnosis; and in Vienna and Switzerland, psychoanalytic techniques were being developed to explore mental functioning.[5] In his examination of progressivism in the United States, historian Daniel Rodgers has argued that despite the great variety in their ideologies, methods, motivations, and even "social languages," so-called progressive reformers shared visions for directing and strengthening society.[6] Similar to US reformers, Brazilian psychiatrists used a variety of social languages at their disposal as they worked to expand the topography of psychiatry within and beyond institutions of confinement.[7] Armed with new theoretical and therapeutic arsenals, they maneuvered for the political mandate they needed and then broke out of the asylum and turned their clinical gaze to the public sphere. Although psychiatrists who worked in the National Insane Asylum had, since before its formal opening, invoked a public whose selves and spirits required defense, their interest in serving those outside the asylum walls reached its apogee in the between 1903 and 1937. Influenced by north and south Atlantic professional trends that embraced mental hygiene, or the science of maintaining mental health and preventing mental disorder, a growing number of Brazilian psychiatrists began to seriously consider the sociocultural and political environment as a key factor in shaping human character.[8] As they ventured out in the public sphere, they managed to cast off, at least temporarily, the therapeutic pessimism that had plagued their practice in the asylum. The objective of the new psychiatric medical model of subjectivity was to understand and to cultivate "normalcy" in order to improve the health of the population, thereby significantly lessening the professional burden of managing—while attempting to cure—the already mentally ill. Psychiatrists had once again begun to believe that they might significantly "solve" mental illness, this time by addressing its cultural roots through a sort of sociotherapeutics reminiscent of public health campaigns of the time. The physical move away from the asylum therefore engendered a new social program, a mental hygiene movement, which sought to promote mental health by treating patients who were not yet fully insane and which, further, sought to prevent mental illness and social deviance. Mental hygiene consisted of a social-surveillance model of preventative medicine that focused on environment and sanitation issues as well as the critical minutiae of social life.

This four-part chapter then chronicles the evolution of Brazilian psychiatry at the height of its power and influence, as psychiatrists straddled both the asylum and the public sphere. It explores psychiatrists' attempts to deepen and to expand the profession's reach. The first part looks at Juliano Moreira's appointment as the director of the National Insane Asylum as a critical turning point in Brazilian psychiatry. Under his watch, asylum facilities were modernized, and transnational intellectual links between Brazilian and German psychiatrists were forged; this not only bolstered the public profile of psychiatry in Brazil but also raised the confidence of its practitioners. Following Kraepelin's promulgation of observation and research, psychiatrists introduced new initiatives within the National Insane Asylum in order to craft a body of knowledge based on the scientific method that would ultimately interrogate the social lives of Brazilians, identifying the habits therein that failed to contribute to good mental health.

The second part looks at how this professional confidence led psychiatrists to take an activist stance toward the curtailment of mental illness. They had been tasked with managing an asylum in which alcoholism was a contributing, if not predominant, factor in the commitment of most of the patients. This section focuses on psychiatric campaigns geared toward the deterrence of alcohol consumption, both as objects in themselves and in order to understand psychiatry's larger foray into the public sphere. They formalized alliances with public health officials through the creation of commissions, conferences, and institutes as they sought to do battle with environmental realities and social practices they identified as threats to sound mental and physical hygiene. The third part looks at how these efforts were institutionalized with the creation of the Brazilian League of Mental Hygiene in 1923. Although many historians of Brazilian psychiatry have studied this professional organization as a powerful Neo-Lamarckian-influenced eugenic institution, this chapter investigates how Freudian psychoanalysis also greatly informed the intellectual development of league members.

The 1920s were an era of political and cultural ferment in Brazil. There was much sociopolitical activity undermining the traditional footings on which public senses of security had rested upon: rapid urbanization, mass urban strikes, broadening opposition to political rule by the coffee oligarchy, political polarization as manifested in the rise of a conservative Catholic movement and the founding of the Brazilian Communist Party, feminist activism, and artistic innovation as expressed during Modern Art Week held in São Paulo in 1922, combined with the arrival of foreign technologies, images, and styles. Both elite and ordinary people, whether young or old, man or woman, expressed anxieties about what it meant to be Brazilian and what it meant to be modern. Could Brazil, in its newness as a nation, turn its racial heritage, abundant natural resources, and moral culture into the civilization of the future, or even into a nation that could act as a peer to France, England, or the United States? In short, could Brazil be one nation, African, mixed, and modern? As psychiatrists wrestled with these questions, they turned to psychoanalysis for responses to the "impasses of Brazilian liberal professionals in the beginning of the 20th century who believed it was their duty, specifically, to resolve the issue of the construction of a national identity."[9]

Brazil's elites saw psychoanalysis as an innovative solution for a national backwardness that they primarily credited to problems stemming from the country's African cultural heritage. To this end, Freudian sublimation was considered in terms of its applicability to the education and reorientation of sexual impulses to promote "civilization." An emblematic icon of the German psychiatric tradition, Kraepelin's organicist model was compatible with Freud's psychodynamic approach to the mind, which enabled psychiatrists to selectively appropriate both Kraepelin's and Freud's works to escape the pessimism of racial degeneration theory, which characterized Brazilians as doomed to suffer from poor mental health.

This part examines how psychiatrists Juliano Moreira, Júlio Pires Porto-Carrero, and Arthur Ramos used and elaborated on these theories to advocate for public policies and to create new public institutions. As representative members of a vanguard that rejected a national narrative of racial pessimism, they still understood degeneracy as an acute social crisis, but one based on a learned series of cultural processes that improvements in health, culture, and (most importantly) education could mend.[10] To address this crisis, these psychiatrists directed institutions, conferences, and leagues, among other public structures that could potentially teach Brazilians about the proper cultivation of sound mental health habits. They found supportive ears on government committees as they argued for the nationwide provision of psychologically based social assistance services to remedy pervasive underlying mental ailments within the populace. They publicized their project; Moreira even hosted German physicist Albert Einstein's tour of the National Asylum during his visit to Rio de Janeiro in 1925 and later opened the reception in honor of Einstein at the Brazilian Academy of Science (Academia Brasileira de Ciências), of which Moreira was president (1925–29).[11]

Lastly, the fourth part looks at the application of psychoanalysis in the creation and management of the Euphrenic Clinic (1932) and the Orthophrenology and Mental Hygiene Service (1934). These institutions served as prescriptive tools, outlining appropriate conduct and morals to instill proper mental hygiene for the individual self and the family. They also functioned as instruments of public relations for psychiatry in Rio. When the ideological underpinnings and practical workings of these institutions were laid bare, it became clear that they did not muster enough popular (and arguably as a result) state support for their continued maintenance. The doctors who administered public psychiatric programs remained disinterested in the will of the city's poor majority, reasoning that opposition to government policies (and to the republic itself) arose from the ignorance of the masses and demonstrated their incapacity for self-government. This dismissive treatment of the population they hoped to serve ultimately proved deleterious. As the clinics catered to a dwindling clientele, psychiatrists would find themselves unable to rationalize their reliance on public coffers to state officials. With the announcement of the Estado Novo in 1937, the Vargas regime, against the backdrop of the economic crises of the Depression-era 1930s, began a truly ambitious campaign of cultural consolidation. The government withdrew its support of European-influenced cultural programs elaborated by psychiatrists and supported by other professional elites. Instead, the Vargas dictatorship sought to co-opt all functional centers of culture to the state (aided by censorship if necessary).[12] It also attempted to promote cultural practices (*candomblé*, *carnival*, etc.) previously marginalized by psychiatrists and other elites, as the bedrock of national identity.

The application of medico-scientific techniques to the enforcement of social order was characteristic of a new "scientific" ideology of public administration that arose in many major Latin American cities at the end of the nineteenth century. Urban professionals and intellectuals influenced by positivism administered city governments such as Buenos Aires after the defeat of the dictator Juan Manual de Rosas in 1852; Mexico City during the Porfirio Díaz presidency (1876–1910); and Rio de Janeiro during the First Republic (the period of republican government started by a military coup that ousted Emperor Pedro II in 1889 and was then overthrown by a coup that brought Getúlio Vargas to power in 1930). These liberal professionals argued that their policies would accelerate progress, understood as a linear process through which both urban space and the often culturally, racially, and ethnically diverse Latin American populations would come to resemble, in behavior at least, those of (white) industrialized Europe. What made Brazil, and specifically Rio, unique in comparison to its Latin American counterparts was the great extent to which a new group of modern rational and scientifically grounded members of Brazilian society employed public health as the dominant lens through which to understand and carry out national development in a new way. Psychiatrists, along with other policymakers in Rio, identified public health as the paramount framework through which they could address the "deficiencies" they believed it necessary to overcome in order to ease the genetic burden of racial mixture, the cultural hangover from slavery, and the ongoing lethargy encouraged by Brazil's tropical location. The deficiencies they cited, like some of the public health solutions for which they advocated, had surfaced in arguments by Europeans such as Count Arthur de Gobineau since the mid-nineteenth century.[13] The Europeanization of the local population, either through cultural or biological whitening, was accepted as an appropriate strategy to invigorate the Brazilian masses—people who, in their "un-whitened" present, were thought to lack sufficient intellectual ability, moral constitution, and physical capacity for modernization. That strategy was reified in the first immigration policy of the First Republic in 1890, a policy that barred the "further entry to Brazil [for] descendants of the African race."[14] In the frontlines of public health, psychiatrists played an essential part in systematic attempts by public officials to "modernize," "civilize," and "whiten" Carioca society. The "Europeanization" project for Rio entailed destroying the urban spaces created by the poor, many of whom were of African or mixed descent, and clearing them out for space designated for "respectable" society, generally defined as whiter and of the upper class. The search for the modernization of the city was conditioned not only by diverse mentalities but also by differing pacts between the municipal authorities, the central government, and influential elites. Aside from the infrastructural modernization and hygienic reasoning behind public works and public health measures, the norms and impositions of the municipality were also tinged by a desire to curtail popular culture, especially manifestations of what was, in barely coded racist language, referred to as "low" culture (read Afro-Brazilian) in an attempt to instill a model of Europeanized bourgeois civility. Historian Jeffrey D. Needell's characterization of the late nineteenth and early twentieth centuries as Rio's Belle Epoque is apt.

In the early decades of the twentieth century, Brazilian cities, and most emblematically Rio de Janeiro, were reshaped by urban reforms constructed in order to create an image of civilized cosmopolitanism. In a nation that was largely agricultural, dependent on coffee exports and ruled by oligarchic elites, Rio de Janeiro was not only the political and cultural center of the nation but was also Brazil's iconic city where new forms of socialization, consumption, and modernization were essayed. Reforms in Rio sought to constitute a bourgeois ordering of public space by dictating to the public the norms of behavior, appropriate dress codes, and hygienic use of space. Modeled on the Haussmannization of Paris, urban planners began to eliminate configurations of urban space dating from the colonial period as well as working-class uses of the city that elites saw as disorderly.[15] As Rio almost doubled in size between 1890 and 1906, growing from five hundred thousand to eight hundred thousand residents,[16] the overtaxed modern systems and public services it had, such as transportation, lighting, sanitation, and policing, were largely due to efforts implemented by Mayor Pereira Passos

(1902–6), dubbed the "tropical Haussmann." Passos, along with federal government officials, made deliberate efforts to alter the image of Rio as a pathogenic port. President Rodrigues Alves selected sanitation and public health doctor Oswaldo Cruz to undertake a comprehensive assessment of the infectious diseases that afflicted residents living in the city of Rio de Janeiro. Alves had firsthand experience with foreigners who had chosen to invest elsewhere rather than take their chances with the tropical diseases associated with Brazil. His platform for the presidency was linked to sanitation reforms, which were increasingly seen as indispensable in the effort to win European investment dollars. As a result of his efforts to eradicate epidemic diseases in the city of Rio de Janeiro, Oswaldo Cruz was often hailed a national hero. As his vaccination programs had a substantial impact on controlling the spread of disease, they also amplified the discourse on the pathologization of the poor. Disease was so common among the poor that popular perception viewed the impoverished as not just lacking in proper hygiene but also guilty of larger moral shortcomings.[17] Favelas were perceived as little more than havens for disease. Their existence appeared to exemplify ambivalence toward the hygienic practices adopted and advocated for by members of the upper classes. Further, the dwellings of the poor were perceived as housing the criminal element of Rio de Janeiro, prompting journalists of the period to campaign vigorously for programs that protected "good citizens" from the "savage elements residing among the poor."[18] One solution to the problems, real and perceived, of rampant crime and disease in the city of Rio de Janeiro in previous years was the founding of correctional colonies for the criminals and the quarantine of the seriously ill.[19] Though attempted, the segregation of the majority of the presumed unfit populations from the wealthy was seen to be impractical.[20]

Juliano Moreira and the Emergence of a New Psychiatry

The National Insane Asylum, the foundational structure of the extraordinary proliferation of the new early twentieth-century clinics and legislation, functioned as a malleable object in service of modernism. Moreira, like Brandão, sought to alter the asylum into a hallmark of exemplary care and a monument to the psychiatric profession. Moreira's reputation as both an able psychiatrist and a scientific reformer made him an ideal candidate to direct the National Insane Asylum and to transform it into the nation's leading model for the new scientific medicine. The institutional power, resources, and prestige he wielded at the asylum validated and advanced his determination to establish psychiatry as a clinical discipline.

State officials recognized that the asylum's leadership had always been a target for controversy, and their decision to appoint a person with Moreira's personal attributes was calculated. Raised in an impoverished household in Salvador, Bahia, the psychiatrist of African descent's personal-professional life served as an emblematic rags-to-riches narrative that ostensibly highlighted the social possibility of overcoming both poverty and racism. After matriculating at the Medical School of Bahia at the age of thirteen and completing his doctoral thesis on malignant syphilis praecox with the highest mark in his class five years later, this serious and talented young man went to Europe, where he would study under a number of famous doctors such as Rudolf Virchow, Paul Gerson Unna, and Hermann Nothnagel. Under the doctors' tutelage, he developed a profound interest in mental illness. Upon returning to Brazil, he became professor of psychiatry at the University of Bahia in 1896 and established the Clinic for Neurology and Psychiatry at St. Isabel Hospital, the first of its kind in the state. Unlike other multiracial Brazilian public elites that emphasized their links to whiteness, Moreira unapologetically claimed blackness as part of his identity.[21] When he publicly accepted the position of professor, he used his speech to condemn racism, saying that in "days with more light and nobleness of character" dark skin would no longer occasion prejudice, calling "negligence and carelessness that petrify" the true "blackness."[22]

Moreira seemingly did not use his accomplishments as an aspirational model of black personhood that individuals of Afro descent should mimic nor as an example of Brazil's racial democracy.[23] Nonetheless, this did not stop others from using him as a normative representative of Afro-Brazilianness. For example, Dr. Thomas Watkins, who had called South America "an everlasting joy to the [black] race as there is no evidence of color prejudice,"[24] cited Dr. Moreira as evidence of Afro-Brazilians' full potential, and to a degree, as evidence of the openness of the society to the full realization of that potential. In a report to the American College of Physicians and Surgeons, the sponsor of his visit, he referred to Moreira as

> a negro of high intelligence, culture, and ability. He is generally considered one of the representative men of Brazil. He has a very keen and intelligent knowledge and interest in the individual inmates of his institution. He has been the state representative to many countries, and to congresses on psychiatry. He has a very large library and reads and speaks fluently in five languages, viz., French, Spanish, Portuguese, German, and English. He speaks English so fluently he would easily be taken for a native of England or the States. He is an exceptional man, but well illustrates the possibilities of the negro in South America.[25]

Moreira traveled extensively in Europe before taking leadership of the National Insane Asylum and was one of the few Brazilian doctors to achieve international prestige. In 1899 he would travel to Europe once again in order to examine psychiatric clinics in various countries and to study the work of pioneering doctors such as Richard von Krafft-Ebing, Eduard Hitzig, Ernst Viktor von Leyden, Paul Emil Flechsig, and Maurice Fournier. He took part in the International Medical Congress at Paris in 1900 and was elected chairman-of-honor in absentia at the 1901 IV International Congress of Assistance to the Mentally Ill in Berlin.[26]

Moreira became a great admirer of the German psychiatric tradition and paid admiring visits to the psychiatric clinics of Halle (1901), Leipzig (1901), and Wurzburg (1902). The free roaming of patients without straightjackets or use of confinement cells impressed him. However, the German government's commitment to psychiatrists and the resulting commitment of psychiatrists to their profession, their patients, and their research impressed him the most.[27] Public health inspector and psychiatrist Dr. Júlio Afrânio Peixoto, a student and follower of Moreira's from Salvador, Bahia, suggested that his esteemed mentor assume the directorship of the National Insane Asylum to Minister of Interior and Justice José Joaquim Seabra. Seabra was Bahian, and the administration of President Francisco de Paula Rodrigues Alves (1902–6) strongly supported Moreira's nomination. His personal and professional identities resonated on multiple levels with statesmen who sung the praises of scientific modernism and rejected the intractability of racial degeneration.

The nomination and appointment of Moreira as asylum director coincided with a pivotal period of national rejuvenation. With federal support, Mayor Pereira Passos (1903–8) modernized the port of Rio de Janeiro, turned historical hills into large boulevards, and reclaimed land from the bay. He moved low-income populations from downtown to the outskirts of the city, creating large public buildings inspired by French architectural aesthetics in their place.[28] During the inauguration of the Central Avenue, the main city artery built during the Passos Reforms, the newspaper *Jornal do Brasil* likened it to Brazil's Independence Day, calling it

> the beginning of [the capital's] physical reform, of its aesthetical rebirth, from which, as we have stated several times, will necessarily follow intellectual enhancements, [and] moral improvement. . . . [The reforms are] an urgent and pressing need, for this municipality that is the heart and brain of the country to raise to the importance and grandeur that befits the country, and then it will not shame the nation before its residents, nor before the rightly fair eyes of the foreign [world].[29]

Historians associate the Haussmannization of Rio de Janeiro under Passos with Alves's dreams of urban modernism. While critics at the time objected to Alves's investing most of the federal budget for public works in the capital, Alves's administration hoped that by altering the built environment, it could "transform, by force, the unruly, 'barefoot' masses into citizens shaped according to the stereotypes that served the European bourgeoisie in exercising its domination."[30] State officials sought to reform social practices such as "carnival, serenades, bohemian gatherings and candomblé" in the city,[31] and they used the public health lexicon to effect structural and symbolic transformations. Born out of the exigencies of the smallpox and yellow fever epidemics of the late nineteenth and early twentieth centuries, which crippled Rio's economic and social life, public health greatly expanded its categorical palette and sociopolitical reach during Alves's administration.[32] Rather than continuing as a mere instrument of governance recruited to abate the spread of infectious diseases, it emerged as a multifaceted civic project, a multitool of reform, of state building, and of nation building. It follows then that it also emerged as fodder for political controversy. Various enterprises became staple investigators on behalf of Brazilian political culture, but scope and comprehensiveness set public health apart. Public health had society at large in its viewfinder. It signified both the unity and disunity of the nation, purporting to defend the public by demarcating specific social groups as threats.

Public health's reliance on a discrete methodological process with sophisticated tools to study, identify, and treat a population coalesced well with Moreira's intellectual training. Upon assuming the position of asylum director, Moreira spearheaded the construction of a series of laboratories and otherwise expanded the physical and intellectual contours of the National Insane Asylum. During the early years of his twenty-seven-year tenure (1903–30), he oversaw the creation of the Bourneville Pavilion for Children (figs. 5.1 and 5.2), a surgical ward, and an optometry department, as well as laboratories for bacteriology, biochemistry, and experimental psychology (fig. 5.3). New occupational therapy clinics and two new farm colonies became part of Rio de Janeiro's mental health system.

In 1905, he and Afrânio Peixoto launched the *Arquivos Brasileiros de Psiquiatria, Neurologia e Ciências Afins*, the first Brazilian periodical specializing in psychiatry, neurology, and related sciences.[33] With the purpose of "record[ing] the national contributions" and "[encouraging] national experts to the careful study of their patients,"[34] the first national journal dedicated to the medical study of mental illness "would . . . elevate the good name of Brazil before the most notable scientific centers abroad."[35] The journal was produced inside the Seabra Pavilion of the National Asylum by "sick printers, who, in this manner, would not forget their profession, but who could use work as a distraction" from their mental ailments.[36] It was a journal focusing on the mentally ill, typeset by confined madmen and madwomen. By publishing articles on different approaches to the treatment of the mentally ill in Brazil and other countries, the journal served as an intellectual clearinghouse whose publications greatly raised the profile of the National Insane Asylum. Two years after its founding, the journal served as the main organ of the Brazilian Society of Neurology, Psychiatry, and

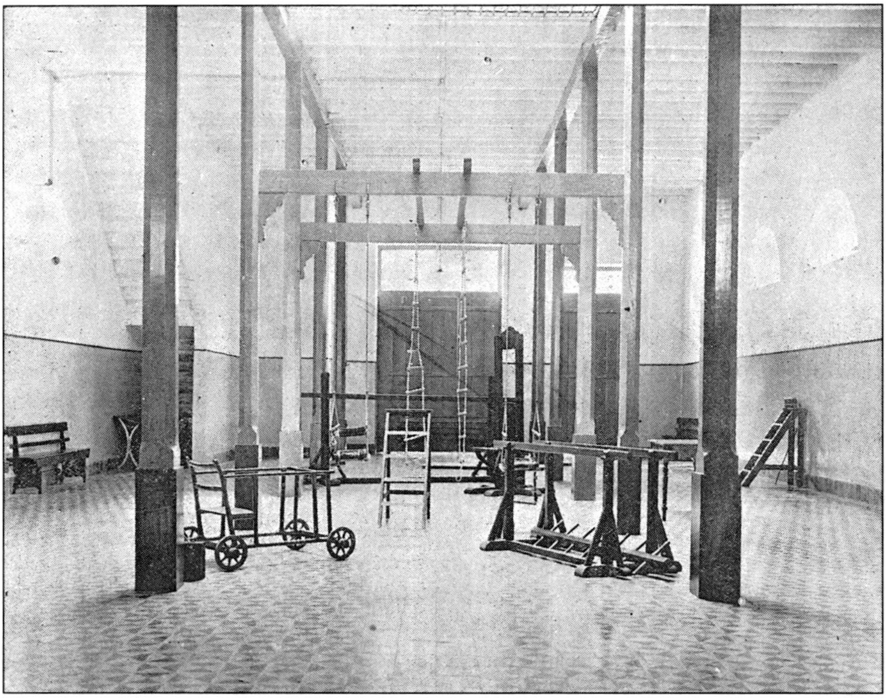

Figure 5.1. Bourneville Pavilion, Hospício Nacional de Alienads, Recreation Room," c. 1905. Olavo Bilac, "No Hospicio Nacional—Uma Visita á Secção das Creanças," *Revista Kosmos* 2, no. 2 (1905): 46.

Legal Medicine (1907–28) (Sociedade Brasileira de Neurologia, Psiquiatria e Medicinal Legal). This professional organization saw its beginnings at a November 1907 meeting of the Academy of Medicine, where approximately forty doctors in attendance, including Moreira, all devoted to helping the mentally ill, sought to collaborate and establish links among themselves.[37]

In a 1910 report presented to the Fourth Latin American Medical Congress, Moreira explained his vision for the asylum, seeking to elevate the patient to the category of "sick of the brain" by transforming the asylum "little by little from a deposit prison to a [mental] hospital."[38] He cited the German model of assistance to the mentally ill as the best model due to the complementarity of its varied parts. This model of a modernized asylum system included an open-door asylum, attached agricultural colonies, loosely supervised at-home treatment, and associated "villages of the insane" working together in an expansive system. Moreira highlighted that "the old closed asylum tends to disappear by transforming itself into a modern asylum."[39] He argued that Brazil should emulate this constellation model of specialized, decentralized, but controlled mental illness treatment.

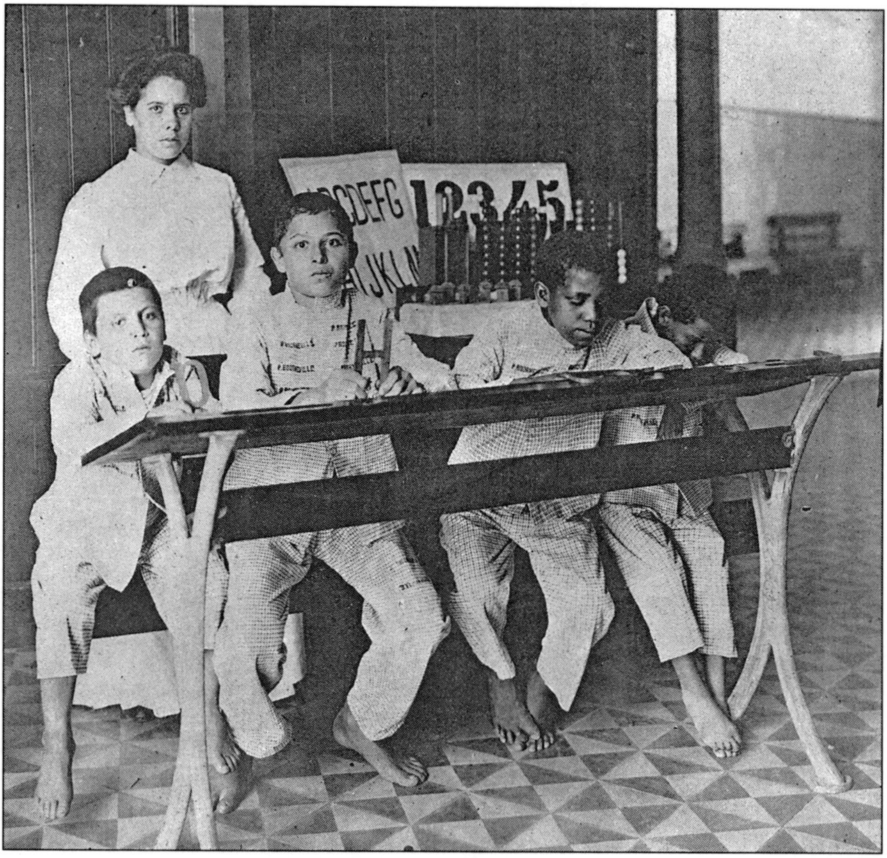

Figure 5.2. "School," c. 1905. Olavo Bilac, "No Hospicio Nacional—Uma Visita á Secção das Creanças," *Revista Kosmos* 2, no. 2 (1905): 47.

Brazilian psychiatrists' engagement with German psychiatric thought went beyond a superficial adaptation of ideas and methods. During the early twentieth century, psychiatrists from each country visited the other, and in so doing, forged intellectual links, creating, among other things, collaborative courses and lectures. The first German doctor to come to Brazil was Max Nonne (1861–1959), the noted neurologist, who traveled to Latin America in 1922 to visit Argentina; Chile; Uruguay; and, finally, São Paulo and Rio de Janeiro. Received by Brazilian psychiatrists Juliano Moreira, Henrique Roxo, and Antonio Austregésilo, among others, the neurologist was impressed by the asylum and noted later from Germany that his "colleagues overseas [Moreira et al.] are perfectly aware of the progress of neurology and German psychiatry" while recognizing that the opposite did not apply.[40] That same year, doctors of the Brazilian Society of Psychiatry,

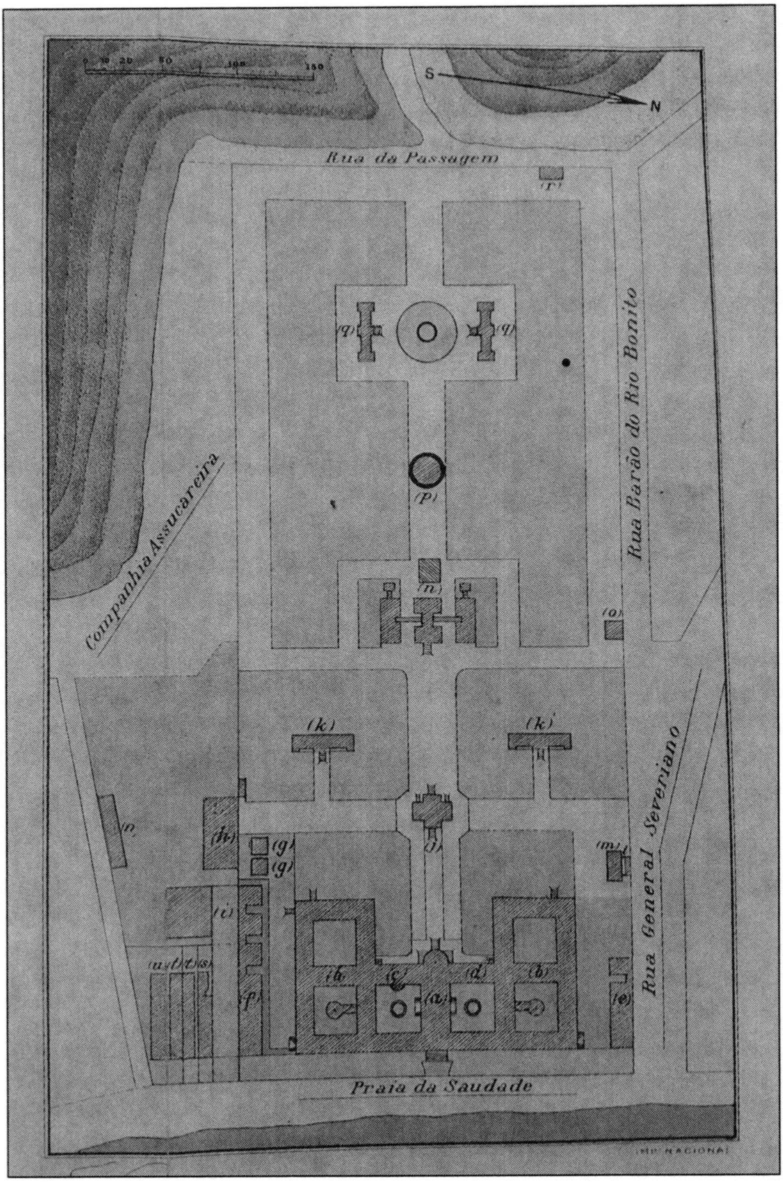

Figure 5.3. Hospicio Floor Plan. Legend: (a) administration and sanitary service; (b) indigent and pensioner patients; (c) surgery services; (d) pharmacy; (e) pavilion for the invalids (men); (f) pavilion for the invalids (women); (g) shelter sheds; (h) laundry; (i) Bourneville pavilion for children; (j) kitchen; (k) pavilion for epileptics; (l) storage; (m) electrical power plant; (n) observation pavilion; (o) morgue; (p) offices; (q) pavilion for intercurrent infectious diseases; (r) guard residence; (s) intern residence; (t) doctor of the observation pavilions; (u) residence of the hospício director; (v) residence of the hospício administrator; (w) roofing machine. *Archivos Brasileiros de Psychiatria, Neurologia e Sciencias Affins* (Rio de Janeiro, 1905), n.p.

Neurology and Legal Medicine received Wilhelm Weygandt (1870–1939), psychiatrist at the University of Hamburg and the Friedrichberg Hospital,[41] who praised Moreira because of his dissemination of German clinical psychiatric methods in South America.[42] During German psychiatrists' interaction with their Brazilian counterparts, many extolled Moreira's role as a model representative of an aspirational Brazilian psychiatry. The German journal in Rio de Janeiro, *Deutsche Rio-Zeitung*, described Moreira as "one of the most prestigious names of Brazilian science."[43] Citing his receipt of an invitation to deliver lectures at the University of Hamburg, it mentioned that Moreira was

> without a doubt, the leading authority in the field of psychiatry in Brazil [who] has also received great recognition from his European colleagues. . . . Mr. Professor Juliano Moreira is not only an alienist of excellence that does everything to elevate his profession. He is also a man of noble character, ready to help whenever needed. And he is, moreover an admirer of Germany and greatly appreciates German science, as we already know.[44]

Moreira enjoyed a professional camaraderie with Kraepelin; in their ongoing correspondence, Kraepelin displayed interest about the pathologies of indigenous peoples (which was part of his larger work on comparative psychiatry),[45] and Moreira expressed interest in how scientific clinical methods could aid psychiatric research during the early twentieth century. Moreira's inquiries focused on Kraepelin's best-known legacy: the classification of psychiatric disorders. In opposition to the leading theories of his time, Kraepelin understood the relationship of symptoms to specific illnesses, and by extension, courses of treatment as complex. Based on clinical observation, he believed that a symptom could occur across disorders and that different disorders could possess varied patterns of symptoms. Kraepelin was the first nosographer to systematically apply a longitudinal approach to mental illness.[46] He reinforced the primacy of the clinical method as the terra firma of psychiatry but went beyond its confines by actively seeking and building alliances with the auxiliary sciences of psychology, neuropathology, pharmacology, and genetics. As one of the leading figures of early twentieth-century global psychiatry, Kraepelin spoke a social language that celebrated applied research methods and the cross-fertilization of the human sciences. Unlike psychiatrists who followed the French empathetic psychiatric tradition, Kraepelin did not advocate for a close working relationship with patients based on the psychiatrist's kindness and persuasion. A staunch believer in objective evidence gathering, he considered observation the prime tool of diagnosis and therapeutic prescription.[47] In contrast to the popular mid-nineteenth-century Pinelian impulse that placed the charismatic Brazilian psychiatrist dutifully tending to patients in the asylum ward,

Kraepelin's work called on them to also carry out research in newly created specialized asylum laboratories. Moreira cited the Munich clinic's investment in modern facilities and medical-laboratory equipment, as well as the courses Kraepelin and his collaborators offered, as an inspiration: "It had a truly cosmopolitan character. During the summer course of 1906, I saw in the Munich Clinic amphitheater, listeners of various nationalities, many of whom already bear the title of psychiatrist."[48]

Soon after that trip, Moreira and trusted colleague Afrânio Peixoto engaged in an extensive study of Kraepelin's classification system in order to apply it to Brazil. In their 1905 article, "Classification of Mental Illnesses of Professor Emil Kraepelin," they highlighted the evolution of Kraepelin's fifteen-group classification system.[49] By 1908 psychiatrist Antonio Austregésilo proposed the establishment of a Kraepelin classification system of mental illnesses as the standard in all Brazilian institutions of mental assistance. The Society of Psychiatry, Neurology, and Legal Medicine was tasked with reviewing the proposal, and Moreira and Peixoto served on a five-person commission to investigate the matter specifically in relation to the National Asylum. By 1910 the society essentially approved Austregésilo's proposal, and Kraepelin's nosology became the standard in all the national public institutions that served the mentally ill.

Kraepelin's ideas about degeneration also influenced Brazilian psychiatrists. Less well-known now than his work as a nosologist, his work as a Neo-Lamarckian epidemiologist likely influenced them as well. Kraepelin's article "On the Question of Degeneration" (1908) calls for "extensive, careful, decades-long studies" of entire regions by "specially trained commissions" to engage in epidemiological research more reliant on widespread clinical observation than on population statistics.[50] Rooted in a complex network of social relationships and administrative jurisdictions, Kraepelin's epidemiological research project's implementation demanded close cooperation and coordination between psychiatrists and various other interest groups, including hospital administrators, public health officials, as well as select professionals within institutions like schools, courts, and military recruitment offices. As this multidisciplinary model brought psychiatrists together with other professionals from outside their usual institutional milieu to work synthetically to inculcate a new mindscape, it helped them identify broader risk and protective factors related to mental illness. The large scale of Kraepelin's epidemiological model, including the prescriptive measures it suggested to abate threats to sound mental health, created an aspirational paradigm that expanded the professional field of the psychiatrist. Brazilian psychiatrists' use of Kraepelin's epidemiological modeling coincided with their denouncement of biological degeneration and the promotion, instead, of a social and environmental deterministic model.

In many ways, these Kraepelinian reforms represented a bulwark against degeneration theory. Political-ideological debates about Brazil's capacity for development and the nation's destiny have been inextricably tied to race. As historian Dain Borges claims, "degeneration" itself was the most common diagnosis given to the mentally ill between 1880 and 1930.[51] He calls degeneration "never far from colour" in Brazil but also "more than colour," and indeed also "a psychiatry of character, a science of identity, and a social psychology."[52] Further, he says, after the 1870s, "There was also a medical-psychiatric strand to 'race' that can be unravelled from the rest of the skein." As the project of nationhood was primarily an intra-elite preoccupation, the selection of whiteness as a key defining feature of the nationality they aspired to create in a country with a predominantly mixed-race population provoked a deep malaise within an elite class. As historian Mariza Corrêa astutely observes, Brazilian intellectuals

> somehow alienated themselves from the society they lived in when they chose race as the primary criterion of nationality, in a process that someone called schizophrenic. Whether schizophrenic or paradoxical, the result of the choice did not depend completely on the Brazilian intellectuals' will: living in a social context that the prevailing science of the day defined as incompatible with "civilization" or "progress"; and having at the same time to account for the condition of citizens of that nation and members of that scientific universe, it was difficult for them not to be ambiguous.[53]

Within the national psychiatric community, ambiguity about the role of race and its influences on mental illness took on two forms. Dr. Raimundo Nina Rodrigues, a figure most commonly known to non-Brazilian audiences for his work on Afro-Brazilian religions,[54] best encompassed the acceptance and adoption of scientific racist strains of thought. As an ardent follower of European eugenics and, in particular, Italian criminologist Cesare Lombroso, the Bahia doctor-ethnologist-anthropologist elaborated a system of thought that linked racial mixture to degeneration and stressed black inferiority.[55] Within this schema, the majority of Brazilians had little hope of achieving truly sound mental health. But Moreira articulated a strident counterpoint that ultimately sought to redeem Brazilians. Rejecting deterministic racist scientific-medical ideas that obstructed Brazilian development and the basic notion that race marked destiny, Moreira stressed social and environmental factors as both units of analysis and sites from which to effect change.

In a discussion of Brazilian nationality, Moreira stressed that, "Apart from blacks, thousands of Europeans landed . . . within them an unwanted population that Portugal sought to relieve from their prisons."[56] With them came syphilis, leprosy, tuberculosis, and most importantly, alcoholism, a vice Moreira considered to be a principal cause of mental degeneration.[57] Within his reasoning, the campaigns of mental hygiene could not be limited to "ridiculous prejudices of color or caste."[58] Moreira also railed against theories of environmental determinism that rendered the tropics synonymous with underdevelopment and moral turpitude. According to colleague Afrânio Peixoto, "The climate does not influence anything about the various symptoms of psychoses. It is within the individual's degree of instruction where the question of differences may present themselves. The descendant of two pure Caucasians, equally pure, raised in the midst of ignorant people have the same rudimentary deliriums that individuals of color devoid of instruction have."[59] In this manner, Moreira and other like-minded psychiatrists argued for increased focus on the social environment and the creation of preventative measures in order to abate mental ailments. While Moreira and Peixoto did not utterly negate degeneration theory, they argued it was overused to explain mental illness:

> This doctrine of degeneration, ever since presented by Morel [has] in recent times come to take possession of psychiatry, [it] has not yet found but thoughtless speculations, that others continue to imitate, because it is easier to think as others than to observe for oneself. . . . It must be said immediately, the indisputable truth cannot be denied: [degeneration] exists, it is profound, it is a great part of our miseries. But it is no less true that its fame has been abused, its actions thoroughly exaggerated.[60]

They stressed that "every child born is comparable to the first man; the 'I' will become hypertrophied, and, judging by the possible expansion, without modifying restrictions, each would be comparable to a madman or a criminal, it is the education, the discipline, the culture, that submits, modifies, and assimilates them; finally giving them a social identity."[61] Years later Peixoto would refer in terms far less flattering to the relevance of degeneration for psychiatry: "In the sciences, as in homes, it is necessary to have a dark corner where one [deposits] provisionally things, that cannot be properly placed in other departments."[62] While he did not subscribe to the supposedly perilous effects of miscegenation itself, Peixoto's writing reflects how he retained many racist assumptions even long after this dismissal of degeneration. In his 1938 book *Climate and Health: A Bio-Geographical Introduction to Brazilian Civilization*, Peixoto observed that

> Gobineau predicted that "children are dying in such high quantities that in the matter of a few, negligible years, there will be no more Brazilians." Not only is the Brazilian population growing enormously . . . but racial mixture is also rapidly increasing. The white albumen is purifying the national molasses. . . . Pure blacks do not exist anymore; mestizos disappear, either because they die prematurely due to somatic weaknesses, sensuality, nervousness and sensitivity to tuberculosis, or because they interbreed with whiter elements: thus the race whitens. . . . In Brazil, the great race—that has assimilated and depurated the other two races, *which are only undesirable due to their uncultured condition and*

> *ugliness*—is the white race. Every day morbidity and mortality surrender to the sanitation of housing and of urban settings, in such a way that currently our mortality rate has a very dignified standing among the best in the world.[63]

The portrayal of the "white race" as undeniably superior to other races in terms of intelligence, culture, beauty, and health did not preclude the celebration of miscegenation as the hallmark of Brazilian national identity. As historian Lilia Moritz Schwarcz cogently argued, Brazilian intellectuals of the early twentieth century constructed a paradoxical new theoretical framework whereby they could argue for an optimistic national project of "perfectible" Brazilian populations, while reinscribing old racial hierarchies through a social Darwinist view of racial difference.[64] This vision of the world is less social Darwinist, as Schwarcz contends, than it is Neo-Lamarckian, because it puts faith on the capacity of self-improvement rather than on the idea of eliminating "undesired" hereditary traits by force. The positive form of eugenics that Neo-Lamarckism embraced, therefore, represented a significantly different approach from that of the negative form of eugenics, popular at the time in Germany and the United States (forced sterilization of women of undesirable ethnic groups is an example), espoused to prevent the reproduction of the unfit.

The central precept of Neo-Lamarckian discourse was the belief that human bodies were not bound to a hereditary destiny but could incorporate external influences such as the environment, upbringing, and social condition. In turn, future generations could inherit these acquired characteristics. This framing of inheritance understood the nation as a collection of populations "perfectible" by controlling the social and environmental milieus, which would improve the nation as a whole. The renowned historian of science and medicine Nancy Leys Stepan argues that Latin American intellectuals embraced Neo-Lamarckian eugenics as a defensive reaction to the negative assessments European intellectuals made about the region. Neo-Lamarckism was able to counter explicit racist ideas because it "came tinged with an optimistic expectation that reforms of the social milieu would result in permanent improvement, an idea in keeping with the environmentalist-sanitary tradition that had become fashionable."[65] Neo-Lamarckism in effect created an alliance between public hygiene and eugenics, whereby "improving the conditions surrounding reproduction" through "hygiene, dietetics, puericulture and preventive medicine" promised to deliver healthier and fitter generations in the future.[66]

Breaking Out of the Asylum

Brazilian psychiatrists drew upon a deep ideological well that was imbued with Neo-Lamarckism, psychoanalysis, and Kraepelin's nosology and theories. Their campaigns against syphilis, epilepsy, and above all, alcoholism, strongly reflected these influences. Alcoholic psychosis, as a mental disorder, operated as a window through which to view the workings of organicist and environmental notions of degeneration in addition to their sociopolitical and cultural underpinnings. Asylum patients presented an overwhelming number of alcohol-related psychoses, and psychiatrists gave alcoholism fastidious attention. "Alcoholic madness,"[67] which was asylum patients' most frequent diagnosis, caused the majority of readmissions. For example, of the 1,508 patients that were reinstitutionalized from 1894 to 1907, 547 were alcoholics.[68] A critical discussion emerged among psychiatrists at the turn of the twentieth century on the etiological relationship between alcohol and insanity—whether alcohol directly caused madness or was a trigger in those with vulnerable states of mind. Afonso Henriques de Lima Barreto, the acclaimed writer who was institutionalized at the National Insane Asylum due to alcohol-related psychosis, noted that "some have asked: do we drink because we are already crazy or are we insane because we drink?"[69]

Psychiatrists arrived at a set of solutions for these patients to deter the high incidence of alcohol-related mental ailments and at medical consensus about the evils of alcoholism as a "social gangrene." Expressing with certainty that alcoholism was a form of decomposition and decay and decrying alcohol even as a beverage, Dr. Artur Alves Bandeira asserted that alcohol was a prime example of society's decline and called for a rigorous campaign against its existence: "Addiction draws; it is like the abyss that fascinates. To resist addiction, as to flee the abyss, requires man to exercise a powerful force of inhibition. . . . The existence of alcoholism is a testament to the backwardness of modern societies that aspire to cultured and civilized forums."[70] In 1904, at the Second Latin American Medical Congress, Dr. Peixoto, in a presentation titled "The Social Defense against Alcoholism," discussed at length the association between alcoholism and madness, criticizing the facility with which Brazilians consumed alcohol, the lack of preventative education measures, and the state's failure to tax the industry. He called the fight against alcoholism in Brazil passive, saying it lagged behind other civilized countries.[71] He proposed higher taxation on the alcohol industry to support antialcohol campaigns and colonies for alcoholics. From 1907 to 1915, Moreira pressed the Ministry of Justice and Interior Affairs office to increase the taxation of alcohol and to create alcoholic reformatories by stressing the dangers of alcohol and its chronic overrepresentation in the asylum.[72] Although neither ever came to fruition, psychiatrists' emphasis on the issue led to state participation in international conferences such as the 1921 Protocol on Opium Conference, which required Brazil to create a commission to create legislation for narcotic substances. Moreira served alongside famed doctor Carlos Chagas, director of the Oswaldo Institute (1917–34) and the Department of Public Health (1920–26). Chagas, a disciple of Oswaldo Cruz, gained national and international prominence when he discovered in 1909 the clinical features of American trypanosomiasis (Chagas disease), a feat unique in medical history.[73] The collaborative impulse between psychiatrists and public health officials gained momentum following this commission and the 1923 creation of the Brazilian League of Mental Hygiene formalized it.

The Brazilian League of Mental Hygiene and Its Dissemination of Psychoanalysis

Founded in Rio de Janeiro by psychiatrist Gustavo Riedel,[74] the Brazilian League of Mental Hygiene (LBHM) was a civil entity, although it was publicly supported through federal grants. It included twelve permanent sections or committees, each with ten members, as well as twelve regional representatives, and met monthly. The league's membership never reached beyond two hundred members, but they included leading psychiatrists such as Juliano Moreira, Afrânio Peixoto, Júlio Pires Porto-Carrero, Antonio Austragésilo, Henrique Roxo, among others.[75] Many of the members came from the staffs of the state and municipal mental asylums and reformatories. The league was a notable addition to the scientifically oriented societies in the federal capital that received subventions from the municipality of Rio and the federal government, which registered the league as a public utility in 1923 and gave support to its free ambulatory clinics.[76] The LBHM's emergence was not an isolated occurrence; a range of organizations such as the Liga de Defesa Nacional (1916), the Liga Pró-Saneamento (1918), and the Ação Social Nacionalista (1920) that sought to remedy the nation's social and sanitary ills arose in the interwar period.

According to its bylaws, the league's purpose was to "realize a program of mental hygiene and eugenics in individual, school, professional and social life" and to publicize the pathological conditions caused by syphilis, alcohol, and other diseases.[77] However, the means by which the league as an organization, and its psychiatrists, respectively, accomplished these goals were eclectic, as *eugenics* became a multifunction term employed to different ends. The *Archivos* journal was one of the league's main tools. As psychiatrist Caldas noted, "The *Archivos*, as the official organ of the LBHM, has a great and noble mission to accomplish: organ of doctrine and combat, [it] propose[s] to open, in our midst, a path by which [psychiatrists] can embark, grow and fructify the ideals of mental hygiene and eugenics, which substantiate the program of that institution."[78] Apart from the journal, the league relied on the lay press to promote its free ambulatory clinics and to launch publicity campaigns in order to educate the public about mental illness prevention and mental hygiene.

While the historiographic literature has documented the influence of Neo-Lamarckian eugenics orientation on league psychiatrists, the impact of Freudian psychoanalysis has not received as much scholarly attention, even though Brazilian psychiatrists used it as a clinical technique, interpretative lens, and developmental theory in the 1920s. Influential among Brazilian psychiatrists was a psychoanalysis that elaborated a theory of the unconscious that inextricably linked sexuality and subjectivity by ultimately disclosing the ways in which unconscious drives influenced symbolic structures beyond the purview of individual agency. As theorist Julia Kristeva would put it, "Freud's discovery designated sexuality as the nexus between language and society, drives and the socio-symbolic order."[79] Brazilian psychiatrists found invaluable both his seminal insight that sexuality played a critical role in the process of social interaction and the distinction Freud drew between human drives and instincts. Particularly, the characterization of drives as having, unlike instincts, no pre-given aims and no adherence to pre-set biological paths, gave psychiatrists a powerful tool against the inalterable biology of the antiblack logic of degeneration theory.[80]

Freudian psychoanalysis was an explanatory tool that would shine a bright spotlight on sexuality within the discourse of racial-cultural miscegenation.[81] Centrally rooted within the narrative of national decline based on miscegenation was a rampant sexuality. As anthropologist Richard Parker observed, "Because of the emphasis Brazilians have put on the three-race mix . . . as the key to their historical constitution, the question of sexuality, of sexual intercourse as a concrete mechanism of racial mixing, took on an unprecedented importance in modern Brazil thinking."[82] Psychoanalysis's rendering of sexuality as a fundamental component of the self, on one hand, and the possibility of its sublimation, on the other, resonated strongly with psychiatrists who adhered to the idea that primitivism and an excessive sexual drive supported the national bane of miscegenation. Instead of denying or pathologizing sexuality's role in the formation of both the personal and the national self, they sought to demystify it and render it a field of critical intervention. Given that Freud's theory of psychosexual development posited that childhood was the foundation of subjectivity, rigorous psychiatric scrutiny centered on the child, and by extension, the institutions and people that surrounded children. In considering psychoanalysis's use value for Brazil, psychiatrist Franco da Rocha asserted,

> There is in psychoanalysis a pedagogical point of view that is of great advantage. It considers as a central issue the psychic determinism of the individual [in addition to] the regular development and the harmonic components of infantile sexual instincts. It is in our defective and harmful manner to ignore the demands of the libido, to hide them completely, instead of looking for the cause of ailments and the degeneration of the species. Psychoanalysis has, in

> this manner, an undeniable value for eugenics science that today occupies the attention of the medical class.[83]

The historiographical record credits Moreira as the first advocate of psychoanalysis in Brazil, based on references to Freud's ideas in his 1899 classes at the Bahia School of Medicine and his presentations on Freud's methods to the Brazilian Society of Neurology in 1914. Others such as Henrique Roxo, Maurício de Medeiros, Antônio Austregésilo, Arthur Ramos, and Júlio Porto-Carrero also heavily incorporated Freudian theories into their courses, studies, and books.[84]

Infancy and childhood were already prime subjects of medicine and philanthropy in Rio de Janeiro during the early twentieth century, which was fertile ground for psychoanalysis's popularity in psychiatric and other professional enclaves. As in other Western countries, the care of children was not only the concern of their families in Brazil during the late nineteenth and early twentieth centuries. It took on a political dimension of control rationalized by the imperative of not only defending and saving children but of preserving social peace and order. Júlio Pires Porto-Carrero was arguably the most significant figurehead of Freudian thought in Brazil; he seized upon sexuality and childhood as both a way to understand what elites often characterized as Brazilian atavism and as the means to treat it.[85] A psychiatrist by training, he held the chair of forensic medicine at the University of Rio de Janeiro and offered lectures, courses, and consultancy services on psychoanalysis through the LBHM, an organization that he had helped create. His wide-ranging objectives included working with schools and the Juvenile Court for the correction of minor offenders while providing sex education to primary teachers and parents.[86] As the psychoanalytical voice of the league, Porto-Carrero argued for a strong interventionist state to guide public psychoanalysis initiatives carried out by experts:

> The state should take between its hands, the child after birth. He is not the property of parents, who pervert the shadow of state power. The healthy child is, like any citizen, an economic value that matters to the collective patrimony. If it is difficult to perform comprehensive education during the early years, [the state should take] control [of] domestic education through experts and to take charge of educating children whose parents are unable to do so.[87]

A strong advocate of the role of psychosexual development in the formation of personality, Porto-Carrero emphasized that sexuality should not be ignored, dismissed, or censored. Indeed, in his view, society should acknowledge and naturalize sexuality's potent power to control and channel it toward productive ends. Within this intellectual schema, Brazilian sexuality was not an abhorrent impulse but more an aberrant one; it was a drive that had been improperly governed. According to Porto-Carrero, ignorance of infantile sexuality coupled with religious beliefs that silenced any discussion of sexuality led to inappropriate behavior with children that included excessive physical contact and promiscuity between adults and children. In his "Notes given to one section of the Brazilian Association of Education" of October 1928, he cautioned against "disordered breastfeeding," which resulted in a "sucking entertainment that goes beyond the needs of feeding." In the same paper, he offered guidelines on how to properly take care of an infant as he warns of excessive contact between adults and children:

> From a very early age, the whole cutaneous surface is a source of pleasure, an example of which is tickling. This pleasure is caused both by the friction of clothes against the baby's skin and by the handling of its body; sometimes when lulling it to sleep or by excessive stroking or while rubbing it during the bath.
>
> This is why the proscription of rocking, as long recommended by pediatricians, is justified. Babies should not be carried in the arms: the best place for them is a small, fixed, individual bed; no cradles or hammocks. Loose airy clothes are recommended. The child should take baths when he reaches an age at which he can wash himself. I have heard of cases of children being strongly sexually aroused when being washed by ladies; this habit is not unrelated to the genesis of some neuroses that surface when they grow up.[88]

In order to appropriately repel improper habits, Porto-Carrero argued for the sublimation of sexual energy. As Freud asserted it in his essay "On Narcissism," "Sublimation is a process that concerns object-libido and consists in the instinct directing itself towards an aim other than, and remote from, that of sexual satisfaction; in this process the accent falls upon deflection from sexuality."[89] Within the wide spectrum of sublimation, Porto-Carrero found physical exertion such as manual labor and physical exercise the most useful followed by intellectual labor and artistic activities. The least useful was religious sublimation, since "its consequence is the strong restraint of sexual impulses and the strong application of the death impulse to the Ego."[90]

Extrapolating on the idea of opposition between the ego and drives (i.e., libidinal instincts), Porto-Carrero articulated a gendered analysis that reified patriarchy. He posited that civilization was a masculine force, upheld by sublimation of sexuality and dominated by the instincts of the ego. It consequently oppressed women as the targets of violence and forms of taboo. Far from rallying for gender parity, Porto-Carrero highlighted that each sex had "real" sociocultural roles that men and women should ultimately perform. Within his gendered framework, women should strive to be good mothers who governed the private sphere and men good breadwinners who operated in the public sphere. Porto-Carrero offered a redefinition of the maternal role, raising the status of the housewife, but in ways that were less in line with gender equality and more in line with the liberal political commitment to gender complementarity and the "equal-but-different," team-oriented, companionate marriage. The modernization of the family made the fulfillment of "proper" gender roles and roles for children possible. Within the patriarchal familial unit, he stressed that authoritarianism should be eschewed, egalitarianism promoted, and children respected. Women, in their roles as mothers, were held responsible for instilling moral values in society; by failing in this capacity, they were responsible for its demoralization and degeneracy. When diverted from their natural functions in the home, women easily degenerated and influenced men to commit antisocial acts; the women also birthed and raised retrograde children unable to reach positive, mature adulthood. Porto-Carrero even expressed a seamless continuum between the family unit and the nation: "The concept of the nation, irrationally limited to the scope of borders, largely reproduces the evils of the miserable position children occupy within their families. Patriotic arrogance is both an imitation and a derivation of the authoritarianism of parents."[91] Thus, a strong family unit corresponded to a strong and fair state; a family that failed to nurture children was akin to an authoritarian nation. As a crucial foundation for healthy national and international life, children's sound psychological development in family environments became a sociopolitical and moral necessity. A wide range of state-supported mental health initiatives that made family relationships into concrete objects of psychopathological knowledge and subjects of therapy emerged and circulated in the 1920s. The model bourgeois nuclear family, which had originated in Europe and borrowed by Latin American social reformers, was a rational and disciplinary social unit that adhered to contemporary precepts of mental and physical health as linked to social hygiene. Nineteenth-century medicine and psychiatry secularized and naturalized the idealized gender norms and moral values of this family model.[92] Following this logic, the healthy and moral woman, naturally docile and submissive, was driven primarily by her mothering instinct, natural modesty, and emotions. Her influence was essential as a civilizing force, for it was the wife and family that tamed the male's aggressive sexual instincts by channeling his energy into productive social tasks. As an ideal model appropriated by the upper and nascent urban middle class, this construction of the Brazilian family came to supplant the earlier extended households and kinship networks of upper-class Rio by the end of the empire.

The diffusion of psychoanalysis as a fulcrum for public psychiatric programs reached a new tenor in 1930–37 with the first presidential administration of Getúlio Vargas. Vargas aimed to regenerate the nation through intense educational, public health, public assistance, and economic reforms. The emergence of what he and his administrators imagined as the "new Brazilian man" depended on the reproduction of healthy, productive citizens.[93] With the inception of Vargas's regime, public health and social assistance became a key feature of the state's development and nation-building agenda. Federal and state-level officials' biopolitical prerogatives coalesced with psychiatrists' attitudes toward mental health and social assistance reforms. This confluence resulted in the creation of a new federal department, the Ministry of Education and Public Health, to oversee Care for Psychopaths in the Federal District department.[94] During the 1920s, the Ministry of Justice and Internal Affairs reorganized the services of Care for Psychopaths in the Federal District, the regulations of which included the administration of various care units, among them the Jacarepaguá colony; however, in 1930 policies of political administrative centralization alone did not motivate the Vargas administration's creation of a new department. As historian Cristina M. Fonseca's work shows, the institutionalization of public health served as a means of nation building due to the ways in which Vargas-era paternalistic health and welfare policies symbolically unified Brazil's territory and people under the idea of a national family.[95] Brazilian psychiatrists found the institutional support, funding, and statecraft to advance their mental hygiene campaigns within this ideological context. In the interests of constructing a nation and instilling a sense of national identity, state institutions increasingly took on the responsibility of regulating social relationships and enforcing cultural norms alongside sexual morality.

The Clinics of Mental Hygiene: The Euphrenic Clinic (1932) and the Orthophrenology and Mental Hygiene Service (1934)

Apart from Porto-Carrero's public announcements praising the virtues of psychoanalysis to children in general, a number of mental hygiene institutions for children were created throughout the country in response to psychiatric attention to childhood as a prime locus of professional activity. Psychiatrists Mirandolino Caldas and Arthur Ramos respectively managed the best examples of these childcare clinics in Rio de Janeiro—the Euphrenic Clinic (1932) and the Orthophrenology and Mental Hygiene Service (1934).[96]

The LBHM created the Euphrenic Clinic, which sought to foster "the eugenic improvement of the mind."[97] Caldas's "euphrenic" was a neologism that stemmed from his desire to strategically situate the care of infancy within the fields of eugenics and mental hygiene. Located in the well-to-do São Cristóvão neighborhood of Rio de Janeiro, the clinic served children from their early months of life to the age of twelve, with particular attention to the ages between two to six, which was considered "a critical time for the formation and internalization of the infantile personality."[98] Like child guidance clinics and child gardens in the United States at the turn of the twentieth century, the clinic sought to remediate and prevent unhealthy mental habits and behaviors in children through the use of Freudian psychoanalysis.

Composed of three technical services (social, psychological, and clinical), the clinic investigated children in all their aspects through visitations and observations of the home and the school. Children were subjected to a series of physical and mental exams as well. Officially, the first child to attend the clinic was a thirteen-year-old boy brought by his mother due to muteness. After tests and observations, psychiatrists diagnosed him as an imbecile. They blamed the diagnosis on his parents—the father, a military engineer, had been retired for over twenty years as a result of a psychopathy that led to ideas of persecution, and clinical notes stated that "the mother was a 'nervous, irritable' person so that the son (possessed) a bad neuropathic inheritance due to his hysterical mother."[99]

The clinic's project of social normalization reflected a Freudian psychoanalytic framework that considered a child's misbehavior as a symptom of mother-child conflicts. A 1932 pamphlet articulated this framework. Simultaneously praising mothers for suffering for their children and admonishing them for not taking preventative steps to head off disastrous futures, the text alarmingly promotes the clinic's use value:

> Doting Mother!
>
> Your children are the most precious relics that you possess.
>
> The small physiological disturbances bother you and make you suffer and lose sleep night after night.
>
> Your son grew up, became a man; your daughter also became a woman.
>
> It was the moment to feel joy and happiness as you had worthily fulfilled your role as mother.
>
> It is not uncommon, however, for terrible disappointments to appear: your son, since infant, was a stubborn and pugnacious boy, turned into a criminal and finds himself in prison; your daughter, always full of oddities, was admitted to a psychiatric hospital.
>
> Much sadness! Much disillusion!
>
> Many deviations from psychism are the fruits of a bad education. And it is the Parents, not rarely, those responsible for these serious anomalies. And almost all, even the most enlightened . . . and unintentionally, by their feelings leaving them unable to see the defects in their youngsters.
>
> You can find in the Euphrenic Clinic the advice that you lack. . . . The main purpose of these clinics is not to treat psychopaths and degenerates: it is, above all, to improve, increasingly, the delicate mechanism of psychic elaboration.[100]

As the pamphlet illustrates, the Clinic's therapeutic practices were geared toward the transformation of women into productive workers. Transforming "instinctive" motherhood into skilled emotional "work," clinic psychiatrists thus hoped to bestow medical expertise onto mothers. At the center of the clinic's work was an important set of psychosocial innovations that focused on mothers' great responsibility in producing emotionally healthy citizens.

Although psychiatrists influenced by psychoanalysis during the 1920s and 1930s identified the middle-class nuclear family as a prime site for the cultivation of children's healthy social and emotional development, they also targeted the education sector as a crucial landscape from which to foster sound mental health. The work of psychiatrist-anthropologist Arthur Ramos in Rio de Janeiro's public school system refuted the causal relationship between race, degeneration, and mental abnormalities. Arthur Ramos was an anthropologist who worked on Afro-Brazilian culture's supposedly stunted development, a role scholars have emphasized. His thesis *Primitivo e Loucura* (1926) rendered Afro-Brazilians pre-modern and pre-logical due to their presumed inability to differentiate between reality and the supernatural through rational thought, but he argued against a biological model of degeneration. In a 1934 pamphlet, Ramos observed, "The racial inferiority complex has blocked our progress. . . . There are no superior or inferior races. But there are social groups that are culturally advanced or retarded."[101] He maintained, of an Afro-Brazilian child, "give him good physical and mental hygiene and the alleged inferiority will disappear."[102] Along with anthropologist Edgar Roquette-Pinto and sociologist Gilberto Freyre, he organized the nation's First Afro-Brazilian Congress in Recife, Pernambuco (1934), which specifically countered the 1929 eugenics conference by celebrating African contributions to culture and society. Freyre, who presided over the event, told the local press that the 1934 conference took a stand against the "official Aryanism" among Brazilian intellectuals in the 1930s.[103] Although Ramos, Freyre, and Roquette-Pinto's discourse was not completely devoid of eugenic principles, they emphasized the influence of culture over biological race. By favoring culture rather than biology, these intellectuals focused their attention on how education and health care could improve the Brazilian race.

Although this work provides context, Ramos's efforts as a psychiatric educational reformer who greatly relied on psychoanalysis as a means to counter degeneracy deserves more scholarly attention. In 1933 he became chief of the Mental Hygiene Service of the Institute of Educational Research in the school system of Rio de Janeiro under the directorship of Anísio Teixeira, director of the school system who launched a massive program of educational reform during his tenure.[104] Ramos was already well acquainted with the work of fellow Bahian Anísio Teixeira; Teixeira served as director of the Bahian State Education Department during Ramos's medical education.

Ideologically, Teixeira represented a network of social scientists and doctors who, like Ramos, viewed infancy as a formative area of direct action to abate degeneracy. Ramos described infancy as "the main field of action of mental hygiene," saying that childhood characteristics are "the nuclei of adult life character" and that preventing mental illness requires adjusting children "to their environment" as "the basic objective, the initial work, to be continued after, in the adjustment of the individual to the successive circles of life."[105] According to him, schools were ideal sites to help children "escape the insidious influence of hoax and superstition[,] combat the slow and invisible effect of macumba and fetishism that infiltrates our lives [and] focus on proper spiritual growth, guided towards the currents of true scientific values."[106] Ramos described a poverty of culture wherein children's psychological problems stemmed from culturally stagnant environments. His psychoanalytic studies from 1926 through 1933 noted that racial degeneration was not genetically inevitable and could be eradicated through methodically executed education policies founded upon psychiatric (i.e., psychoanalytical) principles; as he took his position within Rio's school system, he found a sample of nearly one thousand schoolchildren from numerous sociocultural and economic backgrounds to test his theories. He had free rein to conduct observations and experiment with remedies for the students' abnormalities as he saw fit because Teixeira was an ardent follower of psychoanalytical methods and techniques.

Ramos fashioned a multifaceted plan to monitor and transform "problem children." Preschools called habit clinics (clínicas de hábito) became initial centers of observation and diagnosis, designating students as "normal" or "abnormal," with gradations in the latter category although not in the former. Ramos created a child guidance clinic for school-age children and orthophrenic clinics in six schools. At the clinics, psychiatrists-educators created several records on children, involving the physiological aspects of personality and the primordial instinctive activities (such as hunger, thirst, elimination functions, sleep, rest, and sexual activities) in addition to affective manifestations (e.g., the unfolding of the intelligence, etc.). Once the necessary evaluations were made, and the cases that required specialized treatment were separated, it was the psychiatrist's job to advise parents and educators on how to properly impart the formation of normal habits and how to correct maladjustments. The clinics prioritized action within the social environments of both the family and the school and indicated only secondarily direct interventions on the children.

Mental hygienists worked closely with the schoolchildren, teaching them "normal" cognitive behavior and "correcting the earliest maladjustments found." When the children reached elementary school, mental hygienists continued the "double task of prevention and correction." The clinics closely monitored the subjects while treating their perceived deficiencies.[107]

Demographically, Ramos's sizable laboratory of schoolchildren consisted of both poor blacks and poor whites, as wealthy families were apt to seek private education. This heterogeneity enabled Ramos to detach his work from overtly racial connotations. He pioneered a distinct methodology, embracing Freudian psychoanalysis and Neo-Lamarckian eugenics to challenge the myth of racial degeneracy, thereby contributing to widespread social reforms. Ramos considered spreading hygienic reforms outside of the school to be vital to the process of improving society, and he executed his plan on several levels. Placing propaganda in movies, public bulletins, and the radio, he hoped to diffuse the tenets of good hygiene and exemplary morality to the public.[108] Specifically, he hoped that the improved children would transplant their lessons to their homes, thereby helping to educate their immediate families. In addition, he published instructional guidebooks such as *Saúde do Espírito (Higiene Mental)* (1939), which was written "in simple language, accessible to everyone."[109] After four years of methodical research in the Rio school system, Ramos reasoned, "The grand majority . . . ninety-percent of those deemed 'abnormal' [or] 'problems,' [are in fact] victims of a series of adverse circumstances [including] maladjustment in the social and familial environment." He affirmed his conviction that human intervention could reverse the trend, extolling its capacity to "alter the facts of the problem."[110] However, by the end of his tenure as chief of the Mental Hygiene Service of the Institute of Educational Research in the school system of Rio de Janeiro, he became cynical about his ability to effect socially transformative change, which he blamed in part on the political austerity of the Estado Novo.

Between 1930 and 1937, Getúlio Vargas's project to build an economically robust, politically unified, and socially harmonious Brazil was predicated upon a number of elements, including the expansion of social assistance to the mentally ill. But the corporatist authoritarian political tightening of the Estado Novo in 1937 resulted in a series of state divestment in mental health services. According to Ramos,

> With the advent of the Estado Novo, a false nationalist education, of impositions and restrictions, began to replace the concept of supervised freedom, essential condition for the establishment of true mental hygiene rules. The education and human understanding . . . was replaced by classical pedagogy of rigid discipline bans and constraints. The service still tried to survive this period of shadows. But a holy inquisition of angry censors, although [it did not] openly formulate any allegation against the Service, it did not allow [the Service] the perfect functioning/operation in an atmosphere of freedom, which is the one where science can actually be done.[111]

Ramos blamed the Estado Novo for hindering his mental hygiene program. In 1939, Ramos lamented,

> The generating causes of problems expanded tragically, in Rio de Janeiro. First, are the conditions created by [World War II] the very war, that for the second time in this century, came to convulse the world and to complicate the problem of adjustments, peace between men. Secondly, there are the very deficit conditions, in Brazil, and especially in Rio de Janeiro. Food crisis. Housing crisis. Frightful indices of infant mortality and morbidity. Deficient factors in every manner, that tremendously complicate the problem of assistance to minors. . . . Never had mental hygiene [services] had to deal with so many problems, that left the unprotected of the nation's capital left to rely on their own luck. . . . A mental service with such challenges, [was] so loathsome and so depressing.[112]

Others joined Ramos in recognizing that a robust public psychiatric program necessitated a progressive state attuned to the complexities of providing widespread social assistance to the disadvantaged. Such a state needed to situate the marginalized as its core constituent, and in so doing, strengthen its internal structures. Although Ramos's political ideals might have clashed with the Estado Novo, its emphasis on the centralization of political power did seek to improve the care and bureaucratic management of the mentally ill. With the advent of the new corporatist state, all organs of the Ministry of Education and Public Health (from the then–Ministry of Education and Health) related to health care became part of the Departamento Nacional de Saúde (DNS; National Department of Health). The National Department of Health was composed of four divisions: the Public Health Division, the Hospital Care Division, the Support to Maternity and Child Division, and the Psychopath Care Division. The Psychopath Care division was responsible for the "services relating to care for psychopaths and mental prophylaxis of national character, as well as those of local character that are run by the State, being further responsible for promoting the cooperation of the State on local services by means of federal grants and assistance to monitor the use of funds granted."[113] In a notable lecture presented to the Society of Medicine and Surgery, Dr. Adauto Botelho, director of the Care for Psychopaths of the Federal District, outlined various changes, such as the creation of more asylums, agricultural colonies outside urban centers, and juvenile detention centers, among other programs the organization of psychiatric care in the country required. In order to carry out such tasks the newly created the Serviço Nacional de Doenças Mentais (SNDM, National Service for Mental Illnesses) replaced the Care for Psychopaths in 1941. The state directed its resources and energies to the large custodial asylum model, and the proliferation of state-supported clinics independently managed by psychiatrists increasingly subsided. The rapid creation of national departments that attested to the supposed potency of a large government removed the autonomy of state medical and scientific institutions and subordinated them to federal ones.

These centralizing processes also eroded the autonomy of psychiatrists, who were not offered an active part in the reorganization of mental health services. As state bureaucrats dictated the organizational structure of state institutions and oversaw the management of therapeutic programs for the mentally ill, psychiatrists and their expert knowledge no longer functioned as critical state resources. The steady erosion of their authority led many psychiatrists to enter private practice while others retreated back to large state asylums. Indeed, the political climate of the mid-1930s marked the recession of public psychiatry and mental hygiene initiatives.

Conclusion

This chapter has surveyed some of the key ways in which psychiatrists during 1903–37 diligently sought to safeguard the future of their profession and its works. They hoped to redeem the National Insane Asylum from its tarnished reputation with modern innovations and carried out a wide array of public programs to counter Brazilian degeneracy. Their voracious consumption of the then-popular German psychiatric school, led by Kraepelin, marked the early twentieth century. Kraepelin's ideas bore rich fruit in Brazilian soil by appealing to a psychiatric profession longing for ways to effect transformative change in the asylum. Dr. Moreira's appointment opened the door for the proliferation of new techniques such as laboratories and new pavilions geared toward serving the mentally ill. While the efficacy of these tools in the treatment of mental illness remains generally unknown, these measures certainly emboldened Brazilian psychiatrists to stretch the epistemological boundaries of Brazilian psychiatry. The reception of Kraepelin's ideas and their diffusion in Rio de Janeiro, primarily among psychiatrists associated with the National Insane Asylum during the early twentieth century, cannot be overstated. Psychiatrists found Kraepelin's emphasis on new structures, both material and symbolic, and the rendering of the mentally ill as a "population" within a longitudinal methodological approach to the study of mental illnesses, compelling in light of the problems they diagnosed. Kraepelin's epidemiological approach complemented the Neo-Lamarckian ethos embedded within the logics of urban public health during Alves's administration.

The socioeconomic, political, and social damage wreaked by epidemic diseases had created a muscular public health infrastructure during the early twentieth century. This infrastructure also generated a language of reform that united intellectuals, politicians, and psychiatrists in a common crusade against degeneration socio-medical ailment. As the league's members used publicity campaigns and other means to carry out programs to educate the public about the dangers of alcoholism (and other dangers to the psyche), they also turned to Freudian psychoanalysis as a formidable weapon against cultural and environmental degeneracy. By the 1930s, there was a groundswell of interest in psychoanalysis and, specifically, the variant that focused on infantile sexuality and childhood.

While psychiatrists such as Porto-Carrero at times uses the academic and lay pulpit to praise and instruct the public on the virtues of psychoanalysis in the domain of childhood, Caldas and Ramos, among others, practiced direct action by managing ambulatory clinics as a means to not only diagnose and treat potential mental pathologies in children but also as a preventative resource for families and schools. The psychiatric renaissance that marked psychiatrists' experimentation with new therapeutic innovations that began in the early twentieth century and peaked during the 1920s saw a gradual decline during the late 1930s. The Estado Novo's emphasis on consolidation and centralization ultimately left many social assistance policies in the hands of state administrators as opposed to expert psychiatrists.

While it would be easy to understand the marginalization of psychiatrists as a consequence of a mercurial state seizing control of the public sphere, by this time the limits of the efficacy of their therapeutic regimes were evident, as were the limits of the popularity of their public projects. Unable to craft and propagate a compelling narrative of mental health to the Brazilians they hoped to serve, psychiatrists saw some of their clinics close due to disuse. Most notably, after just two years municipal authorities asked the LBHM to relocate the Euphrenic Clinic so the site could be put to better use. As the indignant clinic director declared, municipal authorities in search of "immediate results based on gaudy statistics" were incapable of "understanding the complexity of the effects of the work of that genre . . . as if the utility of a clinic could be gauged by the number of clients served and not by the results obtained by the client and the acquisition of new experimental data for science."[114] While the clinic ultimately left city property for a pavilion in the Engenho de Dentro Colony of Psychopaths, the exchange between the clinic director and city officials reveals both the lack of consistent public interest in the clinic and, perhaps consequently, the diminution of state support.

During the early twentieth century, state officials and the elite classes generally expressed consistent and enthusiastic support for social assistance initiatives geared toward the mentally ill and focused on mental hygiene. Nonetheless, these programs never garnered significant participation from their main targets of social reform. The pathologization of social habits enshrouded in these initiatives, the stigmatization of participation in them, and possibly even psychiatrists' alignment with a state that employed violence to achieve public health ends at all costs (e.g., the compulsory vaccination effort that led to the 1904 Vaccination Riot),[115] did not endear them to the public they hoped to serve. Despite high hopes of using novel ideas and techniques to promote new conceptions of the self, psychiatrists failed to win the hearts and minds of the Brazilians they hoped to transform. Historian Maria Alice Rezende de Carvalho suggests an insightful analysis of Rio de Janeiro's modernizing process during the Old Republic by underscoring the tensions between the role and the actions of the state, often authoritarian and at the service of a Comtean positivist economic and technical modernization that was not concomitant with the modernization of social relations. Although psychiatrists and other liberal professionals were compelled to assert their "messianic redemption of the people,"[116] many of their efforts met considerable obstacles. Apart from the lackluster appeal their measures garnered, they also had to contend with formidable cultural institutions such as Kardecist spiritism and candomblé during the first part of the twentieth century. Their protracted battles with practitioners and leaders of these mediumistic religions, the subject of the next chapter, would ultimately reveal their successes and failures.

Chapter Six

Mad Spirits of Progress, 1927–44

> "The Mediums' Book" by Allan Kardec is the cocaine of nervous enfeebled individuals . . . and with one aggravation: it is cheaper, reachable, and for those reasons results in the hospitalization of a lot more people than "devil's powder." . . . The hygiene and prophylaxis rely exclusively on burning all Spiritist books and shutdown of candomblés, high, medium, and low, that, for now, infest Rio de Janeiro, Brazil and the entire western part of the world.[1]
>
> —Dr. Antonio Xavier de Oliveira, *Espiritismo e Loucura* (1931)

Psychiatrist Xavier de Oliveira's elision of spiritism with insanity is emblematic of early twentieth-century Brazilian psychiatry's alarmist preoccupation with spiritism as a public health threat. Between 1917 and 1928 he observed, in a sweeping hyperbole, that while alcohol and syphilis were the most common causes of psychosis among patients at the Psychiatric Clinic of the University of Rio de Janeiro, all the rest suffered from spiritism. This condition as a form and cause of psychopathology dominated the Brazilian psychiatric imagination during the early twentieth century as psychiatrists wrote medical and pseudo-medical treatises about it, dedicated entire medical journals to it, and made it a key topic of conversation at asylums and sanatoriums. As an organized profession confronted in Brazil with a popular, modern competitor—one with a radically different view of the self and of rationality—psychiatry was in a state of panic. Xavier de Oliveira and others placed both the doctrines of Kardecist spiritism and candomblé, in their diversities of form and practice, under the conceptual umbrella of "spiritism" to refer to religious-philosophical systems of thought that postulated life after death through the viability of the spirit and the living's communication with spirits through human mediums. In the course of this chapter, I will use "spiritism" or "the spiritisms" to refer to the entire field of possession religions, including Kardecist spiritism and candomblé as the two major branches within spiritism, while recognizing that there was, and remains, a diversity of belief structures between the two and within each.

Brazil's colonial history is replete with instances where communication with the spirits of the dead was fundamental to the sociopolitical and cultural cosmologies of indigenous populations, African slaves, and Portuguese colonists. As the structures of Kardecist spiritism and candomblé each, in very distinct ways, became increasingly formalized and legible over the course of the nineteenth and early twentieth centuries, psychiatrists became more entrenched and yet more frantic in their criticism.

Psychiatrists, with their Freudian focus on the "self," and their hopes of winning the hearts and altering the culture of everyday Brazilians, were vociferous critics with a special antipathy toward possession by either gods or spirits. The radical permeability and durability of the self so implied in spiritism was in direct conflict with Freud's relatively unitary self. Raimundo Nina Rodrigues (1862–1906), an eminent Brazilian psychiatrist, anthropologist, and ethnographer, interpreted possession as "a provoked sleepwalking-like state with fragmentation and substitution of personality,"[2] while psychiatrist Arthur Ramos (1903–49) believed "that trance does not reveal any characteristic beyond what is already established by Psychiatry as mass hysteria."[3] As defenders of a modernity founded upon an aspirational, but real commitment to rationality and the promulgation of, at most, a restrained religiosity, these psychiatrists and others railed against spiritism. To them, it represented an attachment to a primordial time that disassociated Brazilians from the fast trot of modernization. Psychiatrists considered spiritism as dangerously close to the "superstitions" of the lower classes. Indeed, for the barely postcolonial modernist psychiatrists, spiritism evoked an array of deep historical struggles, chief among them competition and conquest histories with black and indigenous pagan belief systems, institutional and chauvinist fears of continued barbaric resistance, and documented disruptions from unruly forms of folk religiosity, and the religious feminine. For these modern secular authorities of science and state, spiritism tapped into fears of antimodern, atavistic, and anarchic tendencies within the populace. When they called for the extirpation of Kardecist spiritism and candomblé, they undoubtedly feared that objectionable practices, especially those that appeared African derived, could give rise to unorthodox versions of citizenship. Although some psychiatrists seem to have exaggerated the threat of spiritism to advance their professional and cultural goals, many appear to have been genuinely panicked by spiritism's practices and popularity. Although the simultaneous proliferation of spiritisms and their persecution in the early modern period has been insightfully explored by a number of scholars, this chapter investigates how and why Rio de Janeiro's psychiatrists moved to form the vanguard of the antispiritist movement that would reach its apogee the late 1920s and 1930s and its denouement during the 1940s.

In order to understand psychiatrists' histrionic responses to spiritism, the frameworks of panic and crisis become useful theoretical tools. Panic has been understood as a psychological state or an emotionally charged group response (generally construed as irrational) to some external menace, whether natural or manmade, actual or imagined.[4] It denotes "a collective flight based on a hysterical belief."[5] The history of panic is closely related to the history of crisis as co-occurring phenomena; moments of crisis hold panicked people and expose sociocultural fissures. As scholar Janet Roitman claims, "Crisis moments are defined as instances when normativity is laid bare, such as when the contingent or partial quality of knowledge claims—principles, suppositions, premises, criteria, and logical or causal relations—are disputed, critiqued, challenged, or disclosed."[6] Spiritism, as a field of practice, posed just that kind of challenge, and Brazilian psychiatrists' characterization of spiritist practices and practitioners as both a form and a cause of psychopathology came in response to just such a moment. This chapter joins a small but growing literature that engages the dynamics of postcolonial sociocultural rule through the study of affect. Privileging emotion, context, and culture is both new and not new; many of the questions driving the folding of emotion into historical investigations were first posed in the 1930s by historian Lucien Febvre, who considered the study of the emotional life a particularly fruitful method for understanding the "mental equipment" of past generations.[7] In 1941 Febvre invited fellow historians to "reconstitute the emotional life of the past" by undertaking "a vast collective investigation . . . on the fundamental sentiments of man and the forms they take."[8] His invitation to contribute to a history of "affective life" has been extended by Peter Burke's recent work on the links between emotional experience, professed values, and political power.

Applying these paradigms to Brazil, I argue that spiritism generated an institutional overreaction, a moment of crisis, within Brazilian psychiatry that ultimately laid bare a hitherto largely subterranean fault within the profession. Psychiatrists had sought to make better Brazilians with a series of initiatives discussed in the previous chapter. They had hoped to use Freudian psychoanalysis to improve Brazilians' mental health in order to make the nation of their struggles into the nation of their dreams. At the same time that Brazilians were, for the most part, choosing not to attend these psychiatric clinics, they were choosing to attend candomblé or Kardecist spiritist services in larger and larger numbers. Brazilian psychiatric analyses of the time tended to identify spiritism as a discrete and consistent object, yet they recognized to a degree that this was not so. The inability to fully understand spiritist religions' complexities, much less their respective mass appeals, generated a crisis of knowledge about possession specifically, and with it about psychiatry's inability to establish itself as the premier touchstone in the mental health and well-being of Brazilians. Psychiatrists did not understand how their dream of a modern Brazil, with hygienic selves of all races working together in a sober and orderly fashion to make a healthy, sane, racially and economically segregated and well appointed capital city was supplanted in the hearts of Brazilians from all walks of life by religions of possession.

Possession, as a defining and constitutive feature of both candomblé and Kardecist spiritism, contains within it layered significations related to the nature of gods and power, selves and bodies, ownership and freedom, time, history, and progress. Taken holistically, this suggests an ontology of personhood that relativizes and provincializes the premise of the autonomous modern individual, the central unit of presence in the psychiatric worldview. Spiritisms announce that the autonomous individual is a fragmentary composition.[9] This malleability of the self, the notion of its openness to intimate, transformative, and ecstatic submission to either gods or the spirits of the dead, both radically delimits the construct of the self and creates a moving edge beyond which the rational may not successfully venture. Spiritism's logics and logos, when understood outside of the language of pathology, fundamentally upset Brazilian psychiatry's model of the self-possessed citizen and nation bound to the vicissitudes of time, materiality, and territoriality. Further, possession, most notably in the deep context of candomblé, had long performed a richness of polymorphic identities, but by the 1920s both candomblé and Kardecist spiritism had each grown enough that the category of "other" was an expression of the distance between psychiatry's moral panic and the cultural landscape that psychiatry had sought to make its own.

There is a significant body of literature that investigates psychiatric-spiritist contestations by focusing upon Kardecist spiritism exclusively. Notable anthropological texts such as David J. Hess's *Spirits and Scientists: Ideology, Spiritism, and Brazilian Culture* (1991) and Emerson Giumbelli's *O Cuidado dos Mortos: Uma História da Condenção e Legitimação do Espiritismo* (1997) have chronicled why various cross-sections of Brazilian society joined spiritist centers, attended meetings, and became believers.[10] Although these studies examine the role of spiritism as a significant knowledge field that challenged psychiatry and its claims to cure and manage madness, they do so in a cursory manner. Since they focus primarily on spiritism, and not psychiatry, they treat spiritism as a medical, philosophical, and religious imaginary that functioned as a hegemonic discourse. Similarly, the existent literature provides a teleological analysis, rendering psychiatry's "eventual" legitimization as a medical science and Kardecist spiritism as a religion inevitable. These works, while informative, too neatly resolve the critical epistemological disputes between psychiatrists and spiritists. Moreover, these studies eclipse the ways in which psychiatrists homogenized both Kardecist spiritism and Afro-mediumistic religions such as candomblé and umbanda by taking at face value the ways in which Kardecist spiritists, acting out of cultural self-preservation and class and race biases, purposely made distinctions between their form of spiritism as "high," and those of Afro-Brazilians or lower classes as "low." By only examining Kardecist spiritism, they too subscribe to the marginalization of candomblé as a significant cultural player in the arena of the creation of Brazilian selfhood and in the consequent psychiatric panic during the early twentieth century. Furthermore, they leave covered the meaningful connections between Kardecist spiritism and candomblé as "black" and "white" religious-cultural movements connected at their center by possession.

Nonetheless, the typical narrative, which historians apply to Kardecist spiritism in Brazil as well as the United States and Europe, describes a two-stage process. During the first half of the twentieth century, psychiatrists considered followers of spiritism as mentally unstable, the mediums-cum-preachers as frauds, and spiritism itself as a contagion of insanity.[11] During the second half of the century, historians generally characterize psychiatry's approach to spiritism as altered by transcultural and ethnographic approaches that stressed the cultural construction-values of knowledge. This was to lead psychiatry to tolerate and then even embrace spiritism as the rise of ethnopsychiatry normalized a diversity of religious practices as potential resources for psychological well-being. This shift may primarily reflect the influence of French anthropologist Roger Bastide, who studied Afro-Brazilian religions.[12] However, this narrative ultimately overlooks the distinctions between Brazil and other nations where spiritism, in its Kardecist and Afro-Atlantic forms, took hold. Unlike in France, where the Catholic Church was spiritism's main critic, or in the United States, where the practice and its followers' occupation of a marginal, yet faddish space in both civil and state societies, led to its toleration, or in Cuba, where santeria (as a form of spiritism) was heavily regulated and policed, in Brazil spiritism was too popular to be fully marginalized and psychiatry outpaced both the Catholic Church and the police in leading the charge against spiritism. Psychiatrists felt, and legitimately so, that Kardecist spiritism's popularity posed a threat to their dream of cultural hegemony. Further, whereas Kardecist spiritism largely declined in Europe and the United States during the early twentieth century, in Brazil it has flourished, and more than a hundred years later, Kardecist spiritism remains a popular religion. Over the course of the nineteenth century, intellectuals, military officials, and politicians alike were drawn to Kardecist spiritism as it offered them a new framework through which to understand the political, social, and moral life of a nation in transition.

The doctrine's staunch espousal of a teleological view of history that emphasized peaceful evolution as the natural order resonated profoundly with republicans who decried monarchism as an atrophied political system but feared that class, racial, and gender discord could lead to violence and revolution. Many of Rio's educated elite recognized in Kardecist spiritism a philosophical ethos that bridged the apparent divide between religion and science while maintaining social stability. Likewise, candomblé, which also continues to thrive in contemporary Brazil, enjoyed great popularity in nineteenth-century Rio among slaves, free people of African descent, and some whites. Similar to other syncretic Afro-Atlantic religions such as santeria, voodoo, and obeah, candomblé represents a mixing of Yoruba and Bantu spiritualities infused with Catholic tenets. As a form of critical social and political practice, candomblé offered a space and a model for cultural resistance. Where candomblé offered Afro-Brazilians a space from which to reclaim and assert their humanity during enslavement, the religion, after emancipation, continued to provide a safe haven for Afro-Brazilians scarred and marginalized by elite society. Candomblé, in the words of anthropologist Rachel Harding, functioned as an "alternative space of blackness" that offered both a framework of resistance to the dehumanizing institutions of colonial power and a way of revaluing black personhood.

Spiritism, in its polyvalent forms, was and is a complex series of movements that can be rightly understood at the intersection of many practices, traditions, and forces. Kardecist spiritism and candomblé as religions of possession were, however, accepted through Brazil during this time period because, taken as a whole, they came to be constitutive of a loose but powerful modernity founded upon hybridity and mediated through possession. This is not to suggest that the two were generally the same; on the contrary, taken together, they offered a Brazilian modernity in which individuals of all colors could be subsumed into histories or powers across space and time, but in which African- and European-based possession practices would make their own distinct cultural and physical spaces. And although they cannot be fully understood when taken together, it is in combination that Brazilian spiritisms have made the potentiality of possession constitutive of what it means to be a modern Brazilian citizen. Neither Kardecist spiritism nor candomblé were in fact anachronistic religious movements stuck in premodern times; each approached the questions of modernity with a distinct mixture of flexibility and tradition, and they have each endured as popular and growing religions in Brazil in the contemporary period.

The spiritisms compromised the hard-fought distinctions of other ideological systems, such as science, medicine, and religion undermining their borders with an alternative logic in which definitive limits between scientific and religious, erudite and popular, and modern and traditional were generally disregarded and rendered impotent. Since Kardecist spiritist mediums explicitly and candomblé authorities implicitly laid claim to understanding and treating mental illness, they undermined the legitimacy of psychiatry. Psychiatrists wrote sensationalist denunciations of spiritism for both lay and academic audiences and enlisted state officials to close spiritist centers, prosecute spiritist mediums, and burn spiritist materials, including books and sacred offerings. Spiritism not only threatened psychiatric therapeutic and cultural space but also sabotaged the field's cultural logics.

Spiritism, as a psychiatric cynosure, functioned as a representation of national degeneration and revealed the fissures within professional psychiatry's discursive infrastructure. I wish to offer a synthetic analysis of Brazilian psychiatry and spiritism that approaches their conflict as constitutive, in unique ways, of modern Brazil. Budding psychiatric modernism was in conflict with many other forces, and it is a common scholarly trend to understand spiritism through a lens colored by the derision with which elite nineteenth-century modernists approached it. This unfortunate trend creates false parallels between spiritism and other supposed antimodern practices that medical reformers during the first republican period sought to extirpate, such as prostitution, gambling, and alcoholism, among others. Spiritism, in its Kardecist and candomblé forms, will instead be understood in this chapter as a powerful contender for the role of lead cultural contributor to Brazilian modernity. Seeing psychiatry through the emotive lens of the panic will primarily allow a fresh critical look at some of the previously obscure underpinnings of psychiatric modernity and give some insight into the disconnect between psychiatric ideals and the actual choices being made by Brazilians. It is worth noting that the validity of psychic phenomena, the efficacy of spiritist practices, the truth-value, or ontological status of spirit possession, like the parallel validity of Catholic beliefs in prayer and the afterlife in chapter 2, fall outside the scope of this study.

In order to investigate how spiritist religions became an important part of psychiatry's undoing, this chapter first gives mid-nineteenth-century background on candomblé and Kardecist spiritism and then examines possession as a constitutive element of both. It then offers a treatment of the construction and contestation of spiritism as an object of the 1890 criminal code. Following that, it examines psychiatry's antispiritism campaign as a form of professional panic that exposed the profession's vulnerabilities. The chapter closes with the diminution of psychiatry's antispiritist denunciations within the connected context of waning psychiatric influence and authority.

Spiritism's Forms: The Problem of Candomblé

Although the historiographic record suggests that candomblé, in its embryonic forms, was most likely present in Brazil starting with the arrival of the first African slaves in the 1530s, the religion did not really begin creating its formal structures in earnest until the early nineteenth century. The first *terreiros* in Rio de Janeiro were founded at the end of the 1800s, just as the process of abolition was ending slavery and the republic was about to be born. According to Brazilian *babalawo* (diviner) Agenor Miranda Rocha, in 1886 Mãe Aninha of Xangô came to Rio from Bahia with two other women and opened a house in the neighborhood of Saúde, a largely African area of the city center.[13] Around the same time, João Alaba of Omolu opened a terreiro in a shantytown on Barão de São Félix Street. Though neither of these terreiros had authoritative successors and closed after the deaths or departures of their leaders, they formally inaugurated the religion in Rio and set the stage for its growth in later decades. Candomblé, primarily in its Nagô-Jeje variant, would grow and flourish as Brazilians of African descent left rural plantations and, seduced by rumors of easy jobs, migrated en masse to urban centers, especially to Rio de Janeiro. In Little Africa, as this section of Rio was known, former slaves created a social network anchored by houses of worship in the hills surrounding the port. The decline of the sugar industry in the northeast, due to competition from the West Indian colonies, was balanced by the growing macroeconomic importance of coffee; this resulted in the displacement of slaves farther south in the country. For this reason, the slaveowners in the province of Rio de Janeiro, who owned a total of 119,141 slaves in 1844, would more than double that number to 300,000 by 1870. The population of Rio as a whole doubled between 1872 and 1890, then doubled again to more than one million inhabitants by 1920.[14] By the end of the nineteenth century, some of this influx had coalesced into a large network of Afro-Bahian free people who had established themselves as leaders of the black community, organized around candomblé terreiros. Afro-Bahian leaders such as Torquato Tenerê and Tia Dada, who lived in Little Africa, were in high demand. They catered to a huge clientele with a variety of problems in need of resolution.[15] As the state's increasing focus on "sanitization" instigated the demolition of largely "African" and presumed unhealthy districts in the city center, these networks facilitated a cultural continuity as Brazilians of Afro descent were pushed farther toward the city's outskirts.

The formalization of candomblé or disruptive force in the eyes of elite Cariocas began in 1888 with abolition, and grew shortly thereafter, on November 15, 1889, with the declaration of the First Republic and soon after with the constitutional separation of church and state. It is precisely at this juncture that the relation of Afro-Brazilians and their religions to Brazilian national identity became a pressing concern. Hitherto, slaves had been regarded as firmly "Brazilian." However low their status, they had occupied an undeniably important position in the national economy, first in sugar production, then in mining, and by the end of the nineteenth century, on coffee plantations. With abolition, however, and their newly inchoate position, former slaves' provisional status as "owned Brazilians" shifted in the eyes of generally white elites, highlighting their identity as Africans, dangerous and unstable in their foreignness. The liberty of freed slaves to perform religious ceremonies involving drumming, sacrifice, and possession dance was an obvious site of contestation; it was in such ritual performances that difference, perceived as an African anti-Brazilianness, was most radically marked. As suggested by the correlation of the shift from "subjects" to "citizens" with the rise of police forces, it was with the liberation of the slaves and the nearly coeval declaration of religious liberty that the negotiation of such issues in legal practice became a national issue.[16] This conflict was legally addressed by a twofold strategy. First, Decree 528 of June 28, 1890, prohibited Africans and Asians from entering Brazil without special congressional approval, while simultaneously aggressively encouraging European immigration. The Law of Lands (Lei de Terras, passed in 1808 and renewed in 1850) conceded "free land" to European settlers, and the adjacent state of São Paulo between 1890 and 1920 offered to compensate European immigrants for the cost of ocean passage. Brazilian state actors, stuck with a largely African, black, and of-color population, and spinning in the massive and speculative wake left in slavery's passing, sought in many ways to buy a whiter Brazil. Second, the Penal Code of 1890, though largely the same as that of 1830, included three significant additions: the newly written Articles 156, 157, and 158.[17]

The articles addressed the "illegitimate" practice of medicine, magic, and curing. Article 156 prohibited the practice of any medicine or dentistry without the necessary legal certification. Article 157 prohibited the "practice of spiritism, magic and its sorceries, the use of talismans and cartomancy to arouse sentiments of hate and love, the promise to cure illnesses, curable and not curable; in sum, to fascinate and subjugate public belief." Finally, Article 158 proscribed "administering, or simply prescribing any substance of any of the natural domains for internal or external use, or in any way prepared, thus performing or exercising the office denominated as curandeiro."[18] Thus, Article 156 was addressed to illegal medicine, 157 to sorcery, and 158 to curandeirismo (including candomblé). The addition of the three articles to the Penal Code of 1890 set the stage for a legal paradox that would endure for much of twentieth-century Brazilian law. Although the Constitution of 1891 declared the freedom of religion and the separation of church and state, according to state culture, Afro-Brazilian religions were detrimental, and posed a threat to national progress. The solution, therefore, was the repression of Afro-Brazilian religions (or "cults" as they were pejoratively known) under alternative categories to religion. Articles 156, 157, and 158 provided the terms necessary for the ongoing control of former slaves and freedpeople despite their new status as full citizens.[19] Their focus on Afro-Brazilian cultural productions, defined the arena of their concern, and, in the coming years, would give perhaps an undue weight to elite (and psychiatric) concerns about the beliefs and thoughts of Brazilians, and especially Afro-Brazilians.

Brazil's first republican constitution declared the privacy of religion and rendered it a field completely removed from state jurisdiction, following the path of France, the United States, and other modernizing countries. And although the fledgling Brazilian republic followed these constitutional models of religious freedom, formally separating church and state, Brazil left popular forms of religiosity subject to civil and military authorities charged with order and health in the public domain. Of the religious practices that were defined not as religions but as matters of "public health," most incorporated African derived religious elements. This was not accidental, but rather a strategic maneuver and in keeping with the ideological rules elites hoped would inform a growing public sphere. Along with civic improvements like public transportation systems and streetlights the republic had to address communally shared, civic problems like sewage and garbage, disease and public health. It was among the latter that candomblé and Kardecist spiritism were classed. The attempt to make bourgeois refinement and European aesthetics the cornerstone of Brazilian national identity was not a novel creation of the late nineteenth century. Public hygiene had been a stated concern of ruling elites since the arrival of the Portuguese court at the ports of Rio in 1808.[20] It was then that the medical field had begun to play an active role in social reform. In the years after the Prince Regent's arrival, medical universities were built, and by 1851 Rio's municipal administration included the Central Committee for Public Hygiene, members of whom wrote on health subjects in the widest sense, including the intersection of morality, race, and degeneration.[21]

Social science and medical science carried out their procedures in homologous terms. It is not surprising that the first anthropologists to write on candomblé were also medical doctors. Candomblé was initially located at the intersection of strings connecting degeneration, hybridism, criminality, and contagion by the work of psychiatrist Nina Rodrigues. His pioneering in-depth studies of candomblé began to appear in newspapers during the last years of the nineteenth century, lamenting the contagious capacity of "fetishist animism" to turn even the upper classes black.[22] The slight but significant shifts in post-abolition law suggest that government officials shared his concern. In fact, in order to render these measures of control more efficient, in 1904, under Decree 1151, the government created the Service of Administrative Hygiene of the Union. Among other things, this department justified the city's "sanitation" and supervised judgments on Articles 156, 157, and 158 of the 1890 Criminal Code.[23] All of these measures proceeded under the crusading banner of public health. Proper hygiene, from which things African influenced were by definition excluded, was a central criterion of the appropriate, and legal, within the state's view of Brazilian religious practice.

Public health had already become the defined terrain in which the homologues between biology and social health were investigated, as well the central site of conflict between theories of social evolution and degeneration and the empirical laboratory dedicated to recording and mitigating the polluting risk of miscegenation. As such, the field of public health lent a sense of order and coherence to a haphazard assemblage of notions about race, health, and civic virtue. The tone of the period was such that real social issues were addressed abstractly and imaginatively, transformed through metaphors like illness, degeneration, pollution, cleansing, and vitality. Candomblé terreiros were invaded and destroyed in the name of protecting public health, even as freedom of religion was proudly proclaimed the law of the land. Candomblé was also marginalized from the constitutional core of the guarantee of freedom of religion by being relegated to the jurisdiction of the Penal Code's domain of illegal health practices and malevolent sorcery. Nonetheless, candomblé attracted Brazilians across race and class spectra. The interdependence of Afro-Brazilian religions and wealthy white and Creole client patrons was sardonically observed in 1906 by João do Rio in his famous ethnographic work *As Religiões no Rio*,[24] a collection of feature stories on religious sects in Rio: "It is we [the middle and upper classes] who assure her [Afro-Brazilian religions'] existence, like the love of a businessman for his actress-lover."[25] His observation captures the perception of Afro-Brazilian culture as forbidden, exotic, enticing, and potentially habit forming. Displaying his contempt for candomblé, but not Kardecist spiritism, he noted that Kardecist spiritists were "sincere," while the terreiros were "exploitative," noting, "Beyond a few groups that conduct themselves with relative honesty, the agents of (candomblé) are shameless rascals. The mediums exploit credulity, the sessions are a cover for depraved acts, and madness sprouts and hysteria rises from each of these incubators of fetishism."[26] Until the 1920s nowhere in national public discourse was candomblé discussed as a bona fide religion; and even then, as this chapter later explores, it was discussed with an ambiguity more reflective of paternalist tolerance and of Afro-Brazilian culture than of national attitudes on religious freedom. Although not codified in any legal document, freedom of religion was categorically denied to candomblé and other related religions of possession such as Kardecist spiritism.

The Transnationality of Kardecist Spiritism

Like candomblé, Kardecist spiritism came to Brazil from abroad. However, while candomblé, represented a series of creative compromises between religious-cultural beliefs and practices deeply held within the millions of enslaved people taken to Brazil from West Africa, Kardecist spiritism was a self-consciously religious movement that stemmed from France.[27] Its Anglo-American forbearer, spiritualism, refers to a loose constellation of practices centered on communicating with the dead that emerged in the Victorian-era United States and Britain following the early, highly publicized séances of Kate and Margaret Fox in 1848. Kardecist spiritism was the product of a transnational circuit that consisted of a European hermeticism that informed French mesmerism. This, in turn, influenced American spiritualism, which traveled back to France to be recast by Allan Kardec (the pseudonym of Hippolyte-Léon Denizard Rivail) before reaching Brazil circa 1865. Credited with being the creator of spiritism in nineteenth-century France, Kardec defined spiritist doctrine as a "science, which deals with the nature, origin, and destiny of Spirits, as well as their relationship with the corporeal world."[28]

Spiritism and progressive politics in the Atlantic world perfectly dovetailed with one another. Indeed, the Fox sisters' earliest séance followers were local Quakers interested in freedom of expression.[29] Through this connection, American séance spiritualism assimilated a Quaker philosophy of "inner light, inner truth, and outer action to reform society according to the spirit principles of grand connection."[30] In the next decades, the influence of Andrew Jackson Davis, whose philosophy called on humankind to work toward "eternal progress" and mental and spiritual perfection, which, once "properly accomplished," would elevate the "social world," magnified spiritualism's reformist tendencies.[31] Nineteenth-century French spiritism built on spiritualism's reformist tendencies. Unlike British and American spiritualism, both of which were diffuse and loosely constituted, Kardec inspired orthodoxy through his book *Codification*, and *Le Revue Spirite*, the movement's main periodical that reported (and thus legitimized) new doctrinal developments and linked spiritist centers throughout France.[32]

Like US spiritualism, French spiritism gained a following across the socioeconomic spectrum in France. However, its emphasis on hard work, individual responsibility, equality, universal education, fraternity, and positivistic inquiry into the spirit world appealed especially to bourgeois liberals.[33] While Kardec's analysis is thin on political commentary and even militates against it, his *The Mediums' Book* reprints the bylaws of his Parisian spiritist circle, which expressly forbade discussion of "politics, religious controversy, and questions of social economy." Still, historian Lynn Sharp suggests "spiritism's calls for equality and solidarity meant calls for social change."[34] Further, Sharp asserts that French spiritist leaders "waged a strong republican, anticlerical campaign, calling for equality and social reform" in the 1860s and 1870s, and educational reforms in the 1880s.[35] However, this was complicated by the ample room that Kardec's doctrines left for classism: his evolutionary model of spirits implied that souls, living or dead, occupied different hierarchical stations that could be equated to economic or social classifications.[36]

Kardecist spiritism was popular in many countries, but more so in Brazil than in any other Latin American country. Brazil's multicultural eclecticism and the diversity of its population and cultural practices, contributed to the popularity and wide diffusion of the doctrine's synthesis of science, philosophy, and Christian morality. Brazilian Kardecist spiritism shared its French progenitor's emphasis on progress and a carefully modulated equality, and also found its base among the bourgeoisie elite. Although spiritism attracted Brazilians from all walks of life, members of the middle and upper classes grappling with how to reconcile their Catholic faith and the scientific tenets of modernization found it particularly appealing; steeped in nineteenth-century rationalism Kardec articulated a doctrine that offered a union of science and religion in one philosophical ethos. Its teleological approach to history and its law of continual progress fit bourgeois culture. Its commonalities with positivism also appealed to the city's intellectuals' and upper classes' traditional belief in divine revelation and their emerging commitment to scientific experimentation as a mode of knowledge making. Kardecist spiritism's espousal of the conservation of order and its interest in social utopia also mirrored the order and progress ethos of Brazil's middle and upper classes. Whereas psychiatry in Rio had entered into public and messy boundary disputes with Catholic caregivers, Kardecist spiritism shifted the frame, asking its followers to believe, at most sites of conflict, that both (i.e., medicine and religion) was an acceptable answer.

Since Kardecist spiritist doctrine advocated the continuous improvement of the individual and society according to a "law of inevitable progress,"[37] its followers prized reconciliation in all areas of life. French immigrants who were part of a modern urban population brought spiritism, its easily disseminated texts and its séances, to Brazil's liberal, literate professional class. It first took hold in Bahia, when the Grupo Familiar do Espiritismo, Brazil's first spiritist circle, created a center in September 1865. Soon, it spread to Rio. Director Luís Olímpio Telles de Menezes, professor, journalist, and member of the Instituto Histórico de Salvador, founded the first spiritist journal in Brazil, *O Echo d'Além Túmulo*, in 1879. The journal's national and international distribution would lead Kardec himself to bestow accolades on the journal's attempt to expand spiritism beyond the confines of Brazil.[38] Among Brazil's merchants, lawyers, engineers, and doctors who became Kardecist spiritists, noted figures included Casimir Lieutaud, director of the revered Colégio Francês and Adolphe Hubert, editor of the *Courrier du Brésil*, a city journal well known for its anticlerical stance. Institutions such as the publishing house Garnier, which published four of Kardec's books between 1875 and 1876, proved instrumental to spiritism's spread.[39] Exclusive urban Kardecist circles often required literacy and therefore excluded the majority of the Brazilian population. The first such group in Rio, the Grupo Espírita Confúcio, created in 1873, disseminated the key doctrines of spiritism through the press and through the care of the infirm using homeopathic remedies. In 1876 the group's creation of the Sociedade de Estudos Espiritas Deus, Cristo, e Caridade and its internal conflicts became characteristic of the spiritist organizations that dotted the urban landscape. Within the Sociedade de Estudos Espiritas, a faction developed that emphasized spiritism's religious mysticism while the other segment highlighted the doctrine's scientific principles. Historian Sylvia Damazio highlights the existence of a division within the group's adherents as well—the Kardecists and the Roustainguistas.[40] The Kardecists in particular took Kardec's book *O Evangelho Segundo o Espiritismo* as a guide. The Roustainguistas followed French Jean-Baptiste Roustaing, a lawyer who converted to spiritism and launched a controversial theory that the pregnancy of the Virgin Mary was fiction, and that Jesus Christ did not inhabit a material body, but a fluid form, or rather he was immaterial.[41] In Rio, however, Kardecist spiritism proved the more popular of the two.

Urban elites had established at least thirty heterogeneous and formal spiritist circles, or societies, in Brazil by 1893. Groups such as the Sociedade Acadêmica Deus, Cristo e Caridade (1879), the Grupo Espírita Fraternidade (1880), the Grupo dos Humildes (1880), and the Grupo Espírita Humildade e Fraternidade (1881) created a panorama, each with slightly different memberships and interests. By the beginning of the twentieth century, there were an estimated one hundred thousand spiritists in Rio alone, and nearly twenty journals that dealt with spiritist matters nationwide.[42] The famed chronicle writer João do Rio noted at the time, "One does not know the number of orthodox spiritists, one can tell of the attraction of our more lucid brains by the science of revelation. The Navy, the Army, the law, medicine, the professoriate, the big world, the press, business have millions of spiritists. There are men who do not make mysteries of their faith."[43] According to historian Ubiratan Machado, João do Rio observed as late as 1912, "It is not only bourgeois families that are conducting Spiritist sessions, but the masses as well. The Spiritist sessions are like improvised dance parties. The true pastime of this age is conversation with those from beyond the grave."[44]

As Machado and others have argued, Kardecist spiritism's popularity in the eighteenth century was in part a reaction against the ascendancy of reason, scientific rationality, and the Cartesian notion that all things could be explained. While Comtean positivism left an ingrained imprint on Brazilian intellectuals, Brazilian culture had long been imbued with mysticisms ranging from a traditional Portuguese Sebastianismo (King Sebastianism) to the variety of African based religions of possession. Machado further observed that, in Brazil particularly, religious syncretism did not gravitate in one direction; religious practices of Afro-Brazilians and the Catholicism of European Brazilians drew thoughts and practices from each other. "The mazombo, or white population born in these 'Brazils,' gradually absorbed the blacks' superstitions, practices, and magical customs. This influence on the white master's religiosity, on top of Iberian superstitions, practices, and magical customs, shaped Brazilian popular Catholicism in an undeniable way."[45] The Brazilian Spiritist Federation (Federação Espírita Brasileira, FEB, 1884) became the de facto flagship institution of Kardecist spiritism in Brazil.[46] The FEB's mission was to publicize spiritism through the "active propaganda by the press and by public conferences."[47] They, like previous European spiritist groups, offered free social assistance to the needy, but the FEB was best known for its doctrine of spiritist mental health and for the programs it put in place for the treatment of mental illness. Their "Servico de Assistencia aos Necessitados" sought to help people both spiritually and physically.[48] As close readers and students of Kardecist spiritist thought, the organization was founded on the theory that there were only two potential causes for madness: either physical damage to the brain, or the presence of unyielding malevolent spirits.

Historians refer to Adolfo Bezerra de Menezes Cavalcanti, the politician, medical doctor and president of the FEB (1889–90, 1895–1900), as the Brazilian Kardec.[49] As a high-profile progressive Carioca, Menezes Cavalcanti's announcement of his belief in spiritism before a large gathering of Rio's elite in 1886, captivated the city's attention, both legitimizing public elite conversions and generating city-wide interest in Kardecist doctrine. In Cavalcanti's most influential Kardecist work, Insanity through a New Prism (1897), he framed Kardecist conceptualizations of insanity and advocated for the practice of disobsession, the procedure of conversing with errant spirits who disturb the living and cause physical and mental illness, as a means to alleviate the suffering of the living. The three-part book provided a new paradigm to guide doctors' and psychiatrists' interpretation of mental illness. In the first part, the author defended the existence, in man, of a spiritual principal. He reinforced Kardec's ideas, attacking materialism and affirmed that men were spirits that possess bodies of flesh to temporarily exist on earth. The second part develops the idea that the brain is only a material instrument to reproduce the thought that is originally in the spirit. According to Cavalcanti: "The function of the body, in general, and of the organs, in particular, is to be a simple apparatus or instrument of the soul, because that never ceases even if the body stops."[50] In the third section of the book, he analyzed obsession as a cause of insanity, stating, "If it is easy to explain mental disturbances, when the transmitter organ of thought is injured, the same does not occur in the cases noted by famous French psychiatrist Jean-Étienne Dominique Esquirol, to match it with the perfect integrity of the brain."[51] He articulated the claim that when madness did not have an organic cause, its source was "inferior" spirits. He conveyed that these influential spirits did "not hurt or injure the body, but they inspire bad thoughts, bad feelings, terrible resolutions. They come to dominate our will, to the point of turning us submissive as if entranced."[52]

Thus, Kardecist spiritism championed the existence of malevolent spirits and their influence on the mind, whereas psychiatry defended a social and biological paradigm. The inefficacy of much psychiatric treatment at the time contributed to the popularity of the Kardecist spiritist psychiatric asylums, meeting centers, and generally, the Kardecist theory of mental illness. Psychiatry's influence was perhaps just past its peak, and the problem posed by the chronically insane that they had once laid at the feet of the Santa Casa was coming back to haunt them as well. Since antipsychotic and other pharmaceutical drugs were not yet available, psychiatrists' tool kit was small and ineffective. Even four decades into running the asylum, they could not actually back up their curative claims. Madness, as a real object in culture and as a tragic personal reality had remained largely untouched through their Pinelist fervor, their passion for systems, their utopic attempts at antialcoholic and antisyphilitic social engineering. Moreover, the scandals associated with the National Insane Asylum's failures as an institution of confinement and the subsequent barrage of criticism did much to discredit psychiatry and open what had been psychiatric professional ground. Brazilian spiritisms, both Kardecist and candomblé, took over much of that sociocultural terrain, while challenging the monopolistic religiosity of the Catholic Church. In so doing, both gained adherents, but they also attracted much criticism.

Denunciations of Spiritism

The republican penal code of 1890 outlawing "malevolent" forms of spiritist practice effectively codified the liminality of spiritism's various forms. Providing context is the role of the criminal code in state efforts to assert Brazil's place in an international Atlantic order long dominated by northern, abolitionist, and progressive powers, in spite of its being the last country to abolish slavery in the Americas. From this debased position, government and elite sectors of Brazil sought to assemble a dossier of evidence of Brazil's right to a place among the ranks of civilized nations. The administration of Marshal Deodoro da Fonseca, the first republican president, advanced that cause by supporting the European-inspired penal code, which as historians Carlos Aguirre and Ricardo Salvatore have noted was by no means isolated among popular juridical models of the post European-enlightenment Atlantic. Across post-independence Latin America, as legislators "enacted an array of new laws, codes, and constitutions . . . many legislative pieces were selectively cloned from French, British, and other European sources which were usually considered the non plus ultra of juridical science and progress."[53] In prohibiting spiritist practices, the Brazilian state sought, in part, to provide evidence of its own civilizing offensive and political modernity. Paradoxically, the Penal Code of 1890 may have done more to cement spirtisms' place in Brazilian culture than to eradicate them. Theorist Jacques

Derrida's observation that "the essence of law is not prohibitive but affirmative"[54] may help to clarify why Brazil's early twentieth-century detractors seized on these laws and the court proceedings that sprang from them as evidence of a backward nation with a possessed, even Africanized, population. The code allowed for the creation of positive, even official, proof of the reality strength of practices that the state, through prohibition, sought to discredit.

At this juncture, it becomes pertinent to explore the significance of the criminalization of spiritism for spiritist followers, both at times when they were strictly enforced and also when they were not. The work of anthropologist-historian Yvonne Maggie convincingly argues that the Brazilian legal structure at the outset of the republic never sought to extinguish spiritism and forms of magic but rather only to administer and regulate them, making it likely that the Brazilian people and state had more in common on the subject of spirit possession than either had with the psychiatric establishment.[55] Unlike British colonies in Africa, which outlawed not witchcraft but rather the accusation of witchcraft, discrediting witchcraft as a legitimate legal claim, Brazil's laws entertained such accusations as a viable area of jurisprudence. In agreeing to let the state's courts be used to adjudicate claims of this kind, the government validated the existence of (and belief in) spiritism—along with magic, witchcraft, and sorcery—and the need to control it.

At the time of the penal code's passage, the FEB press began a campaign to support Kardecist spiritism and to undermine its critics. For example, the *Reformador*, the FEB's publication, stressed that the republican government had adopted a retrograde attitude toward Kardecist spiritism in comparison to the progressive tolerance of other countries. According to the *Reformador*, there were eight periodicals in England, one in Norway, one in Russia, two in Holland, three in Belgium, three in Germany, two in Austria, one in Hungary, one in Turkey, fourteen in France, twelve in Spain, one in Switzerland, four in Italy, one in Egypt, one in Australia, seven in the United States, five in Mexico, one in Venezuela, one in Peru, two in Chile, four in Cuba, one in Uruguay, four in Argentina that focused on Kardecist spiritism. In naming these various countries with their corresponding number of Kardecist periodicals, the *Reformador* sought to prove that Brazil, "a nation that intended to put itself on par with the civilized,"[56] was in fact not as advanced as its advanced counterparts, given its criminalization of Kardecist spiritism. When Kardecists were not disparaging Brazil for going against global "modernist" trends, they publicly articulated spiritism's social conservatism and reconciliatory ethos as compatible with the republic's Comtean positivism.[57] A month after the code went into effect, the *Reformador* published an article addressed to the Ministry of Justice contesting Article 157's alignment of Kardecism with magic and other forms of superstition. It read in part, "Spiritism [Kardecist], Sr. Minister, is the most complex negation of all superstitions: It battles the most powerful cause of delays in the human spirit, it affirms that one should only believe in what observation, illuminated by modern scientific processes, can verify with the acquisition certain by the patrimony of knowledge."[58] In a competition for modernist legitimacy, Kardecists accused of retarding progress saw themselves as agents of moral advancement. Imagining themselves as partners with the state to combat forces of disorder, Kardecist spiritists stressed that it was unnecessary and unjust to criminalize their spiritism as a crime against public tranquility:

> It is very surprising that the authorities intend to dispense with one of their best collaborators in the enormous work of raising the moral level of society. The guarantee of the security of public order and peace anchor themselves more in the elevation of character and in the moral precepts than in any coercive laws. . . . Spiritism folds in all the shades of humility, selflessness, the fulfillment of civic duty. Is it, thus, the enemy of society and deserving of punishment? Or is it one of the most powerful civilizing factors of the homeland.[59]

While the FEB, through the *Reformador*, did not stop the criminalization of spiritism, it did elicit a response from João Baptista Pereira, one of the principal legislators of the penal code. The jurist emphasized in a *Jornal do Commércio* article that his objective was to curb the practice of illegal medicine and to end charlatanism. According to him, Kardecists had adopted practices that sometimes fell under those parameters, and as such, should be limited. He observed:

> Article 157 and its two paragraphs, referring to crimes against public health, brought to the (fore) some supporters of spiritism that, with access to impotent rage, swore against the Code and with insults . . . lunged against its author who, very Christian, pardons them because he is convinced that, they, being hallucinatory, do not know what they say and should be treated with charity. . . . We will not . . . censor those who embrace it: as a speculative science without descending [to] their experimental practices . . . we know to respect the liberty of faiths, even the most extravagant.[60]

His condescending manner persisted throughout his response, as he characterized followers of spiritism as unfortunate victims who were superstitious, and likely to enter the asylum:

> Spiritism has intrepid believers. These gullible followers are fooled, like Cassandras of comedies, by shameless charlatans and their ridiculous practices, which are almost always to blame for both enriching those who exploit

> others, and for driving true believers straight to the asylums. . . . The research led by men of proven science and unblemished professional moral certainty concluded that the spiritist doctrine is a superstition . . . it is proved, not by one, but my many judiciary surveys that have proceeded, in various countries, and all crowned with success, that the fervent believers of spiritism are some unfortunate victims, who are fleeced of their money and judgment. How can a sect speaking in the name of science, of morality, and of religion request for itself a letter of security allowing it to explore the lucrative industry without [recognizing the] risks and dangers.[61]

Baptista stood by the creation of Article 157, saying he could not be "indifferent" to a "defenseless public powerless to combat an industry that attacked the purse and compromised health."[62] His stance, and the stance of the progressive republican state in general, mirrored the model of the patron-client relationship, with the responsibility for, and patronization of, the Brazilian masses implied therein. In response, FEB representatives put forth a series of refutations in a set of articles in early January 1891. They stressed that while Baptista claimed not to condemn Kardecist spiritism as a speculative science, but nonetheless stood by a vaguely worded Code that blurred the difference between spiritism and superstition.[63] They pointed out that Article 157's strategic economy of generalization criminalized an entire field of ritual practices. The argument for specificity on the part of Kardecist spiritists and their deployment of "superstition" was racially coded language for candomblé and the practices of the largely Afro-Brazilian lower classes. This relatively transparent moment of Kardecist spiritists willingness to use race and class politics should be read back into the debate in which the word "spiritism" was generally understood by both sides to refer to Kardecism, and yet, was legally directed toward a racial continuum of congregations ranging from the "whitest" Kardecist circle to the "blackest" of candomblé terreiros. In the name of Euro-aspirational modernity, state actors wished to whiten black Brazilians through an anticandomblé and antipossession campaign of cultural engineering. At the same time, Kardecist spiritists argued persuasively that Kardecism (and therefore possession) were accepted parts of scientific European modernities. Although jurists made a fine distinction between "high" and "low" forms of spiritism, Kardecist spiritists argued that the law did not and therefore produced, in religion scholar Theophus Smith's terms, both "tonic" and "toxic" effects.[64] Kardecist spiritists engaged with juridical law and attempted to shape its enforcement as a potential social curative (against low forms of spiritism) even as they opposed and resisted its more general attack on spiritism as toxic. Kardecist spiritists' defense of their own brand of spiritism did not repel denunciations, much less the outpouring of psychiatric moral panic that would be leveled against Brazil's religions of possession.

Psychiatric Persecution of Spiritism

The confrontation between psychiatry and spiritism in its Kardecist and candomblé forms was perhaps inevitable given the secularization of institutions, the value attributed to science, the emergence of new theories about human and social behavior, and the fundamental cultural and demographic heterogeneity of Brazil. Both spiritisms and psychiatry sought to explain the same questions in different ways: the origin of mind, the relationship between mind and body, and the treatment and prevention of mental illness. Franco da Rocha's 1896 text was one of the first psychiatric texts to make an explicit link between insanity and spiritism.[65] Using an 1895 São Paulo Juquery Asylum report as a springboard, he noted that Kardecist spiritism was a rising factor of insanity, stating that it would be "an unfortunate and entirely useless imprudence to permit this new religion, that only serves to increase the number of insane people."[66] The 1895 report made numerous references to an alarmist 1885 article titled "Collective Madness in a Spiritism Session in Taubaté," which described "an event worthy of the deepest regrets resulting in hallucinations by the various people in this city who follow spiritism."[67]

At approximately the same time, Nina Rodrigues's groundbreaking work *O Animismo Fetichista dos Negros Bahianos* (1896), likewise characterized candomblé as a cause of collective madness. Rodrigues stressed that Africans, criollos, and mestizos who practiced candomblé were susceptible to suggestion and mass hysteria. He also doubted Afro-Brazilians' ability to adapt to Brazilian political and cultural systems, stuck as they were between fetishism and idolatry in a religion that involved spirit possession.[68] Positing that candomblé functioned as a political institution for Afro-Brazilians and therefor a rival to the formal state, he argued that this made Afro-Brazilians unstable political subjects. Nina Rodrigues argued that candomblé had taken possession of the country by embedding itself in the public spirit ("no animo publico") and that this posed a danger of further expansion via contagion. His reimagined use of the connection between possession and contagion echoed some of psychiatry's earliest fears about what were then marginal slave religions. Police reports of illegal religion cases in the late nineteenth and early twentieth centuries borrowed his language; terms such as "possession" and "somnambulant spirit," among others, became commonplace. As anthropologist Paul Johnson astutely notes, Rodrigues's "studies and their vocabulary provided the grammar for legal control of religion during the first decades after emancipation as slave religion was reformed as part and parcel of a civil religious project."[69] The civil religious project of candomblé, then, served as the foundation upon which the enforcement of new public health laws prohibiting all forms of spiritism were constructed.

In the early twentieth century, conferences, publications, and theses about the prejudicial character of spiritism (both Kardecist spiritism and candomblé) at the Colleges of Medicine in Rio de Janeiro and São Paulo increasingly cemented the medical and psychiatric strategy of linking spiritism and insanity.[70] Despite medical and early psychiatric characterizations of spiritist phenomena as forms of fraud, or delusions that could lead to madness, the professional psychiatric community did not perceive it as a critical threat until the late 1920s. As their assessment of the threat changed, psychiatrists began to malign spiritism and accuse mediums of various forms of malevolence. As a group they advocated for its regular prosecution and censorship. At the same time, the state response to spiritism was erratic and uncommitted; prosecutions were the exception, and the resulting convictions were accompanied by minimal penalties.

While psychiatric opinion was still gravitating toward a concerted emotional aggression toward spiritisms, and particularly Kardecist spiritism, in the early 1910s, there remained some nuance within the profession. They did not try to use the police as a lever to enforce Article 157 of the Penal Code. Examination of the landmark 1909 October-November session of the Rio de Janeiro Society of Medicine titled "The Dangers of Spiritism," offers insight into their mindset. Conference convener Dr. Felício dos Santos, psychiatrist and self-declared "Catholic, apostolic, Roman" fired the opening salvo against spiritism by affirming that the "asylums were always filled with victims of spiritism. Spiritism and alcoholism are the biggest proponents of insanity."[71] However, Dr. Nascimento Gurgel, who spoke after Dr. Felício dos Santos, disagreed with his colleague and stressed the need for more research on spiritism, pointing out that the topic had garnered international attention as a worthwhile research area from prominent doctors, such as French physiologist Charles Richet, who had a year earlier presented a lecture on a different subject to the academy.[72] Soon after this exchange, Dr. Fernando Magalhães proclaimed he believed the development of spiritist practices posed no danger to society and asserted that the medical field was vast enough to accommodate spiritism. He asserted that the Penal Code should be used to punish doctors with medical degrees who acted in criminal or ignorant ways as zealously as it might be used in the repression of medicine practiced by those without a medical degree. Dr. Teixeira de Souza also spoke at the session, declaring:

> We must not persecute (spiritist) centers. There are no healers who have no cures! And there are no doctors who do not have setbacks! Moreover, the time does not lend itself to such intransigence within the medical profession. Medicine has traversed a period of anarchy, of which any/no therapy does not exempt itself. Lies of yesterday appear today as truths; theories, now decadent, may rise again victorious tomorrow. Therefore there is no need to

> systematically reject those that heal by this or that means. Is there in spiritism some dogma that attacks public health? No.[73]

In an uncomfortable compromise, doctors in this session ultimately decided, for the time being, not to pursue a vigorous campaign against spiritism.

By the time that the Society of Medicine met again on April 19, 1927, spiritism had become a much bigger and more contentious issue for the doctors. This time, psychiatrist Leonídio Ribeiro led the charge against spiritism, directly advocating for state action against "the abusive practices of the religious sect, known as spiritism." He stressed: "The intervention of spiritism in treating any neurosis is always harmful. The spiritists who most dedicate themselves to these treatments, are, generally, uncultured and illiterate individuals, without any notion of the dangers that they expose to the mentally ill. Spiritism, is, it can be said . . . without exaggeration, a veritable factor in the [production of] mad people. . . . Among the insane, who everyday enter the Asylum, the majority come from spiritist centers."[74] He claimed that there were "Two reasons, one which was most serious and important, that would justify a vigorous campaign [against spiritism]; to defend the dignity of our profession, today by all so disregarded, and to prevent the ills that these practices always bring to public health."[75] This depth of concern about the professional integrity of psychiatry was new as psychiatrists publicly employed the language of self-preservation, and boundary defense. Dr. Sebastião Barroso, agreeing with Ribeiro, noted that spiritism had spread from "the lower classes" to "people of high society"[76] and hence should be stopped. The evocation of contagion from "the lower classes" to "people of high society" underscores the extent to which the upper classes, as the symbolic representatives of Brazilian modernism, had to be policed to ensure proper behaviors and habits.

It was not by happenstance that psychiatrists' slow-burning anxiety toward spiritism reached a fevered pitch during the 1920s. Although the increasing growth of both Kardecist spiritism and candomblé had much to do with the timing of the mental health profession's antispiritist panic, movement in other strains of elite culture in Brazil also played a large role. Psychiatrists, with reason, felt boxed in. The 1920s saw the emergence of a Brazilian artistic and cultural modernism that, like similar emerging aesthetic modernisms elsewhere in Latin America, sought to undermine many of the beloved bastions of elite culture from which it had sprung. This culturally rebellious modernism was officially born in February of 1922, when avant-garde intellectuals and artists met for "The Week of Modern Art" in the Municipal Theater of São Paulo as part of the centenary celebration of independence. This event proved to be a major rupture in Brazilian thought. The First World War, with its opaque provenance and staggering death toll, had been over for four years. Disenchanted with a Europe that had dutifully marched into and through a devastating, and apparently pointless war, the aesthetic avant-garde in Brazil's major cities revolted against European influences that had hitherto dominated the arts in Brazil. Mario de Andrade, the often-proclaimed father of this new artistic modernism, recognized the movement as a rebellion against French and Portuguese aesthetics and a celebration of Afro-Brazilian and indigenous cultures. Elites proclaimed themselves the cultural heirs and avengers of indigenous and Afro-Brazilian figures as they "cannibalized"[77] those elements of European cultural traditions that they wished to adapt to the Brazilian context (e.g., Italian futurism) while incorporating indigenous and African elements with the self-conscious goal of creating something organic to the nation. Within this new cultural movement, intellectuals and artists "discovered" indigenous and Afro-Brazilian cultures as they appropriated cultural artifacts into a new, more diverse national iconography and origins story. While Brazilian racism pervaded this new modernism, the architects of the new iconography simultaneously insisted on a new openness to the products of African and indigenous cultures as sources of authenticity and identity. The intellectuals and artists of the time saw little contradiction between the valorization of indigenous and Afro-Brazilian cultures alongside the exclusion and subordination of actual indigenous and Afro-Brazilian people. Indeed, this modernism should not be seen as an activist movement against the status quo, except in cultural terms. Many of the appropriated symbols from the African or indigenous past were brought into this frenzied culture making uncoupled from actual African- or indigenous-descended people. One of the few exceptions to this was a commitment to attending candomblé, and to a lesser extent, Kardecist services.

Furthermore, the 1927 meeting reflected the failure of their mental hygiene programs. As discussed in chapter 5, in the 1920s psychiatrists sought to disseminate Freud's doctrines to the general public by issuing recommendations and prescriptions in the popular press, on the radio, and through a series of largely failed clinics. Their fundamental experience of failure in the public sphere included the reiteration of a stinging encounter with citizens, who were consistently choosing not to enter psychiatric clinics but rather to attend candomblé terreiros or Kardecist centers. By 1927 it was clear that many Brazilians did not see psychiatry as holding the answers to the pressing questions related to the well-being of the mind. Seeking to establish a formal consensus among their colleagues in response, the doctors present at the 1927 meeting created a "Survey among Brazilian Experts." Far from rigorous and extensive, the "survey," directed by Ribeiro in addition to four other doctors, consisted of four questions sent to twelve professionals.[78] The questions included:

1. Is Your Excellency of the opinion that there exists fundamental science in what is called spiritist phenomena?
2. Does Your Excellence know of facts or experiences that scientifically document spiritism?
3. Can the practice of spiritism cause damage to the mental health of the individual?
4. Can the abusive exercise of the art of curing by spiritism entail dangers to public health?[79]

Leonídio Ribeiro's and Murilo Campos's 1931 book *O Espiritismo no Brasil* listed the near unanimous survey results that naturalized the relationship between spiritism and insanity.[80] The one distinction, perhaps without a difference, among the respondents was whether or not mediumistic spiritist sessions spontaneously created madness in the attendees or whether it only affected the predisposed, sort of uncovering latent insanity. For example, Henrique Roxo and Faustino Ezpozel defended the idea that spiritism could incite insanity in any person, whether he or she was predisposed to mental illness or not. Roxo created a new diagnosis, "Episodic Spirit Delirium," which he presented at a 1936 medical conference in Paris, to encapsulate the purported psycho-pathogenic qualities of spiritism.[81] In contrast, Franco da Rocha argued that "Many, when they seek spiritism, are already half crazy," and therefore spiritism alone did not cause their mental problems. He affirmed that the "simple practice of consulting spirits should not, by itself, constitute a great evil, provided that the individual does not possess a predisposition for insanity."[82]

Many psychiatrists believed that low levels of education and tendencies toward mysticism were risk factors for mental illness.[83] While there had been a formal psychiatric rejection of simple biological race theories of madness, sociocultural theories undergirded by racism often took their place. Despite their formal, profession-wide statements to the contrary, many psychiatrists believed that those of African descent were especially vulnerable to the vicissitudes of spiritism. Furthermore, as men whose personal and professional identities rested on the Apollonian promise of taming madness, they consistently espoused that women, irrespective of race and ethnicity, were deeply susceptible to the spiritist siren's call. Indeed, psychiatrists conjured evocative scenes of disorder where spiritism unleashed multiform irrationality. Rocha envisioned spiritist proceedings and their effects: "Together in a poorly lighted room, everybody in silence, and an intense emotional state, no wonder the consequences. The emotional state, the collective excitement, and surrounding modifications evoke, especially in women, hysterical outbreaks, and the abnormalities go even further—to complete loss of reason."[84] The popularity, and the perceived intimacy of spiritist gatherings, as well as the perceived suggestibility of the attendees unnerved psychiatrists as they hyperbolically proclaimed that spiritist practices induced the disintegration of the family,[85] suicide,[86] and rape.[87]

By the late 1920s, the pressure of psychiatric panic, expressed through the histrionic language surrounding spiritism, motivated state officials to act. Even though Article 157 of the 1890 penal code already outlawed "malevolent" forms of spiritism, the 1920s would see state officials undertaking a series of tense prosecutions against the FEB and its president. Similarly, the Redemptor Spiritist Center of Rio de Janeiro (Centro Espírita Redemptor), another landmark spiritist institution, faced prosecution throughout the late 1920s. Psychiatry's adversarial relationship with spiritism peaked when psychiatrists pressed for state censorship of spiritist print materials, including the burning of existing spiritist books, journals, pamphlets, and material goods.[88] In 1927 the Rio de Janeiro Chief of Police, in an attempt to subdue critics of police inactivity against spiritism underscored that spiritism was indeed a matter taken seriously by the police: "Crimes against public health are of great interest for the police. There is much to be done in the sense of eliminating the practice of low Spiritism, cartomancy, and other forms of public exploitation. Mysterious cults of Oriental origin, residues of African esoteric beliefs of the African tribes, such as Macumba and Candomblé, distorted by ignorance and bad faith freely existed in the Federal District because of the failure in applying the penal laws."[89]

Despite psychiatric condemnation and consequent state action against their faith, acts, and meeting places, spiritists of all kinds continued their practices. Kardecist spiritists even inaugurated their first radio program, Hora Espírita Radiophonica, in June of 1939. Psychiatrists, concerned at the inefficacy of their antispiritist movement and aware of radio as a powerful dissemination tool among the city's largely illiterate population, sought to ban the radio program. At the behest of Dr. Carlos Fernandes, the Rio de Janeiro Society of Medicine and Surgery passed a unanimous motion to ban the broadcasting of the radio program and sent its proposal to the president of the Republic and the Ministers of Justice and Education. On the day the motion was sent to state offices, Dr. A. L. Nobre de Mello, director of the Rio de Janeiro Assistance to Psychopaths of Mental Hygiene and Prophylaxis Service in reference to the proposed radio ban stated in an interview with the journal *Diário da Noite*:

> I believe it is the unanimous opinion of the medical profession to emphasize the dangers that come from the collectivity of spiritist practices. I cannot, therefore, cease to applaud warmly, the motion of the worthy Society of Medicine and Surgery in this social health campaign. . .
>
> In our environment, spiritism has not been an inoffensive religious sect. To permit its expansion and growth through the radio is to cultivate a superstition that has already enslaved, regrettably, millions of civilized men.[90]

Nobre de Mello, like many of his peers, focused his critique on Kardecist spiritism's threat to the "civilized," while in the same breath subtly deployed the words "superstition" and "enslaved" to evoke candomblé, complete in its spellbinding power but also in its Africanness. Furthermore, his syntax suggested that candomblé, akin to a contagion, was extending its influence to a civilized Brazil. The journal also interviewed Kardecist spiritist doctor Seraphim Lobo who defended and celebrated the charitable aspect of the free medical care provided by Kardecist spiritists in the "Dispensary Antônio de Pádua (1929)," of which he was the director. Stating that the dispensary treated more than ten thousand people in two years, free of charge, he contrasted this figure with the Society of Medicine's claim to having treated 1,372 mentally ill suffering from spiritism in ten years.[91] The intertextual exchange between Nobre de Mello and Lobo illustrates clearly the therapeutic and institutional conflict between Kardecist spiritists and psychiatrists. Ultimately, psychiatrists failed in their attempts to ban the radio show and curtail the broadcasting of spiritist doctrine.[92] Indeed, none of their attempts to eradicate spiritism, Kardecist or candomblé, from the urban landscape during the 1920s and 1930s met with success. But spiritism thrived despite the successful disruption of spiritist centers, terreiros, dispensaries, and asylums, as well as the maligning of mediums, spiritist doctors, and lay adherents alike as insane or criminal actors. Brazilians from a variety of class, racial, ethnic, and socioeconomic backgrounds disregarded the prescriptions of psychiatrists about the medical and socio-moral hazards of Kardecist spiritism and candomblé as they flocked to spiritist gatherings.

Psychiatrists' inability to impede spiritism's growing popularity reflects a series of sociopolitical and cultural factors worth unpacking. According to historian Artur César Isaia, Kardecist spiritists steadfastly sought to showcase that they held the values of the elite classes. Nonetheless, they had their practices rendered illegitimate by those who "Africanized" them."[93] Although they attempted to highlight, to potential adherents, the differences between Kardecist spiritism and Afro-Brazilian forms of spiritism, their strident defense of Kardecist spiritism was also a defensive reaction to psychiatrists' purposeful elision of Kardecist spiritism and Afro-mediumistic religions. Psychiatrists knew the differences between the two, but they persistently conflated them in seeking to discredit Kardecist spiritism, banking on the currency of "African" as a pejorative. Kardecist spiritist mediums' persistent claims to cure and to treat mental illness directly undermined the professional standing of psychiatrists. Since mediums were often educated men who went to the same schools as psychiatrists, and they were often of the same socioeconomic and racial background of psychiatrists, they represented a formidable challenge to psychiatrists' legitimacy. Unlike candomblé, situated beyond the edge of psychiatric sociality, Kardecist spiritism was in no way liminal to the psychiatric elites' Atlantic world. It is with a greater degree of social purpose than veracity then, that in the preface of Ribeiro's and Campos's *O Espiritismo no Rio*, psychiatrist Afrânio Peixoto declared, "Low spiritism has only, by difference, the gradations of culture and morality. . . . I have attended, out of scientific curiosity, spiritist sessions, in various social contexts. The same background, the same methodology, the same results, only variations of rudeness and manners."[94] In another instance, psychiatrist Xavier de Oliveira not only fused macumba with Kardecist spiritism but also established a causal links between spiritism, blackness, immorality, and mental illness when describing the ritualistic elements and practices of a macumba session:

> Pieces of candles, of cigars, rosemary leaves, and of other herbs, rosary beads, cornmeal manioc flour with bad smelling olive oil and a whole series of proper ingredients are consecrated and used, all to be placed in any crossroads, late at night. Other times, playing at the home of the victim, only the medium healer can disable its harmful effects. . . . The sexy dances that always close these assemblies of exploiters and exploited who lack even the stain of filthy lust that is one of its main characteristics. In the mannerisms of their sensual steps one can see the brutal instinct of the beast living within each one of these macabre orgies. An eternal satanic carnival with all its train of miseries and with all its unfortunate consequences. And this is that they call a science, some and a religion others! Spiritism, epidemic madness that now devastates humanity, I say.[95]

The psychiatric vision of social progress that animated Brazilian intellectual life in the early republican period was deeply invested in the construct of a degenerate "other," of which candomblé had long been partially constitutive, and into which psychiatry sought to subsume Kardecist spiritism. In the narrative that psychiatry had developed, public health served as the theater in which psychiatry's eventual defeat of atavistic foes (i.e., candomblé and Kardecist spiritism) would play out. In a strategic sleight of hand, psychiatrists deliberately lumped candomblé, as the indelibly African and often maligned repository of black illogic and barbarism, and Kardecist spiritism together, seeking to render both as forces of disorder. In response, Kardecist spiritists championed distinctions between "high" and "low" forms of spiritism, partly in keeping with their own classism and antiblack racism, and partly as a way to avoid the classism and racism that others, including psychiatrists and the police, sought to deploy against spiritism writ large. In many ways Kardecist spiritists' rhetoric during this time can be seen as an attempt to ensure that antiblack, anti-African, nostalgic antislave, and antipoverty prejudice would not mark Kardecism on its way to impacting candomblé. This had a paradoxical effect. Inadvertently, the argument for a deliberate distinction between Kardecist spiritism as "high" and Afro-mediumistic religions as "low," made most legibly by Kardecists, became a productive type of affirmation for all forms of spiritism in that their unique and clearly culturally compelling identities were articulated publicly from the streets to the halls of government. This was not, however, a balanced or bloodless process. Kardecist spiritism and candomblé did not receive equal levels of repression. Afro-Brazilian spiritists bore the lion's share of the antispiritist backlash instigated by psychiatrists and their state allies. Undoubtedly contributing to this imbalance were Kardecist spiritists' employment of whiteness as a marker of self-identity, class standings, social connections, and cultural affinities—all of which resembled those of state representatives who judged them.

However, when Kardecist spiritists used criminal trials, newspaper articles, radio broadcasts, and other performative spaces to defend their doctrine and to delegitimize other "spiritists," they also made spiritism into a national spectacle, and in so doing, popularized it, etching it deeply on the Brazilian imaginary. Inscribed as a single Janus-like cultural entity within the legal framework of spiritism, "high" and "low" spiritism became, inside that exaggeratedly broad legal frame, culturally constitutive of each other. Not only did the "Africanness" of the one mirror the "Westerness" of the other, but the two grew inextricably intertwined in many important ways. The persistent public recitation of spiritism's particulars (whether Kardecist, candomblé, or a more minor sect) engendered its constant circulation as a stable trope in public life. Spiritism's circulation then lead to its framing as a mainstay feature of popular culture and daily life.

Spiritism's Revenant

The impetus within psychiatry for the diminution of their attacks against spiritism can be identified as early as 1935. Odilon Galloti, professor of psychiatry in Rio de Janeiro, broke publicly with his brethren in asserting in the newspaper: "In my opinion, spiritism is scarcely ever a straight cause of psychopathy . . . in 10 years of my practice, I had 6,400 patients and in only one case could I make a diagnosis of spiritist-related delusion. I confess I don't know whether the evolution of the case confirmed my hypothesis or not."[96] By the early 1940s psychiatric panic and the drive to persecute all things spiritist had been replaced by the more tolerant zeitgeist that would characterize psychiatric attitudes going forward. Most notably, Osório César, who worked in the Juquery Insane Asylum in São Paulo, renounced his previous claims about spiritist mediums as charlatans who caused madness in his 1929 book *Misticismo e Loucura.* He declared in 1941, "Most mediums did not present any kind of mental pathology" and acknowledged having made a "serious mistake."[97] He admitted that "psychiatrists are mistrustful of people and they have the bad habit of frequently classifying ideas [and] facts that conflict with common sense of the time with a hint of madness."[98]

Historian José Leme Lopes attributes this psychiatric toleration of spiritism and its practices to an anthropological cultural reorientation and credits the French sociologist and anthropologist Roger Bastide, who studied Afro-Brazilian spirit possession practices for many years and criticized the ethnocentric prejudice that led to its condemnation.[99] By the mid-twentieth century, Brazilian psychiatry developed a greater sensitivity toward cultures outside the traditional European diasporic biomedical hegemony influenced by the emergence of transcultural psychiatry.[100]

The gradual tapering off of psychiatry's battles with spiritism had, up until this point, been a result of their similarly gradual somber recognition and acceptance of the basic fact that the "mystical" was a cherished, central, and non-negotiable part of culture for a Brazilian populace who had simply combined an enchanted worldview with modernity. Indeed, psychiatrists' inability to curb spiritism's popularity not only challenged the Weberian thesis that modernity is "disenchanted" but also showed the often contradictory ways spiritism belonged to, connected to, or could co-exist with modernity.[101] Historian Michael Saler's dialectical approach that recognizes "unresolved contradictions and oppositions, or antinomies" of "Janus-faced" modernity is most compelling in understanding psychiatric-spiritist encounters.[102] The pillorying of spiritism by psychiatrists was undoubtedly tempered by the rise of a centralized interventionist state that sought to institutionalize culture and centralize social welfare. Accustomed to their roles as expert allies of the state committed to the project of order and progress through the execution of their professional labors, under the Vargas regime, psychiatrists had to grapple with how to legitimize their work as a necessary public good. Confronted with institutional setbacks in the National Asylum, lackluster mental hygiene clinics, and the popularity of competing therapeutic approaches such as Kardecist spiritism and candomblé, psychiatrists were faced with a daunting task.

The ascension of President Getúlio Vargas to power in 1930 presented another factor that contributed to psychiatric antispiritism abetment. Vargas took office in 1930 as the leader of approximately thirty million Brazilians. When he was forced from power in 1945, there were fifty million Brazilians, and the meaning of that national designation was more powerfully enunciated than it had ever been before.[103] He rose to power during the Great Depression, which had greatly undermined the traditional coffee bean oligarchy. With the support of an alliance of states outside of the coffee triumvirate of Rio de Janeiro, São Paulo, and Minas Gerais and the support of the tenentes (lieutenants), a group of liberal reformers in the military, Vargas's arrival inaugurated a concept of the nation and the public sphere that was both progressive and reactionary. It was progressive as a rejection of the old political oligarchy of landowners, seeking instead a coalition of workers, a rising urban middle class, and regional leaders from outside the main agricultural engines of Brazil. It was progressive in creating for the first time an overt public sphere of institutions devoted to meeting shared national needs: a minimum wage to solidify a working class, emergency drought measures for the northeast, electrical service expanded in the cities, a federal university system, women's suffrage (1932), national hydroelectric capacity (1939), petroleum (1938) and steel projects (1941), and nationally broadcast radio programs of popular music.[104] Not insignificantly, generating a populist platform also entailed diminishing, at least rhetorically, the canonical Brazilian stratification between *gente de cor* (people of color) and *gente decente* (decent people).

In coming to power in 1930, the populist authoritarian Vargas regime marked critical redefinitions of Brasilidade (Brazilianness) as the ideology of racial-cultural mixture received state support as a new a priori in Brazilian political culture. By the time the Estado Novo (1937–45) was established, the federal government had established itself as the center of cultural authority, intervening in all levels of culture production and set on promoting "Brazilianness" as the primary binding value for all of Brazil's classes. During the consolidation of Vargas's dictatorial regime, the Estado Novo, the administration (specifically via the Department of Press and Propaganda and the Ministry of Health and Education) made popular culture an indispensable element in the state's production of a new model of authenticity.[105]

Viewed in its totality, the Vargas regime (1930–45) cemented a shift in the official position toward spiritism. The 1934 constitution declared all to be equal before the law, without distinctions based on birth, sex, race, profession, country, social class, wealth, religious belief, or political ideas. Soon after the inauguration of the Estado Novo, under the familiar model of the benevolent dictatorship, Vargas made a speech in July 1938 about his desire to "organize public opinion so that there is, body and soul, one Brazilian thought."[106] In this new climate, the unpredictable arrests and general harassment of spiritist mediums lessened as state officials adopted the broad national policy of accommodation and co-optation. Displacing psychiatrists as bureaucratic experts, the federal government required spiritist centers to register with municipal alongside state authorities and closed noncompliant centers. In this manner, they effectively incorporated spiritism into a bureaucratic framework to facilitate psychiatric and state regulation of the practice and its practitioners. The legal regulation of spiritism illustrates the extent to which the state made the practice, its leaders, and practitioners what political theorist and anthropologist James Scott calls "legible" or visible.[107]

The institutionalization to regulate spiritism took form when, in 1934, the Polícia de Costumes was instituted, followed in 1937 by a special section within this division—the Department of Toxins and Mystifications—under which such regulation could more efficiently be carried forward.[108]

During the same period Vargas approved the presidential Law Decree 1202, which not only recognized the legitimacy of traditional houses of candomblé and Kardecist spiritist centers but also permitted them to practice. Shortly thereafter, in the Penal Code of 1940, Article 208 further protected some terreiros, regarding as a crime the disturbance or insult of religions, including religious acts and objects.[109] The state, therefore, exhibited intolerance toward antispiritist actions and clearly frowned on divisive fulmination. Psychiatrists, in their panicked overreach, and in what may have been an inevitable result of the cultural disconnect between them and the public they hoped to serve, lost their place as creators and managers of public culture. Their time of ascendency was to be replaced in the public sphere by a muscular state that allowed nearly all forms of pluralism, demanding only loyalty and support of the nation and its keeper, the state. The heroic era of public psychiatry ended not with a bang but rather with the state moving psychiatrists to advisory roles within the institutions that they had, in many cases, created and managed. In many ways, it was fitting that their legacy includes a slate of institutions devoted to a populism that they themselves were among the last to adopt and that saw them as marginal institutional players.

Conclusion

On Saturday, August 31, 1940, President Getúlio Vargas visited the Juliano Moreira Psychiatric Colony to inaugurate two new pavilions designed with more than 840 beds for the mentally ill. During his tour of the institution, Vargas conversed with patients and listened to them attentively. The inauguration ceremony was deliberately scripted to celebrate the state, and in particular, Vargas's patronage of the institution. It formally began with a speech by Minister Gustavo Capanema exalting the social assistance program of the Vargas administration, followed by psychiatrist Adauto Junqueria Botelho's generous appraisal of the colony's various therapeutic services that would not have been possible without the Vargas administration. Botelho, a psychiatrist who was a student of Juliano Moreira's, was the newly appointed director (1941–54) of the National Service for Mental Illnesses. The third and final part of the ceremony consisted of a patient presenting the president with an ornate, hand-carved wooden box on the behalf of all the mentally ill patients. The iconic photograph, used by the major newspapers of the day, captures the passing of the present over a table filled with food and a large flower arrangement. It is arresting not only for what it reveals but also for what it renders enigmatic. Behind the mentally ill man is a woman whose identity is unknown. Behind Vargas, standing conspicuously in front of two Brazilian flags, is a cohort of state officials.[1] The colony's psychiatrists are absent. While the divide between sane-insane, citizen-state, black-white had ostensibly been breached by the mentally ill man and Vargas for a moment, the facilitators of these breakthroughs were ontologically silent. In many ways, this photograph marks the extent to which Brazil had entered a new era. Although still a productive good for the use of both nation and state, at this new juncture psychiatry was to play a supporting role rather than a lead role, giving way to the state to facilitate and manage mental health care more directly.

This book traces the emergence of psychiatry in Rio de Janeiro by focusing on the ways in which psychiatrists created initiatives and programs to address mental illness and to serve the mentally ill. The professional itineraries of doctors in and out of institutional settings, and through changing political, bureaucratic, intellectual, and cultural terrain challenge the notion of psychiatrists as experts who enjoyed broad and unquestioned authority. It chronicles the developmental arc of psychiatry in Rio de Janeiro from its first incarnation as a theory and a movement for therapeutic change, through the heroic, if aspirational, arc of psychiatry, to the profession's denouement as a formidable force in the public sphere during the 1940s. Psychiatry's work toward curing the mentally ill during the long nineteenth century was, in many ways, admirable. It was largely unsuccessful, but it did result in notable direct improvements for the institutionalized. The creation of the asylum and the promulgation of the moral treatment as a therapeutic ideal were two of psychiatry's foundational and most lasting accomplishments. Although psychiatrists' belief in the promises of the moral treatment as a cure to madness was never realized, they were able to move treatment away from the corporal punishment of the mentally ill previously prevalent in religious hospitals. The creation of a specialized asylum, albeit a hybrid religious-medical one, allowed lay people, police officers, and other state officials to construct the mentally ill as a population apart among those that frequented the city streets. By underscoring their flight from normative proscribed behaviors and practices as a direct result of illness often beyond their control, psychiatrists rendered the mentally ill as a population apart from those in need. By underscoring their flight from normative proscribed behaviors and practices as a direct result of illnesses often beyond their control, psychiatrists rendered the mentally ill as one of the premier populations deserving of social assistance. Legislative measures supported by psychiatrists during the course of the early twentieth century underscored the mentally ill's incapacity to assume full responsibility over their own civil affairs and their violations against the public and the state. In raising the profile of the mentally ill based on their inability to fully exercise their citizenship, psychiatrists made themselves temporarily indispensable to not only a system of mental health care but also to a political infrastructure of relative and partial rights and privileges that continues to inform conversations about the state, care, welfare, mental illness, dependency and culture.

The deeper significance of study of Brazilian psychiatry's development as a profession stems from the ways it provides a foil for understanding Brazilian nation-state formation. During the first half of the Old Republic (1889–1930), psychiatrists reflected the ideals of state officials. Simultaneously, they refracted what the majority of Cariocas valued. Most glaringly, psychiatrists' embrace of Freudian psychoanalysis over the course of the 1920s and Brazilians' benign neglect of Freudian-inspired clinics showcased in sharp relief the ways in which the cultural matrix that undergirded the psychiatric profession was at odds with Brazilian culture. What in Brazilian culture fostered and favored disregard for psychiatry? Psychiatry in the Americas rode the wave of professionalization, scientism, and the growth of a mass culture characteristic of the second Industrial Revolution while these developments were markedly different in Brazil. The substantive difference between the way psychiatric theories and treatment were received in Brazil compared to other parts of Latin America is how psychiatry emerged against deep cultural traditions of psychic and physical care that had dominated the country's long colonial and imperial eras. The late institutionalization of medicine in Rio led to the utility of religions and their institutions as mental health resources. An historian of religions, Charles H. Long, defines religion as "orientation in the ultimate sense, that is, how one comes to terms with the ultimate significance of one's place in the world."[2] Since religion became the means by which one could cultivate an alternative understanding of one's humanity in the face of modernization's constant affronts and denials during the tumultuous transformations of the nineteenth and early twentieth centuries, it also became the means by which mental solace could be sought.

Psychiatrists' glowing appraisals of their initiatives (e.g., Freudian psychoanalytical—inspired clinics) fell upon deaf ears as potential patients-clients migrated to competitive treatments stemming from candomblé and Kardecist spiritist practices. These religions, systems of care, and modes of subjectivity represented the individual as embedded within a context of place or time, as part of the flow of generations, conceiving each life as a step in a transpersonal, purposeful journey.[3] Psychiatry never linked itself to Brazilian popular culture and vice versa. The field never served as a social tool of the masses, which many practitioners undoubtedly understood as a legitimate badge of the field's status and significance. The extent to which psychiatry never transformed itself into a populist therapy was inextricably tied to its lack of cultural mass appeal. Psychiatrists fundamentally misunderstood their potential patient-client population due to Western cultural biases. Their irrevocable and histrionic rejection of candomblé and Kardecist spiritism was based on the deliberate conjoining and maligning of both with primitivism and Africanness. Ultimately, psychiatry would not be the only field that managed the diagnosis, treatment, and prevention of mental disorders. Nor would it be the premier practical guide in the management of everyday life.

By the late 1930s and early 1940s, psychiatrists recognized that Brazil was not an imagined community that wanted to be on the couch. Simultaneously, technocrats, serving the dictates of the muscular state headed by President Vargas, had not only taken over many psychiatrists' duties but also had diminished their roles in public institutions and the public sphere. This is not to say that psychiatrists did not serve any patients. By the early 1940s, their cultural value was consumed by a postwar middle class that had evolved and grown over the course of the late 1930s and 1940s. Psychoanalysis in particular proved alluring to this class as it ran on a parallel course with the rise of the self, the field both shaping and reflecting the ascent of individualism in society.

Thus, how much had changed at the levels of state and civil society as a result of psychiatrists' attempts to provide medical care and social assistance to the mentally ill?

For Brazilian psychiatrists, in the nineteenth and early twentieth centuries, providing humane care to the insane was a symbol of Brazil's progress which, as long as it went unfulfilled, reflected poorly on society as a whole and particularly on the medical profession and the imperial and then republican states. Yet, much of the impetus to confine the insane did not originate in the state but came from within professional liberal classes and society more broadly as people increasingly demanded from the state medical care and social assistance that once was associated with formal religious institutions.

Efforts to understand how insanity was defined and managed in the past is not only relevant to histories of medicine and society but also has an ongoing significance, since many of the questions that Brazilian psychiatrists grappled with in the late nineteenth and early twentieth centuries remain unresolved. Unlike the other diseases that preoccupied doctors and public health officials throughout the nineteenth century—malaria and yellow fever, for example—whose causes had been clearly identified by the early twentieth century, the causes of mental illnesses remain significantly mysterious. Despite advances in neuroscience, brain imaging technologies, and targeted therapeutic regimes, scientists (far more than laypeople) continue to acknowledge how little they understand about the complexities of the brain and its connection with the sociocultural background of patients and clients. This book acknowledges the importance of the real advances in care, and in some cases therapy, for the mentally ill—both in the time period covered in this book, and today. It also recognizes the complicated motives of all parties involved, certainly including psychiatrists, politicians, and caregivers. Still, this book joins others that explore the ways in which attempts to solve largely insoluble social ills, especially the significantly intractable such as mental illness and the provision of care to those in need can and does change human culture in unpredictable and sometimes serendipitous ways.

Notes

Introduction

1. *Marmota Fluminense*, December 10, 1852, 1.

2. Peter Conrad provides a detailed discussion of "medicalization" as it moved outward from being a process associated with the professionalization of medicine and the application of more stringent standards in teaching and practice to its penetration of society as a whole as medical ideas reshaped consciousness and transformed ordinary emotions into disorders. See Peter Conrad, *The Medicalization of Society: On the Transformation of Human Conditions into Treatable Disorders* (Baltimore: Johns Hopkins University Press, 2007).

3. First recognized in archival texts in the late eighteenth and early nineteenth centuries, candomblé is an amalgamation of the religious ideas and beliefs of the various West and Central African ethnic groups that arrived as slaves in Brazil. Similar to Haitian vodou, Cuban santeria, and other African diasporic theologies and religions in the Americas, candomblé was (and remains) a complex Afro-Brazilian religious tradition whose fabric and multiple layers can be understood as a response to slavery, cultural dislocation, colonialism, and the subaltern position of blacks in Brazilian society and culture. Drawing from scholar Rachel E. Harding's *A Refuge in Thunder: Candomblé and Alternative Spaces of Blackness* (Bloomington: Indiana University Press, 2000), candomblé can be understood "as [a] means to healing; the cultivation of axé (life force) and the creation of alternative orientations in the context of slave-based societies" (79).

4. French mathematician and scientist Allan Kardec (the pseudonym of Hippolyte-Léon Denizard Rivail), the founder of Kardecist spiritism, defined it as a "science, which deals with the nature, origin, and destiny of Spirits, as well as their relationship with the corporeal world." See Allan Kardec, *Introduction to the Spiritist Philosophy* (1859; repr., Philadelphia: Allan Kardec Educational Society, 1999), 6. As a belief system, spiritism seeks a deeper relationship between the material and spirit worlds. Kardec stressed that spirits (like matter) were components of the natural world, thus regulated by laws and suitable for scientific investigation. Brazil currently has the largest number of Kardecist spiritists of any nation in the world.

5. Michel Foucault, "Questions of Method," in *The Foucault Effect: Studies in Governmentality*, ed. Graham Burchell, Colin Gordon, and Peter Miller (Chicago: University of Chicago Press, 1991), 86.

6. Representative works on this social dimension of the reforms include Teresa A. Meade, *"Civilizing" Rio: Reform and Resistance in a Brazilian City, 1889–1930* (University

Park: Pennylvania State University Press, 1997), and Jeffrey D. Needell, "The *Revolta Contra Vacina* of 1904: The Revolt Against 'Modernization' in *Belle-Époque* Rio de Janeiro," *Hispanic American Historical Review* 67, no. 2 (May 1987): 233–69.

7. This concept and the processes associated with it have been less thoroughly developed in the Brazilian historiography than elsewhere. For its elaboration in other national contexts, see Nikolas Rose and Peter Miller, "Political Power Beyond the State: Problematics of Government," *British Journal of Sociology* 43, no. 2 (1992): 173–205; David Garland, "The Limits of the Sovereign State: Strategies of Crime Control in Contemporary Society," *British Journal of Criminology* 36, no. 4 (1996): 452–55; Nikolas Rose, "Governing 'Advanced' Liberal Democracies," in *Foucault and Political Reason: Liberalism, Neo-liberalism and Rationalities of Government*, ed. Andrew Barry, Thomas Osborne and Nikolas Rose (Chicago: University of Chicago Press, 1996), 50–62; and Barbara Cruikshank, *The Will to Empower: Democratic Citizens and Other Subjects* (Ithaca, NY: Cornell University Press, 1999). These scholars are chiefly interested in how Foucault's concept of governmentality can be used to understand the specific ways neoliberalism has transformed politics.

8. Jeremy D. Popkin, *Press, Revolution, and Social Identities in France, 1830–1835* (University Park: Pennsylvania State University Press, 2002), 9.

9. See Teresa A. Meade's "*Civilizing*" *Rio*; Dain Borges, *The Family in Bahia, Brazil, 1870–1945* (Stanford, CA: Stanford University Press, 1994); Jeffrey D. Needell, *A Tropical Belle Epoque: Elite Culture and Society in Turn-of-the-Twentieth-Century Rio de Janeiro* (Cambridge: Cambridge University Press, 1987).

10. Erwin Ackerknecht, *A Short History of Psychiatry* (New York: Hafner, 1968); Gregory Zilboorg, *A History of Medical Psychology* (New York: W. W. Norton, 1967); Roy Porter, *A Social History of Madness: Stories of the Insane* (London: Phoenix Giants, 1996). A full list of canonical texts in the history of psychiatry is too long to mention here.

11. Andrew Scull, *Museums of Madness: The Social Organization of Insanity in Nineteenth-Century England* (New York: St. Martin's Press, 1979); David J. Rothman, *The Discovery of the Asylum: Social Order and Disorder in a New Republic* (Boston: Little, Brown, 1971).

12. Nancy Tomes, *A Generous Confidence: Thomas Story Kirkbride and the Art of Asylum-Keeping, 1840–1883* (Cambridge: Cambridge University Press, 1984); Gerald Grob, *The Mad Among Us: A History of the Care of America's Mentally Ill* (New York: Free Press, 1994); Anne Digby, *Madness, Morality and Medicine: A Study of the York Retreat, 1796–1914* (Cambridge: Cambridge University Press, 1985).

13. See Jonathan Sadowsky, *Imperial Bedlam: Institutions of Madness and Colonialism in Southwest Nigeria* (Berkeley: University of California Press, 1999); Richard Keller, *Colonial Madness: Psychiatry in French North Africa* (Chicago: University of Chicago Press, 2007); and Sloan Mahone and Megan Vaughan, *Psychiatry and Empire* (Basingstoke, UK: Palgrave Macmillan 2008) are insightful studies in this body of work.

14. Jonathan Sadowsky, "The Reality of Mental Illness and the Social World: Lessons from Colonial Psychiatry," *Harvard Review of Psychiatry* 11, no. 4 (July 2003): 91–112.

15. Marcos Cueto, *Missionaries of Science: The Rockefeller Foundation in Latin America* (Bloomington: Indiana University Press, 1994); Marcos Cueto, *Saberes andinos: Ciencia*

y tecnología en Bolivia, Ecuador, y Perú (Lima: Instituto de Estudios Peruanos, 1995); Marcos Cueto, *Salud, Cultura y Sociedad en América Latina* (Lima, Peru: Instituto de Estudios Peruanos, 1996); and Marcos Cueto, *El Regreso de las Epidemias: Salud y Sociedad en el Perú del siglo XX* (Lima: Instituto de Estudios Peruanos, 1997).

16. Christopher Abel, *Hygiene and Sanitation in Latin America c. 1870–1950* (London: Institute of Latin American Studies, University of London, 1996).

17. Ann Zulawski, *Unequal Cures: Public Health and Political Change in Bolivia, 1900–1950* (Durham, NC: Duke University Press, 2007).

18. Uday Singh Mehta, *Liberalism and Empire: A Study in Nineteenth-Century British Liberal Thought* (Chicago: University of Chicago Press, 1999).

19. Uday Singh Mehta, "Liberal Strategies of Exclusion," *Politics and Society* 18, no. 4 (December 1990): 427–54.

20. On the intersection of medical discourses and exclusionary policies in other contexts, see Ann Laura Stoler, *Carnal Knowledge: Race and the Intimate in Colonial Rule* (Berkeley: University of California Press, 2002), and Aihwa Ong, "Making the Biopolitical Subject: Cambodian Immigrants, Refugee Medicine, and Cultural Citizenship in California," *Social Science and Medicine* 40, no. 9 (1995): 1243–57.

21. The historian, fiction writer, and poet Cristina Rivera-Garza has also problematized the categories of the "normal" and the "abnormal" through the lens of modernization in early twentieth-century Mexico, revealing the "march of progress" that began in earnest during the reign of Mexico's Porfirio Díaz (1876–1911) as largely consistent of subtler and more insidious strategies of social regulation. See the following articles (among others) by Cristina Rivera-Garza: "'She Neither Respected nor Obeyed Anyone': Inmates and Psychiatrists Debate Gender and Class at the General Insane Asylum La Castañeda, Mexico, 1910–1930," *Hispanic American Historical Review* 81, no. 3 (2001): 653–88, and "Dangerous Minds: Changing Psychiatric Views of the Mentally Ill in Porfirian Mexico, 1876–1911," *Journal of the History of Medicine and Allied Sciences* 56, no. 1 (2001): 36–67. Also see her novella *Nadie Me Verá Llorar* (Mexico City: Tusquets Editores, 2003) and her book *La Castañeda: Narrativas dolientes desde el Manicomio General, México 1910–1930* (Mexico City: Tusquests, 2010).

22. Mariano Ben Plotkin, *Freud in the Pampas: The Emergence and Development of a Psychoanalytic Culture in Argentina* (Stanford, CA: Stanford University Press, 2002).

23. See Julia Rodriguez, *Civilizing Argentina: Science, Medicine and the Modern State* (Chapel Hill: University of North Carolina Press, 2006), and Jonathan Ablard, *Madness in Buenos Aires: Patients, Psychiatrists, and the Argentine State, 1880–1983* (Calgary, Canada: Calgary University Press, 2009).

24. See Michel Foucault, *Madness and Civilization: A History of Insanity in the Age of Reason* (New York: Pantheon Books, 1965). The realignment of madness is central to Foucault's explanation of confinement. In the classical period, madness became part of a wider class of social deviancy, which was defined by its relationship to work. Foucault argues that the mad did not really exist as a separate group but only as part of a wider deviancy. Criminals and the idle were inseparable from madmen. In the context of Brazilian historiography, see, for example, the classic works by Jurandir Freire Costa, *História da Psiquiatria no Brasil: Um Corte Ideológico* (Rio de Janeiro: Venou, 1974), and Roberto Machado, Ángela Loureiro, Rogério Luz, and Kátia Muricy, *Danação da Norma: A Medicina Social e Constituição da Psiquiatria no Brasil* (Rio de Janeiro: Edições Graal, 1978). Also see Maria Clementina Pereira Cunha, *O*

Espelho do Mundo Juquery a Historia de um Asilo (São Paulo: Paz e Terra, 1986), and Magali Gouveia Engel, *Os Delírios da Razão: Médicos, Loucos e Hospício, Rio de Janeiro 1830–1930* (Rio de Janeiro: Ed. Fiocruz, 2001).

25. Michel Foucault's "great confinement" refers to a sweeping internment that occurred in mid-seventeenth-century absolutist Europe. While it assumed different forms in diverse monarchies, individuals who offended bourgeois rationality (e.g., prostitutes, beggars, criminals, paupers, etc.) became confined with the insane. Within the asylum, this varied population was rendered epistemologically similar due to their idleness, the exemplar of unreason. See Foucault, *Madness and Civilization*, 43, 49.

26. Silvia Marina Arrom, *Containing the Poor: The Mexico City Poor House, 1774–1871* (Durham, NC: Duke University Press, 2000).

27. This book is part of the post-Foucauldian Brazilian historiographical turn as evidenced by upcoming books, articles and contemporaneous works that are currently in dissertation form in Brazil. See for example, Richard Negreiros de Paula's "Um Doutor contra Doutos Leigos: Teixeira Brandão e suas Opiniões quanto ao Poder de Decisão sobre a Custódia Médica," *Revista de História (USP)* 1 (2009): 169–94; Ana Teresa Venancio, "Da Colônia Agrícola ao Hospital-Côlonia: Configurações para a Assistência Psiquiátrica no Brasil na Primeira Metade do Século XX," *História, Ciências, Saúde-Manguinhos* 18, suppl. 1 (2011): 35–52; Cristina Facchinetti edited a special issue of *História, Ciências, Saúde-Manguinhos* 17, no. 2 (2012), with novel studies on psychiatry in Brazil during the early twentieth century. She also wrote, with Pedro Felipe Neves de Muñoz, "Emil Kraepelin na Ciência Psiquiátrica do Rio de Janeiro, 1903–1933," *História, Ciências, Saúde-Manguinhos* 20, no. 1 (2013): 239–62. Also, see William Vaz de Oliveira's published dissertation, *A Assistência a Alienados na Capital Federal da Primeira República: Discursos e Práticas entre Rupturas e Continuidades* (Rio de Janeiro: Universidade Federal Fluminense [Niterói], 2012).

28. I refer to the doctors who organized the asylum-construction campaign as proto-psychiatrists because they were not formally trained in psychiatry. While a formal chair in psychiatry would not be established at the Medical College of Rio until the late nineteenth century, these doctors, and the ones that followed in their footsteps, were well read on matters related to psychiatry. Apart from avidly reading psychiatric medical texts in Brazil, many traveled to France, where they engaged in transnational conversations about mental illness and its treatments.

29. Emilia Viotti da Costa, *The Brazilian Empire: Myths and Histories* (Wadsworth, CA: Wadsworth Publishing, 1985), 77.

30. For a rich description of various political, economic, and social aspects of the nation's capital, see Adolfo de Morales de los Rios Filho, *O Rio de Janeiro Imperial* (1946; repr., Rio de Janeiro: Topbooks Editora, 2000).

31. The gradual nature of the abolition process in Brazil was a calculated attempt on the part of Brazilian ruling elites to control the conditions of full freedom for slaves. In this manner, gradual abolition included a range of strategies designed to guard the emerging social order and protect the planters' interests in a postslavery society. These measures included a series of strategies to slow and then to stop a thriving internal slave trade, a series of abolition laws that slowly released selected groups of slaves over time, heightened restrictions on the freed slave population, and the construction of a sophisticated array of punitive social institutions. At the

heart of these policies was the construction of programs and instruments that served the dual purpose of mollifying abolitionists while simultaneously creating social conditions that assured not only labor's subservience to capitalists' interests but white supremacy. See Thomas Skidmore, *Brazil: Five Centuries of Change*, 2nd ed. (New York: Oxford University Press, 2009), 67–72.

32. The population grew from 274,972 in 1872 to 522,651 in 1890 and finally reached 811,443 in 1906. Eulalia Maria Lahmeyer Lobo, *História do Rio de Janeiro: Do Capital Federal ao Capital Industrial Financeiro*, vol. 2. (Rio de Janeiro: IBMEC, 1978), 470–71.

33. The positivistic logo "Order and Progress" was emblazoned on the 1890 Brazilian republican flag. See Thomas Skidmore, *Black into White: Race and Nationality in Brazilian Thought* (Durham, NC: Duke University Press, 1993), 11–14.

34. See Directoria Geral de Estatística, *Républica do Estados Unidos dos Brasil, Recenseamento do Rio de Janeiro (Distrito Federal)* (Rio de Janeiro: Officina da Estatística, 1930).

35. See Jeffrey D. Needell, *Tropical Belle Époque: Elite Culture and Society in Turn-of-the-Century Rio de Janeiro* (New York: Cambridge University Press, 1987).

36. See Marcos Luiz Bretas, *Ordem na Cidade: O Exercício Cotidiano da Autoridade Policial no Rio de Janeiro: 1907–1930* (São Paulo: Rocco, 1997).

37. Christine Ritui, "João do Rio: Ombre et Lumière du Rio de Janeiro de la Belle Époque." *Littérature et Modernisation au Brésil*, ed. Jacqueline Penon and José Antonio Pasta Jr. (Paris: Sorbonne Nouvelle, 2004), 32.

38. Although vague, the first attempt to define the term was the criminologist Alexandre Lacassage who, in 1876, saw it as an "art of knowing" the influences that come from the milieu. Then, in 1902 the Pasteurian Emile Duclaux stressed the broader theoretical dimension of the term in which illnesses were seen not as themselves but in relation to their repercussions on society, and later the natalist Just Sicard de Plauzoles saw it as a "science" concerned with the fruits of human capital: production and reproduction. Nevertheless, at the core of every definition was the notion that social hygiene governs the collective body rather than the individual body, in which hygiene was seen as an individual moral attribute. Thus, as part of a late nineteenth-century redrawing of boundaries between the public and private spheres, social hygiene became an important component of the lives of every member of society. Alexandre Lacassagne defined *hygiène social* in his 1876 text *Précis d'hygiène privée et sociale* as "the art of knowing the various influences that come from the milieu in which human beings develop themselves and modify themselves in the way most favorable for their physical, intellectual and moral development" (*L' hygiene est L'art de Connaître les Influences Diverses qui Proviennent des Milieux dans lesquels L'homme Evolue et de les Modifier dans le sens le plus favorable à son Developpement Physique, Intellectual, et Moral*). See Lacassagne, quoted in Alain Drouard, *L'Eugénisme en Questions: L'Exemple de l'Eugénisme Français* (Paris: Ellipses, 1999), 81. For Ducleaux's definition, see Emile Duclaux, *Hygiène Sociale* (Paris: Félix Alcan, 1902), 5; and for Sicard de Plauzoles's definition, see Just Sicard de Plauzoles, *Principes d'hygiène sociale* (Paris: Editions Médicales, 1927), 44.

39. Nancy Leys Stepan, "*The Hour of Eugenics*": *Race, Gender and Nation in Latin America* (Ithaca, NY: Cornell University Press, 1991), 1–20.

40. Contrary to the dominant historiography, not all psychiatrists and social reformers subscribed to this understanding of degeneracy. Most notably, psychiatrist Renato Kehl understood racial and cultural degeneracy as fixed and argued for negative eugenics. See, for example, Robert Wegner and Vanderlei Sebastião de Souza, "Eugenia 'Negativa,' Psiquiatria e Catolicismo: Embates em torno da Esterilização Eugênica no Brasil," *História, Ciências, Saúde-Manguinhos* 20, no. 1 (January–March 2013): 263–88.

Chapter One

1. See Roy Porter, *Madness: A Brief History* (Oxford: Oxford University Press, 2002), and Edward Shorter, *A History of Psychiatry: From the Era of the Asylum to the Age of Prozac* (New York: John Wiley, 1997), for discussions about the preoccupation with the rise of madness during the nineteenth century.

2. Théophile Roussel, *Notes et documents concernant la legislations étrangères sur les aliénénes: Annexe au process-verbal de la séances du 20 mai 1884.* Commission relative à la revision de la loi du 30 juin 1838 sur les aliénés, 2 vols. (Paris: P. Mouillot, 1884), 1:298.

3. Studies that have concisely investigated asylum life include Monique de Siqueira Gonçalves and Flávio Coelho Edler, "Os caminhos da loucura na Corte Imperial: Um embate historiográfico acerca do funcionamento do Hospício Pedro II de 1850 a 1889," *Revista Latinoamericana de Psicopatologia Fundamental* 12, no. 2 (June 2009): 393–410; Marco Antonio Arantes, "Hospício de doutores," *História, Ciências, Saúde-Manguinhos* 15, no. 1 (March 2008): 49–63; Cristiana Facchinetti, Andréa Ribeiro, and Pedro F. de Muñoz, "As insanas do Hospício Nacional de Alienados 1900–1939," *História, Ciências, Saúde-Manguinhos* 15, suppl. (2008): 231–42; and Ana Maria Galdini Raimundo Oda and Paulo Dalgalarrondo, "História das primeiras instituições para alienados no Brasil," *História, Ciências, Saúde-Manguinhos* 12, no. 3 (December 2005): 983–1010.

4. See the introduction of Roberto DaMatta and David J. Hess, eds., *The Brazilian Puzzle* (New York: Columbia University Press 1995), for a discussion of mimicry and cultural imitation.

5. This stems from the title of David J. Rothman's foundational work *The Discovery of the Asylum: Social Order and Disorder in the New Republic* (Boston: Little, Brown and Company, 1971).

6. Eduardo Hoornaert, "The Church in Brazil," in *The Church in Latin America, 1492–1992,* ed. Enrique Dussel (Maryknoll, NY: Orbis, 1992), 191.

7. Philip Curtin, *The Atlantic Slave Trade* (Madison: University of Wisconsin Press, 1969), and Herbert S. Klein, *The Atlantic Slave Trade* (Cambridge: Cambridge University Press, 1999).

8. Klein, *Atlantic Slave Trade,* 198.

9. Robert Edgar Conrad, *The Destruction of Brazilian Slavery, 1850–1888* (Berkeley: University of California Press, 1972), 4.

10. Some reports suggest that the British never stopped much more than 20 percent of slave shipping, the abolition effort's efficacy lying not in directly stemming

the flow but rather in driving the prices high enough for the profitability of the slave trade to suffer. Klein, *Atlantic Slave Trade*, 199–201.

11. Sidney Chalhoub, *Cidade Febril: Cortiços e Epidemias na Corte Imperial* (São Paulo: Companhia das Letras, 1996); Sidney Chalhoub, *Visões da liberdade: Uma História das Última Décadas da Escravidão na Corte* (São Paulo: Companhia das Letras, 1990); Sidney Chalhoub, *Trabalho, Lar e Botequim: O Cotidiano dos Trabalhadores no Rio de Janeiro da Belle Époque* (São Paulo: Brasiliense, 1986). It is important to note that during this period, most free Brazilians in Rio, who were people of color, most likely did not think of themselves or self-identify as "black."

12. Manoel Florentino, "Slave Trading and Slave Traders in Rio de Janeiro, 1790–1830" in *Enslaving Connections: Changing Cultures of Africa and Brazil During the Era of Slavery*, ed. José C. Curto and Paul E. Lovejoy (Amherst, NY: Humanity Books, 2004), 57.

13. Mary Karasch, *Slave Life in Rio de Janeiro, 1808–1850* (Princeton, NJ: Princeton University Press, 1987), 62. In 1834, 97,599; in 1838, 97,162; in 1849, 205,906.

14. See A. J. R. Russell-Wood, *Fidalgos and Philanthropists: The Santa Casa da Misericórdia of Bahia, 1550–1755* (Berkeley: University of California Press, 1968), 1–23.

15. Russell-Wood notes that the captaincies of *São* Vicente, Pernambuco, Espírito Santo, Rio de Janeiro, *São* Paulo, and Porto Seguro all had Misericórdias established nearly contemporaneous with town establishment during the sixteenth century. Ibid., 39–40. A number of issues proved contentious between the Santa Casa and city councils throughout Brazil. Russell-Wood notes, for example, that the Bahian city council impeded the Misericórdia at every opportunity unless it was to its own advantage. See ibid., 101.

16. Luís Vicente de Simoni, "Importância e Necessidade da Criação e um Manicômio ou Estabelecimento Especial para o Tratamento de Alienados," *Revista Médica Fluminense* 5, no. 6 (September 1839): 151.

17. Reginaldo Fernandes, "José Martins da Cruz Jobim: Um Fundador da Academia Nacional de Medicina," in *Revista do Instituto Histórico e Geográfico Brasileiro* 327 (Rio de Janeiro: Instituto Histórico e Geográfico Brasileiro, 1980), 251–53.

18. "Boletim da Sociedade, Sessões da Reunião Preparatória: Sessão de 28 de maio de 1829," in *Semanário da Saúde Publica* (Rio de Janeiro: Sociedade de Medicina do Rio de Janeiro, 1831), vol. 1, p. 4.

19. Boletim da Sociedade, "Sessões da Reunião Preparatória; Sessão de 28 de Maio de 1829," in *Semanário de Saúde Pública*, vol. 1 (Rio de Janeiro: Sociedade de Medicina do Rio de Janeiro, 1831), 5; Reginaldo Fernandes, "José Martins da Cruz Jobim: Um Fundador da Academia Nacional de Medicina," *Revista do Instituto Histórico e Geográfico Brasileiro* 327 (1980): 251–53.

20. Robert Walsh, *Notices of Brazil in 1828 and 1829*, 2 vols. (London: Frederick Westley and A. H. Davis, 1830), 1:401–2.

21. Ibid.

22. See "Do Cholera Morbus," *Semanário de Saúde Pública* 6 (February 5, 1831), 36; "Informações sobre a Cholera Morbus," *Semanário de Saúde Pública* (August 20, 1831): 172–73; "Medidas Sanitariás contra o Cholera Morbus," *Semanário de Saúde Pública*, September 17, 1831, 38, 192–93.

23. "Boletim Universal (Ciências Médicas)," *Semanário de Saúde Pública* 10 (March 5, 1831): 52–53; Claudio Luís da Costa, Antônio Martins Pinheiro, José Martins da Cruz Jobim, Agostinho Tomas de Aquino et al., "Parecer da Commisão da Salubridade Geral, sobre a carta do Sr. Manoel de Valadão Pimentel, relativa as febres da Macacú, remetido ao Governo em 13 do corrente," *Semanário de Saúde Pública* 29 (July 16, 1831): 152–54.

24. David Hothersall, *History of Psychology*, 3rd ed. (New York: McGraw-Hill, 1995), 266. "Moral" treatment refers to the psychological aspects of mental illness and is void of any ethical connotation. In other words, it referred to therapies applied to the mind, and not the body, of the patient.

25. Ann Goldberg, *Sex, Religion, and the Making of Modem Madness: The Eberbach Asylum and German Society, 1815–1849* (New York: Oxford University Press, 1999), 47–48.

26. Doris Sommers, *Foundational Fictions: The National Romances of Latin America.* (Berkeley: University of California Press, 1991), looks at the ways in which politics are inextricable from fiction in the history of nation building in Latin America by locating an erotics of politics in literature during the "Boom" period (the 1960s and 1970s literary period where novelists such as Carlos Fuentes of Mexico, Mario Vargas Llosa of Peru, and Gabriel García Marquez articulated a modernist aesthetics). Sommers's study illustrates how a variety of novel national ideals are all ostensibly grounded in "natural" heterosexual love and in the marriages that provided a figure for apparently nonviolent consolidation. Drawing upon Sommers's use of the term, "foundational fiction" for the purposes of this article can be read as the ways in which Pinel's gesture serves as a genesis narrative for psychiatry. As a fictional text, it formed a common foundation for a professional discipline and its followers.

27. See Dora B. Weiner, *Comprendre et Soigner: Philippe Pinel 1745–1826, La médecine de l'esprit* (Paris: Fayard, 1999).

28. Pinel was greatly influenced by William Cullen's *First Lines of the Practice of Physic* (1777). The first to coin the term *neurosis*, Cullen advocated a more humane attitude toward the mentally ill. Among William Cullen, other physicians who advocated for a moral treatment included Vincenzo Chiarugi in Florence, Italy, and Joseph Daquin, who worked in the French Alps. Also, influenced by Cullen's classification system, Pinel divided mental diseases into five categories: melancholia, nondelirious furor, delirium, dementia, and idiocy. See Mário Eduardo Costa Pereira, "Cullen e a introdução do termo 'neurose' na medicina," *Revista Latinoamericana de Psicopatologia Fundamental* 13, no. 1 (2010): 128–34.

29. Philippe Pinel, "Observations sur le regime moral," 13; "Recherches et Observations sur le Traitement Moral," Memoires de la Société Médicale d'Émulation Pour l'an VI an VII (Year VII): 215–55.

30. Jan Goldstein, *Console and Classify: The French Psychiatric Profession in the Nineteenth Century* (Cambridge: Cambridge University Press, 1987), 64–119.

31. For general historical background information on the Santa Casa de Misericórdias, see Russell-Wood, *Fidalgos and Philanthropists.*

32. José Martins da Cruz Jobim et al., *Relatório da Commissão de Visita das Prisões, Cárceres de Conventos, e Estabelecimentos de Caridade, Nomeada pela Câmara Municipal do Rio de Janeiro* (Rio de Janeiro: Tip. do Diário, 1830), 2.

33. Ibid.

34. Ibid., 3.

35. The young emperor would actually assume the throne at the age of fourteen. See E. Bradford Burns, *A History of Brazil*, 2nd ed. (New York: Columbia University Press, 1980), 169–70.

36. Luís Vicente De-Simoni. "Importância e necessidade da criação de um manicômioo ou estabelecimento especial para o tratamento de alienados," *Revista Médica Fluminense* 5, no. 6 (September 1839).

37. J. F. X. Sigaud, "Reflexões acerca do trânsito livre dos doidos pelas ruas da cidade do Rio de Janeiro," *Diário de Saúde*, vol. 1, 1, April 18, 1835.

38. De-Simoni, "Importância e necessidade."

39. Manuel Duarte Moreira de Azevedo, "A Faculdade de Medicina do Rio de Janeiro: Notícia Histórica," *Revista do Instituto Histórico e Geográfico Brasileiro* 30, no. 4 (1867): 409.

40. Ibid., 206–7.

41. Ibid., 99–101, 189.

42. Roberto Machado, Angela Loureiro, Rogerio Luz, and Katia Muricy, *Danaçao da Norma: Medicina Social e Constituiçao da Psiquiatria no Brasil* (Rio de Janeiro: Graal, 1978), 379.

43. M. J. Barbosa, *Relatorio e Estatística do Hospício de Pedro II de 09/12/1852 até 30/07/1853* (Rio de Janeiro: Tip. Dois de Dezembro, 1853), 14–15; *Relatorio e Estatistica do Hospício de Pedro II desde 1/07/1854 até 30/06/1855*, in *Anais Brasilienses de Medicina*. Rio de Janeiro 10, no. 4 (1856): 118–19.

44. De-Simoni, "Importância e necessidade," 151.

45. To facilitate the development of such a program, Pereira dispatched in 1845 physician Antonio José Pereira das Neves to Europe to study the treatment of the insane by the French, Belgians, Germans, English, and Italians. See Araújo, *A Assistênca Médica Hospitalar Século XIX*, 68.

46. De-Simoni, "Importância e necessidade," 260.

47. Ibid.

48. Ibid.

49. Pedro Calmon, *O Palácio da Praia Vermelha* (Rio de Janeiro: Universidade do Brasil, 1952), 41.

50. Ibid.

51. *Jornal do Comércio*, December 1, 1852, 1, December 6, 1852, 1.

52. José Leme Lopes, "A Psiquiatria e o Velho Hospício" in *Quatro Século de Cultura: Ciclo de Conferências Comemorativas do IV Centenário da Cidade do Rio de Janeiro, aprovado pelo Conselho Universitário em 28 de novembro de 1964* (Rio de Janeiro: Publicação da Universidade do Brasil, 1966), 341.

53. Christine Stevenson, *Medicine and Magnificence: British Hospital and Asylum Architecture, 1660–1815* (New Haven, CT: Yale University Press, 2000), 210.

54. Achilles Ribeiro de Araújo, *A Assistênca Médica Hospitalar no Rio de Janeiro no Século XIX* (Rio de Janeiro: Conselho Federal de Cultura, 1982), 66.

55. Carrara marble is an expensive building material. It gets its name from Carrara, Italy, the city in which this marble is most commonly quarried.

56. Ferreira da Rosa, *Rio de Janeiro* (Rio de Janeiro: Edição Oficial da Prefeitura, 1905), 135.

57. Daniel P. Kidder and Daniel Cooley Fletcher, *Brazil and the Brazilians, Portrayed in Historical and Descriptive Sketches* (Philadelphia: Childs and Peterson, 1857), 114.

58. Louis Agassiz and Elizabeth C. Agassiz, *A Journey in Brazil* (Boston: Ticknor and Fields, 1868), 81–82.

59. Subsequent asylums were created all throughout Brazil: São Paulo (1852), Pernambuco (1864), Pará (1873), Bahia (1874), Rio Grande do Sul (1884), Ceará (1886), and Alagoas (1888). See José Clemente Pereira. Alienados que passaram do antigo hospital e das enfermarias provisórias para o Hospício de Pedro Segundo nos dias 8 e 9 de dezembro de 1852, in Arquivo Nacional, Série Saúde / Ministério do Império, Maço IS 3, 4, 1850–53.

60. J. J. L. da Silva, "Relatório apresentado ao Provedor da Santa Casa da Misericórdia do Rio de Janeiro, de julho de 1866 a junho de 1867," *Gazeta Médica da Bahia* 40, nos. 42–43 (1868): 187.

61. Isabel dos Guimarães Sá, "Catholic Charity in Perspective: The Social Life of Devotion in Portugal and its Empire 1450–1700," *E-Journal of Portuguese History* 2, no. 1 (Summer 2004): 1–19.

Chapter Two

1. Due to Emperor Dom Pedro I's abdication in 1831, and his heir's young age, a Regency ruled Brazil from 1831 to 1840. States pressed for greater socioeconomic and political autonomy in the period, and the regents responded by giving provinces more of that autonomy. Greater freedoms in addition to apocalyptic fears of economic downturns and loss of life from unruly masses led to elite support of the boy emperor, Dom Pedro II, who ascended the throne on July 18, 1841, at age fifteen instead of the constitutionally specified age of eighteen. The second empire was created with expectations that it would serve as a tool of national unity, stability, and prosperity. See Roderick J. Barman's classic text *Citizen Emperor, Pedro II and the Making of Brazil, 1825–91* (Stanford, CA: Stanford University Press, 1999), for an examination of the Regency period and Dom Pedro II's rise to power.

2. In place of "alienists," the nineteenth-century term commonly used to refer to doctors of mental illness, the terms "asylum doctors," "doctors," "proto-psychiatrists," and "psychiatrists" are used throughout this chapter.

3. I frame the state as a space, and not as a subject, in which different social actors converge or as a *field*, in which power relations among other social *fields* are articulated, to use Bourdieu's terminology. See Pierre Bourdieu, *The Field of Cultural Production* (Cambridge, UK: Polity Press, 1993), 34. Employing this definition of the state allows me to render bureaucracy as a material support of the state, and consequently, as a reflection of its processes of expansion, consolidation, or crisis.

4. See Russell-Wood, *Fidalgos and Philanthropists*, 14–16, for an examination of the charity organization's origins. The initiative for the Santa Casa has been variously attributed to Dona Leonor, the widow of Dom João II, the Trinitarian friar Miguel Contreiras, and a group of six laymen.

5. Ibid., 28–29. Except for stewards, who were elected monthly due to their labor intensive obligations. For a detailed examination of the Catholic lay brotherhood's operations in Rio de Janeiro, see Luciana Mendes Gandelman, "A Santa Casa da

Misericórdia do Rio de Janeiro nos séculos XVI a XIX," *História, Ciências, Saúde-Manguinhos* 18, no. 3 (2001): 613–30.

6. Russell-Wood, *Fidalgos and Philanthropists*, 28–29.

7. Miri Rubin, *Charity and Community in Medieval Cambridge* (Cambridge: Cambridge University Press, 1987), 146–47.

8. See Isabel dos Guimarães Sá, *Quando O Rico Se Faz Pobre: Misericórdias, Caridade e Poder no Império Português, 1500–1800* (Lisbon: Comissão Nacional para as Comemorações dos Descobrimentos Portugueses, 1997).

9. The Santa Casa administration sent Neves to Europe from 1845 to 1847 to familiarize himself with and to study the "model psychiatric establishments" in order to learn the best way to care for the insane. As a result of this commission, he published "Relatório acerca do tratamento dos alienados e seus principais hospitais em França, Inglaterra, Itália, Alemanha, Bélgica e Portugal," in *Anais de Medicina Brasiliense*, July 1847–July 1848, nos. 7, 11, and 12, pp. 161–66, 271–74, and 292–95; July 1848–July 1849, no. 1, 12–16, pp. 42–47. Even though the title of the report cites various countries visited, Neves only stayed in France.

10. Saint Vincent de Paul and Louise de Marillac founded the Daughters of Charity in 1633. By the turn of the seventeenth century, they had been established and were managing more than two hundred charitable institutions throughout France (especially hospitals and home relief agencies), as well as outposts in the Polish kingdom. By then, they were probably the most significant nursing order to emerge from the Counter-Reformation. See Sioban Nelson, *Say Little, Do Much: Nurses, Nuns, and Hospitals in the Nineteenth Century* (Philadelphia: University of Pennsylvania Press, 2003).

11. Colin Jones, *The Charitable Imperative: Hospitals and Nursing in Ancien Régime and Revolutionary France* (London: Routledge Press, 1989), 137. By the early eighteenth century, doctors and hospital administrators in Europe seemed to accept the important medical role the sisters had assumed as apothecaries who grew their own medicinal herbs and novice surgeons who performed minor operations. See Jones *Charitable Imperative*, 113, 192–97. War correspondent William Howard Russell complimented the experience and skill of the Sisters of Charity as military nurses in an article that highlighted the disgraceful conditions in British military hospitals. See: A SUFFERER BY THE PRESENT WAR, "Why have we no Sisters of Charity?" *The London Times*, October 14, 1854, 7.

12. John P. Beal, James A. Coriden, and Thomas J. Green, eds., *New Commentary on the Code of Canon Law* (Mahwah, NJ: Paulist Press, 2000), 837–38.

13. Some suggest that the rights of patronage of Portugal during the early colonial era engendered a regalist nationalist ideology which made ultramontanism particularly strong in Brazil in comparison to the Catholic countries of Europe. See C. F. G. de Groot, *Brazilian Catholicism and Ultramontane Reform, 1850–1930* (Amsterdam: CEDLA, 1996). This French missionary phenomenon also appeared in other parts of Latin America. See Claude Pomerleau, "French Missionaries and Latin American Catholicism in the Nineteenth Century, *The Americas* 37, no. 3 (1981): 351–67.

14. The earliest recorded presence of French ultramontane activity in Brazil stems from 1848, when Brazilian bishop Antonio Ferreira Viçoso, and French priest Jean-Baptiste Etienne, superior general of the Daughters of Charity, organized for the recruitment of nuns to help the poor and the sick in Mariana, Minas Gerais. See Ana

Maria Ribeiro dos Santos et al., "A Atuação da Irmã de Caridade Abrahíde Alvarenga no Piauí: Uma História a Ser Contada," *Texto & Contexto Enfermagem* 14, no. 4 (2005): 551–56.

15. Jeffrey D. Needell's *Tropical Belle Epoque: Elite Culture and Society in Turn-of-the-Century Rio de Janeiro* (Cambridge: Cambridge University Press, 2001) captures quite well the influence and dissemination of French culture and ideas during Brazil's long nineteenth century.

16. *Tratado entre a Santa Casa da Misericórdia da Corte e as Irmãs de Caridade* (Rio de Janeiro: Tipografia de Oliveira & Companhia, 1881).

17. The brothers included a scribe, a treasurer, and a prosecutor. The Santa Casa board under the supervision of the director named them annually. See Article 3 of *Decreto No. 1.077, de 4 de Dezembro de 1852 Aprova e manda executar os estatutos do Hospício de Pedro II.*

18. See Articles 4 and 21 of *Decreto No. 1.077, de 4 de Dezembro de 1852 Aprova e manda executar os estatutos do Hospício de Pedro II.*

19. M. A. A. Peres, "A ordem no Hospício: Primórdios da Enfermagem Psiquiátrica no Brasil (1852–1890)" (PhD diss., Universidade Federal do Rio de Janeiro, Escola de Enfermagem Anna Nery, Programa de Pós-Graduação em Enfermagem, 2008).

20. *Tratado entre a Santa Casa da Misericórdia da Corte e as Irmãs de Caridade* (Rio de Janeiro: Tipografia de Oliveira & Companhia, 1881).

21. Michael J. Steiner, *A Study of the Intellectual and Material Culture of Death in Nineteenth Century America* (Lewiston, NY: Edwin Mellen Press, 2003).

22. Nelson, *Say Little, Do Much*, 19.

23. A medical degree at the Rio de Janeiro College of Medicine required six years of schooling and a formal thesis written in Portuguese or Latin. See Lycurgo Santos Filho's *História Geral da Medicina Brasileira*, 2 vols. (São Paulo: Hucitec, 1991), for a general encyclopedic history of Brazil's medical profession. Indeed, the first medical thesis in Brazil on the idea of mental illness, "Considerações gerais sobre a alienação mental," by Antonio Luiz da Silva Peixoto, was published in 1837. Between 1850 and 1880, students at the college produced thirty-five theses on the subject of mental illness, with the majority of them (twenty-six) written during the years from 1870 through 1879.

24. The doctors in charge of the medical service of the Hospício Pedro II during the Second Empire included: Manoel José Barbosa (1852–66 and 1869), José Joaquim Ludovino da Silva (1866–68, 1870–71), Ignácio Francisco Goulart (1872–77), Gustavo Balduíno de Moura e Câmera (1878–81), Nuno Ferreira de Andrade (1881–82), Dr. Agostinho José de Souza e Lima (1881–87), and João Carlos Teixeira Brandão (1887–97).

25. M. J. Barbosa, *Relatório e Estatística do Hospício de Pedro II, de 09/12/1852 até 30/071853* (Rio de Janeiro: Tip. Dois de Dezembro, 1853), 17. Barbosa was aided by Drs. Robert Christian Avé Lallemant (in charge of the female wing), and Dr. Antônio José Pereira das Neves (in charge of the male division). Neves was the only doctor of the three with work experience in mental illness.

26. M. J. Barbosa, "Relatório e estatística do Hospício de Pedro II, desde 1 de julho de 1854 até 30 de julho de 1855, *Annaes Brasilienses de Medicina* 5 (1856): 2.

27. M. J. Barbosa, "Relatório e estatística do Hospital de Pedro II, desde 1 de Julho de 1854 até 30 de Julho de 1855," *Anais Brasilienses de Medicina* 10, no. 4 (1856): 98–104, 118–21.

28. Ibid., 101.

29. Luiz Vicente De-Simoni, "Importância e necessidade da criação de um manicómio ou estabelecimento especial para o tratamento dos alienados," in *Revista Médica Fluminense* 6 (September 1839): 241–46.

30. Barbosa, "Relatório e estatística do Hospício de Pedro II, 100.

31. For example, from 1859 to 1890, the asylum consistently housed more than 300 residents. Afterward, its usual annual occupancy consistently hovered at 350. G. B. de Câmera in Roberto Machado, Roberto Ángela Loureiro, Rogério Luz, and Kátia Muricy, *Danação DaNorma: Medicina Social e Constituição da Psiquiatria no Brasil* (Rio de Janeiro: Graal, 1978), 457.

32. I. F. Goulart, "Carta do médico-director do HP II ao Provedor da Santa Casa da Misericórdia, de 06/02/1874," in *Questões relativas à assistência médico-legal a alienados*, ed. J. C. T. Brandão (Rio de Janeiro: Imprensa Nácional, 1897), 38.

33. See Dora B. Weiner, "The Madman in the Light of Reason: Enlightenment Psychiatry, Part I: Custody, Therapy, Theory, and the Need for Reform," in *History of Psychiatry and Medical Psychology*, ed. Edwin R. Wallace and John Gach (New York: Springer Press, 2010), 255–80; Dora B. Weiner, "The Madman in the Light of Reason, Enlightenment Psychiatry, Part II: Alienists, Treatises, and the Psychologic Approach in the Era of Pinel," in *History of Psychiatry and Medical Psychology*, ed. Edwin R. Wallace and John Gach (New York: Springer Press, 2010), 281–304, for a discussion of how and why French psychiatry became popularized in the Atlantic world during the nineteenth century.

34. Both articles were published in the French medical journal *Annales Médico-Psychologiques* in the section that in each addition describes asylums in different parts of the world.

35. Rey was a medical resident at the Saint-Anne Asylum whose account was the result of a thirty-day stay in the asylum. Between 1874 and 1878, he made trips to South America and the Iberian Peninsula visiting a series of medical institutions and carrying out research. He cited defects in the institution's physical structure and noted that "the strong cells are absolutely primitive and resemble much the dark period of asylum history." After providing information on living quarters, he noted, "Thus, is the current asylum that, unfortunately, was constructed without the administration having received orientation from a psychiatrist." Philippe-Marius Rey, "O Hospício e os alienados no Brasil," *Rev. Latinoam. Psicopat. Fund.* 15, no. 2 (June 2012): 383–84. Rey, like other psychiatrists at the time, subscribed to an environmental determinism that envisioned the asylum's architecture, aesthetic design, and location as critical elements to help restore minds to sanity. See Carla Yanni, *The Architecture of Madness: Insane Asylums in the United States* (Minneapolis: University of Minnesota Press, 2007) for an astute analysis of the environmental determinism that guided the construction of nineteenth-century asylums in Europe and the United States.

36. Rey, "O Hospício e os alienados no Brasil," 386.

37. Ibid.

38. Ibid.

39. Ibid., 402.

40. Ibid.

41. Ibid., 403.

42. François Jouin, "Uma Visita ao Asilo de Pedro II no Rio de Janeiro, Brasil," *Rev. Latinoam. Psicopat. Fund* 15, no. 2 (2012): 411.

43. Ibid.

44. Ibid., 412.

45. For example, see references to Rey's report in T. W. McDowall, "Part Three: Psychological Retrospect," *Journal of Mental Science* 22 (1877): 614–46.

46. See Jeffrey D. Needell, "The State and Development under the Brazilian Monarchy, 1822–1889," in *State and Nation Making in Latin America and Spain: Republics of the Possible*, ed. Miguel A. Centeno and Agustin E. Ferraro (New York: Cambridge University Press, 2013), 79–99; and Steven C. Topik, *Trade and Gunboats: The United States and Brazil in the Age of Empire* (Stanford, CA: Stanford University Press, 2000), for a discussion of these socioeconomic and political processes.

47. Barman, *Citizen Emperor, Pedro II and the Making of Brazil*, 399. Also see Heitor Lira, *História de Dom Pedro II (1825–1891): Declínio (1880–1891)* (Belo Horizonte: Itatiaia, 1977), 126.

48. See Needell, "The State and Development under the Brazilian Monarchy, 1822–1889," 79–99.

49. The first Positivist Association was founded in Rio de Janeiro in 1876. In 1881 Miguel Lemos and Teixeira Mendes founded the Positivist Apostolate. The 1860s marks the beginnings of the reform spirit in Brazil. The most immediate cause of a shift in national mood was the Paraguayan War (1865–70). The need for aid from Argentina and Uruguay to overcome Paraguay, a much smaller and poorer nation, led the Brazilian elite to reexamine their nation. Specifically, Brazil's ineptitude in initial mobilization for the war forced many to acknowledge the great extent to which Brazil lacked modern facilities in basic critical areas such as education and transportation. See Thomas Skidmore, *Brazil: Five Centuries of Change* (New York: Oxford University Press, 1999), 58–64.

50. Clóvis Beviláqua, *Esboços e Fragmentos* (Rio de Janeiro: Laemmert, 1899), 96. In many ways, positivism attracted Brazilians because it mirrored Brazilian culture. Both were paternalistic, hierarchical, corporatist, and socially conservative. Positivism's social reform was geared toward conserving the social order rather than radically changing it.

51. J. J. L. da Silva, "Relatório apresentado ao Provedor da Santa Casa da Misericórdia do Rio de Janeiro," 186–90, 214–15, 225–27.

52. For further discussion of psychiatry's professional status at the end of the nineteenth century, see Andrew Scull, Charlotte MacKenzie, and Nicholas Hervey, *Masters of Bedlam: The Transformation of the Mad-Doctoring Trade* (Princeton, NJ: Princeton University Press, 1996), 268–74.

53. In November 1870, a small group of liberals—mainly teachers, doctors, and lawyers—organized a Republican Club in Rio de Janeiro. A "Republican Manifesto," published in December 1870, opposed the centralization of political power by advocating an end to the monarchy and the establishment of a federal republic based on the model of the United States. Joseph Smith, *A History of Brazil* (New York: Pearson Education Limited, 2002), 60.

54. See Cristiane Silva Melo and Maria Cristina Gomes Machado, "Notas para a história da Educação: Considerações acerca do Decreto Nº 7.247, de 19 de Abril de 1879, de Autoria de Carlos Leôncio de Carvalho," *Revista Histedbr On-line* 34 (June 2009): 294–305, and Marlos Bessa Mendes da Rocha, "O Ensino Elementar no Decreto Leôncio de Carvalho: "Visão de Mundo" Herdada pelo Tempo Republicano?" *Revista Brasileira de Educação* 15, no. 43 (2010): 126–47 on the background to late nineteenth-century educational reforms in Brazilian higher education.

55. M. J. F. Eiras, "Questões Sociais: A Nova Cadeira de Psychiatria-Hospício de Pedro II-organização de novos asylos de alienados e uma legislação apropriada," Parts I, II, III, IV, V, *Jornal do Commércio,* February 17, 18, 21, 23, March 1, 1883.

56. Nuno de Andrade, "Memoria historica dos acontecimentos mais notaveis, occorridos na Faculdade de Medicina do Rio de Janeiro em 1879" (unpublished manuscript, 1879), 17–19.

57. He held this post until 1889.

58. "Carta de Nuno de Andrade para o Sr. Conselheiro Visconde de Jaguary, em 9 de abril de 1882," in *A Santa Casa de Misericórdia e o Hospício de Pedro II.* (Rio de Janeiro: Typ. Imperial e Constitucional de J. Villeneuvre & C., 1882), 3.

59. Ibid., 4.

60. Ibid., 5.

61. Ibid.

62. Ibid., 6.

63. "Carta do Visconde de Jaguary ao Sr. Dr. Nuno Ferreira de Andrade, em 26 de abril de 1882," in *A Santa Casa de Misericórdia e o Hospício de Pedro II.* (Rio de Janeiro: Typ. Imperial e Constitucional de J. Villeneuvre & C., 1882), 14.

64. Ibid.

65. Ibid., 14.

66. Ibid., 11.

67. Ibid., 13–14.

68. "Carta do Nuno," 14.

69. The Viscount of Jaguary appointed Dr. Agostinho José de Souza e Lima as the interim director of the asylum until Dr. Brandão assumed the post. See "Carta do Visconde de Jaguary ao Dr. Nuno Ferreira de Andrade, em 4 de maio de 1882," in *A Santa Casa de Misericórdia e o Hospício de Pedro II.* (Rio de Janeiro: Typ. Imperial e Constitucional de J. Villeneuvre & C., 1882), 14–15.

70. For a biography of Dr. Teixeira Brandão see M. Teixeira, "Teixeira Brandão: O Pinel Brasileiro." In *Psicologização no Brasil: Atores e Autores,* ed. Luiz Fernando Dias Duarte, Jane Russo, and Ana Tereza A. Venancio (Rio de Janeiro: Contra Capa Livraria, 2005), 39–63.

71. J. C. T. Brandão, *Questões relativas à assistência medico legal a alienados e aos alienados* (Rio de Janeiro: Imprensa Nácional 1897), 16.

72. Ibid.

73. Ibid., 17.

74. Ibid., 54.

75. Ibid., 73–75.

76. Ibid., 75.

77. See J. T. Nabuco de Araújo, "Oficio do Min. Da Justiça ao Chefe de Polícia de 14/08/1854," in *Assistência Pública e Privada no Rio de Janeiro—História e Estatistica.* (Rio de Janeiro: Tip. Do Anuário do Brasil, 1922), 448.

78. Faria Lemos, F. Da, "Relatório do Chefe de Polícia ao Min. Da Justiça" (1871), in *Assistência Pública e Privada no Rio de Janeiro—História e Estatistica.* (Rio de Janeiro: Tip. Do Anuário do Brasil, 1922), 449.

79. Ibid., 450.

80. J. C. T. Brandão, *Os Alienados no Brasil* (Rio de Janeiro: Imprensa Nácional, 1886), 50.

81. Ibid.

82. Ibid., 25–26; Phillipe-Marius Rey, *L'Hospice Pédro II et les Aliénés au Brésil* (Paris: Imprimerie de E. Donnaud, 1875), 9. It was commonplace to see announcements in newspapers of the time advertising the services of these casas de saúde. For example, the announcement for the Casa de Saúde of Dr. Eiras published in the *Jornal do Commércio* on May 1, 1892, page 4, read, "Companhia Casa de Saúde Dr. Eiras—Botafogo—continues to receive the alienated, hoping to soon inaugurate a new pavilion, constructed in accord with the most modern psychiatric precepts. Chalet Olinda, annexed to the Casa de Saúde Dr. Eiras, receives convalescents, people suffering from chronic ailments, etc. . . . The use of hydrotherapy and electrical therapy is used daily."

83. Lucidus, "Piedade para o alienado," *Diário de Rio de Janeiro.* January 20, 1871, 10.

84. Brandão, *Os Alienados no Brasil,* 52.

85. Ibid., 16.

86. Julyan G. Peard, *Tropical Medicine: The Idea of the Tropics in Nineteenth-Century Brazil* (Durham, NC: Duke University Press, 2000), 28–29. He was also the founder of the Instituto Pasteur and the Hospital N. S. das Dores, in Cascadura, Rio de Janeiro for the treatment of tuberculosis.

87. J. Moreira, *Relatório do director do Hospício Nacional de Alienados Relativo ao ano de 1905,* Rio de Janeiro: Imprensa Nacional, 1905), 73.

88. "Hospício Nacional de Alienados," *O Brazil-Médico* 4, no. 37 (August 15, 1890): 300.

89. An immediate and important consequence of psychiatric control of the asylum was the institutionalization of secular nursing throughout Brazil. The contraction of lay French nurses by republican officials, at the insistence of psychiatrists, to work in the asylum led to the creation of a professional nursing school annexed to the institution (Decree 791 of September 27, 1890). The Professional School of Nurses prepared women to work in hospices and hospitals (both civil and military). It functioned precariously for many years until it was formally inaugurated in 1905. See Telma Geovanini, Almerinda Moreira, Soraia Dornelles Schoeller, and Wiliam C. A. Machado, *História da Enfermagem: Versões e Interpretações* (Rio de Janeiro: Revinter, 1995). As the national flagship establishment for nursing, the school provided women with an invaluable opportunity to enter the professional sphere.

90. Heitor Resende, "Política de saúde mental no Brasil: Uma Visão Histórica," in *Cidadania e Loucura: Políticas de Saúde Mental no Brasil,* ed. Silvério Almeida Tundis and Nilson do Rosário Costa (Petrópolis, Brazil: Editora Vozes, 1990), 45. For a comprehensive discussion of the links between public health and politics in Brazil, see

Nancy Leys Stepan, *The Beginning of Brazilian Science: Oswaldo Cruz, Medical Research, and Policy* (New York: Science History Publications, 1976). It explores the interaction between public health and politics during the renowned physician and epidemiologist Oswaldo Cruz's sanitary campaign. Also see Nancy Leys Stepan's *The Hour of Eugenics: Race, Gender, and Nation in Latin America* (Ithaca, NY: Cornell University Press, 1991).

Chapter Three

1. Historian Gerald Grob's research confirms a similar situation in the context of the nineteenth-century American asylums. Gerald Grob, *The Mad Among Us: A History of the Care of America's Mentally Ill* (New York: The Free Press, 1994), 85.
2. Henri Lefebvre, *Production of Space* (Cambridge, MA: Blackwell, 1991), 85.
3. Gaston Bachelard, *The Poetics of Space*, trans. Maria Jolas (Boston: Beacon Press, 1994), 15.
4. It was formally known as Decree 206, formally passed on February 15, 1890.
5. Literally the *encilhamento* referred to the area in a racetrack where bets on horses were made. In economic jargon of the nineteenth century, *encilhamento* was the peculiar mix of inflation, financial speculation, and currency devaluation. Antonio Evaristo de Morais, *Reminiscencias de um Rábula Criminalista* (Rio de Janeiro: Editora Briguiet, 1989), 15. Rio's Bolsa de Valores developed out of Brazil's external market for coffee and the new breed of elites made wealthy by the expansion of the crop in the southeast of the country. The gradual replacement of slave with free wage labor beginning in the middle of the nineteenth century liberated capital previously invested in slave labor and increased the circulation of money in Rio's economy. Wage labor increased family consumption and spending, and Brazil's internal consumer market expanded. On the origins of Rio de Janeiro's stock market, see Maria Bárbara Levy, *História da Bolsa de Valores do Rio de Janeiro* (Rio de Janeiro: IBEMEC, 1977).
6. Stuart Hall et al., eds., *Policing the Crisis: Mugging, the State and Law and Order* (London: Macmillan, 1978), 16. The concept of moral panic originated with Stanley Cohen's *Folk Devils and Moral Panics: The Creation of the Mods and Rockers* (London: MacGibbon and Kee, 1972), since republished several times. I have relied principally on the following for theoretical underpinning and comparative purposes: Erich Goode and Nachman Ben-Yehuda, *Moral Panics: The Social Construction of De*viance, 2nd ed. (Malden, MA: Wiley-Blackwell, 2009), and David Garland, "On the Concept of Moral Panic," *Crime, Media, Culture* 4, no. 1 (2008): 9–30.
7. George Reid Andrews, *Blacks and Whites in São Paulo, Brazil 1888–1988* (Madison: University of Wisconsin Press, 1991), 48. Sidney Chalhoub, "Vadios e Barões no Ocaso do Império: O Debate sobre a Repressão da Ociosidade na Câmara dos Deputados em 1888," *Estudos Ibero-Americanos* 9, nos. 1–2 (1983): 53–67.
8. Mary Karasch, *Slave Life in Rio de Janeiro, 1808–1850* (Princeton, NJ: Princeton University Press, 1987), 362.
9. Luiz de Aguiar Costa Pinto, *O Negro no Rio de Janeiro: Relações de Raça numa Sociedade em Mudança*, 2nd ed. (Rio de Janeiro: Editora Universidade Federal do Rio de Janeiro, 1998), 100–114.

10. Thomas Holloway, *Policing Rio de Janeiro: Repression and Resistance in a 19th Century City* (Stanford, CA: Stanford University Press, 1993).

11. Ibid., 289.

12. Lourence Cristine Alves, "Quem Eram os Habitantes do "Cemitério dos Vivos": Uma Análise Quantitativa dos Prontuários dos Pacientes do Hospício Nacional de Alienados (1883–1910)" (unpublished paper, 2011).

13. J. J. L. da Silva, "Relatório apresentado ao Provedor da Santa Casa da Misericórdia do Rio de Janeiro," 190.

14. Barbosa, "Relatório e estatística do Hospital de Pedro II, desde 1 de Julho de 1854 até 30 de Julho de 1855," 98–104, 118–21.

15. Ibid.

16. P. Rey, *L' Hospice Pédro II et les Aliénés au Brésil* (Paris: Imprimerie de E. Donnaud, 1875), 26.

17. Andrew Scull, *The Most Solitary of Afflictions: Madness and Society in Britain, 1700–1900* (New Haven, CT: Yale University Press, 1993), 99.

18. Georges Didi-Huberman, *Invention of Hysteria: Charcot and the Photographic Iconography of the Salpêtrière*, trans. Alisa Hartz (Cambridge, MA: MIT Press, 2003), 6.

19. Using all the scientific resources of the time that included laboratory analyses, photographs, electro-stimulation, drawings, casts, and histological sections, Charcot described the symptoms observed, sought the corresponding anatomical and histological lesions, and analyzed causes and mechanisms. He attracted many students from France and Europe who achieved international renown, such as Sigmund Freud, Eugen Bleuler, Alfred Binet, Georges Gilles de la Tourette, and many others.

20. "Escola Profissional de Enfermeiros e Enfermeiras," *Jornal do Commercio*: *Gazetilha*, October 1, 1890, 1.

21. "Escola de Enfermeiras," *Diário Oficial* (Rio de Janeiro), October 1, 1890.

22. *Brazil-Medico*, October 8, 1890.

23. "Escola de Enfermeiras," *Diário Oficial* (Rio de Janeiro), October 1, 1890.

24. For insightful examinations on gender and modernity in late nineteenth- and twentieth-century Rio de Janeiro, see Sandra Lauderdale Graham, *House and Street: The Domestic World of Servants and Masters in Nineteenth-Century Rio de Janeiro* (Cambridge: Cambridge University Press, 1988); Susan K. Besse, *Restructuring Patriarchy: The Modernization of Gender Inequality in Brazil, 1914–1940* (Chapel Hill: University of North Carolina Press, 1996); and Sueann Caulfield, *In Defense of Honor: Sexual Morality, Modernity, and Nation in Early-Twentieth-Century Brazil* (Durham, NC: Duke University Press, 1999).

25. See Maria Lucia Mott, "Midwifery and the Construction of an Image in Nineteenth-Century Brazil," *Nursing History Review* 11 (2003): 34.

26. On standardization among women, see Lilia Katri Moritz Schwarcz, *O Espetáculo das Raças: Cientistas, Instituições e Pensamento Racial no Brasil: 1870–1930* (São Paulo: Companhia das Letras, 1993). As Antônio Sérgio Guimarães and others have astutely noted, racial motives in Brazil are often hidden beneath complex set of informal rules and processes with a variety of "code words." See Antônio Sérgio Guimarães, *Racismo e Anti-Racismo no Brasil* (São Paulo: Editora 34, 1999), 140–41.

27. Kim D. Butler, *Freedoms Given, Freedoms Won: Afro-Brazilians in Post-Abolition São Paulo and Salvador* (New Brunswick, NJ: Rutgers University Press, 1998), 28.

28. Moreover, state-subsidized immigration from Europe, as a means to whiten the population, led to a de facto preference for white labor. Between 1889 and 1934, 4.1 million immigrants entered Brazil (approximately 56 percent of them settled in the coffee fields of São Paulo). By the time immigration ebbed in 1949, 4.55 million had arrived, mostly Italians, Spaniards, Portuguese, Germans, Russian, and Polish Jews, along with Syrians, Lebanese, and other Arabs from the Middle East in addition to a considerable Japanese community. See George Reid Andrews, *Blacks and Whites in São Paulo, Brazil 1888–1988* (Madison: University of Wisconsin Press 1991), Thomas E. Skidmore, "Racial Ideas and Social Policy in Brazil 1870–1940," in *The Idea of Race in Latin America*, ed. Richard Graham (Austin: University of Texas Press 1990), 7–36. The census of 1872 noted that 38 percent of the population as white and 20 percent as black, with the remainder of the population being pardo ("brown"). Between 1884 and 1893, Brazil recorded 883,668 European immigrant arrivals. Rio de Janeiro had a tradition of hiring enslaved, freed, and free blacks in the skilled trades and factories, which made the participation of blacks and people of color in the state's industrial workforce more significant than in other states. In 1891 Brazilian-born persons made up 57 percent of Rio de Janeiro's industrial workers, and 30 percent of that population was black (but this percentage was still small in relation to the number of Afro-Brazilians in the state). Ana Lucia Araujo, *Public Memory of Slavery: Victims and Perpetrators in the South Atlantic* (Amherst, NY: Cambria Press, 2010), 212–13.

29. Martha Cristina Nunes Moreira, "A Fundação Rockefeller e a Construção da Identidade Profissional de Enfermagem no Brasil na Primeira República," *História, Ciências, Saúde-Manguinhos* 5, no. 3 (November 1998–February 1999), 637. Also see Paulo Fernando de Souza Campos, Taka Oguisso, and Genival Fernandes de Freitas, "Cultura dos Cuidados: Mulheres Negras e Formação da Enfermagem Profissional Brasileira, *Cultura de los Cuidados Año* XI-No. 22 (2007): 33–39.

30. James Holston, *Insurgent Citizenship: Disjunctions of Democracy and Modernity in Brazil* (Princeton, NJ: Princeton University Press, 2009), 5.

31. Olivia Maria Gomes Da Cunha and Flávio dos Santos Gomes, eds., *Quase-cidadão: Histórias e Antropologias da Pós-Emancipação no Brasil* (Rio de Janeiro: FGV Editora, 2007).

32. Giorgio Agamben, *Homo Sacer: Sovereign Power and Bare Life* (Stanford, CA: Stanford University Press, 1998).

33. In terms of residence, 113 resided in the municipality of the court, twenty from the Province of Rio de Janeiro, and seven from other provinces (one from Minas Gerais, one from Santa Catarina, four from Rio Grande, and one from Sergipe). See José Clemente Pereira, "Alienados que passaram do antigo hospital e das enfermeiras provisórias para o Hospício de Pedro Segundo nos dias 8 e 9 de dezembro de 1852," in Arquivo Nacional, Série Saúde / Ministério de Império, Maço IS 3 4, 1850–53.

34. Arquivo Nacional, Série Saúde / Ministério de Império, Maço IS 3 4, 1850–53.

35. Ibid.

36. Mining of documents from 1850 to 1888 resulted in the culmination of 1,835 admission records into the asylum, 1,746 of which documented the social status of patients. Out of the 1,835 records, 1,749 registered their medical diagnoses.

37. Lourence Cristine Alves, *O Hospício Nacional de Alienados: Terapêutica ou Higiene Social?* (master's thesis, Rio de Janeiro, 2010), 85.

38. Ibid.

39. M. J. Barbosa, Relatório do medico director do serviço sanitário do Hospício Pedro Segundo. 1 Julho 1870. Arquivo Nacional, Série Saúde / Ministério do Império, Maço IS3 7, 1864–70.

40. Afonso Henriques de Lima Barreto, *O Diário do Hospício: O Cemitério dos Vivos* (Rio de Janeiro: Secretaria Municipal de Cultura, Departamento Geral de Documentação e Informação Cultural, 1988), 211.

41. However, the history of patient labor in European psychiatry suggests that the notion of an agricultural colony was not a novel idea by the end of the nineteenth century. The first institution of this type was presumably established in France in 1847. See Claude Quétel, *Histoire de la Folie: De l'Antiquité à nos jours* (Paris: Tallendier, 2009); Waltraud Ernst and Thomas Mueller, eds., *Transnational Psychiatries: Social and Cultural Histories of Psychiatry in Comparative Perspective, c. 1800–2000* (Cambridge: Cambridge University Press, 2010); Roy Porter and David Wrights, eds., *The Confinement of the Insane: International Perspectives, 1800–1965* (Cambridge: Cambridge University Press, 2003).

42. Established in the Loire Valley in 1840 and the subject of Foucault's well-known analysis in *Discipline and Punish.* See Michel Foucault, *Discipline and Punish: The Birth of the Prison*, trans. Alan Sheridan (Harmondsworth, UK: Penguin, 1979). John Ramsland, "Mettray: A Corrective Institution for Delinquent Youth in France, 1840–1937," *Journal of Educational Administration and History* 22, no. 1 (1990): 30–46.

43. Ceri Crossley, "Using and Transforming the French Countryside: The 'Colonies Agricoles' (1820–1850)," *French Studies* 45 (1991): 36–54. See also Laura Lee Downs, *Childhood in the Promised Land: Working-class movements and the Colonies de Vacances in France, 1880–1960* (Durham, NC: Duke University Press, 2002). The Mettray agricultural colony for abandoned and delinquent children serves as the most famous example, popularized by Michel Foucault in *Discipline and Punish: The Birth of the Prison,* trans. Alan Sheridan, 2nd ed. (New York: Vintage Press, 1995).

44. Brandão, *Os Alienados no Brasil,* 94. Also in *Arquivos Brasileiros de Neuriatria e Psiquiatria* 39, no. 2 (1956): 60–101.

45. João Carlos Teixeira Brandão, *Relatório da Assistência Médico Legal de Alienados apresentado ao Ministro de Estado Negócios do Interior, Fernando Lobo Leite Pereira, pelo Dr. João Carlos Teixeira Brandão, diretor geral* (Rio de Janeiro: Imprensa Nácional, 1892), 5.

46. Ibid., 96–97.

47. Ibid., 98.

48. Brasil, Ministério do Interior, *Relatório apresentado ao Presidente da República dos Estados Unidos do Brazil* (Rio de Janeiro: Imprensa Nácional 1891), 28.

49. João Carlos Teixeira, *Relatório da Assistência Médico Legal de Alienados apresentado pelo Diretor Geral, Dr. João Carlos Teixeira Brandão, ao Ministro de Estado dos Negócios do Interior, Dr. João Barbalho Uchoa Cavalcanti, em 28 de Janeiro de 1890* (Rio de Janeiro: Imprensa Nacional, 1891), 54.

50. Philippe Pinel, *A Treatise on Insanity* (1806; repr., New York: Hafner, 1962), 218.

51. Michel Foucault, *History of Madness,* ed. Jonathan Murphy and Jean Khalfa (New York: Routledge Press, 2006), 336.

52. See Ann Laura Stoler, *Along the Archival Grain* (Princeton, NJ: Princeton University Press, 2009); Albert Schrauwers, "The 'Benevolent' Colonies of Johannes van den Bosch: Continuities in the Administration of Poverty in the Netherlands and Indonesia," *Comparative Studies in Society and History* 43, no. 2 (2001): 298–328; Stephen Toth, *Beyond Papillon: The French Overseas Penal Colonies, 1854–1952* (Lincoln: University of Nebraska Press, 2006); and Neil Roos, "Work Colonies and South African Historiography," *Journal of Social History* 36, no. 1 (2011): 54–76. While Claire Edington's "Beyond the Asylum: Colonies Agricoles and the History of Psychiatry in French Indochina, 1918–1945," *Proceedings of the Western Society for French History* 39 (2011): 267–77, urges a critical reexamination of labor as a medical tool, it fails to critically assess how different modes of labor (i.e., agricultural manual labor) had sociopolitical and cultural implications.

53. See Ana Teresa A. Venancio, "From the Agricultural Colony to the Hospital-Colony: Configurations for Psychiatric Care in Brazil in the first half of the twentieth century," *Hist. Cienc. Saúde-Manguinhos* 18, suppl. 1 (2011): 35–52.

54. Indeed, harnessing race in asylum records is a difficult task not only due to incomplete patient records but also to the mutability of racial designations. This could most readily be seen in the case of the writer Afonso Henriques de Lima Barreto (1881–1922). When first confined to the asylum in 1914, he was categorized as white whereas he was labeled *pardo* (brown or mixed-race) during his hospitalization from December 1919 to February 1920.

55. The identification of patients with the lower laboring classes (and in some cases with children) is apparent in Andrew Scull, ed., *The Asylum as Utopia: W. A. F. Browne and the Mid-Nineteenth Century Consolidation of Psychiatry* (London: Routledge Press, 1991), 229–31.

56. Freud's *unheimlich*, the uncanny, or "that species of the frightening that goes back to what was once well known and had long been familiar." Sigmund Freud, *The Uncanny* (London: Penguin Books, 2003), 124.

57. Anthony Vidler, *Architectural Uncanny: Essays in the Modern Unhomely* (Cambridge, MA: MIT Press, 1992), 4.

58. Holloway, *Policing Rio de Janeiro*, 231.

59. The term *pavilion* had multiple meanings in the nineteenth century. Asylum builders used it to mean a two- or three-story building within a larger structure. In medical hospitals, the term *pavilion* referred specifically to a long, thin structure, with windows on two sides that remained unencumbered on three sides. Such a pavilion was usually also part of a larger hospital complex. See Yanni, *The Architecture of Madness*, 41.

60. See Adrian Forty, "The Modern Hospital in England and France," In *Buildings and Society: Essays on the Social Development of the Built Environment*, ed. Anthony D. King (London: Routledge, 1980), 32–50; Anthony King, "Hospital Planning: Revised Thoughts on the Origin of the Pavilion Principle in England," *Medical History* 10 (1966): 360–73. While views on miasmatism were to be discarded and superseded in the 1880s by germ theory, the construction of pavilion-plans into the 1930s continued. See Jeremy Taylor, *The Architect and the Pavilion Hospital: Dialogue and Design Creativity in England 1850–1914* (London: Leicester University Press, 1997), to examine England as a case study of the pavilion-plan's continuity into the early twentieth century.

61. Amos Rapoport, *The Meaning of the Built Environment: A Non Verbal Communication Approach* (Tucson: University of Arizona Press, 1990).

62. Donald Preziosi, *Architecture, Language and Meaning: The Origins of the Built World and Its Semiotic Organization* (The Hague: De Gruyter Mouton, 1979).

63. William Whyte, "How Do Buildings Mean? Some Issues on the Interpretation in the History of Architecture," *History and Theory Journal* 45 (2006): 153–77.

64. Much of the historiography focuses on the asylum's built environment as an instrument of control, a therapeutic aid, or a means of segregation. Peter Bishop's "Surveying 'The Waiting Room,'" *Architectural Theory Review* 18, no. 2 (2013): 135–49, an examination of the waiting room as an intermediary zone of passage, is instructive when thinking about the Observation Pavilion.

65. Lima Barreto, *O Diário do Hospício*, 53.

66. Speaking of the panopticon in *Discipline and Punish*, Foucault notes, "Thanks to its mechanisms of observation, it gains in efficiency and in the ability to penetrate into men's behavior; knowledge follows the advances of power, discovering new objects of knowledge over all the surfaces on which power is exercised" (204).

67. See Lindsay Prior, "The Architecture of the Hospital: A Study of Spatial Organization and Medical Knowledge," *British Journal of Sociology* 39, no. 1 (1988): 86–113.

68. Zygmunt Bauman translates Lévi-Strauss's categories of the *anthropoemic* and the *anthropophagic*, two strategies by which we neutralized the unfamiliar into emic space and phagic space to explain contemporary "public but non-civil" zones: "forms of the 'emic' strategy are spatial separation, urban ghettos, selective access to spaces and selective barring from using them. The second strategy [the phagic] consists in a soi-distant 'disalienation' of alien substances . . . if the first strategy was aimed at the exile or annihilation of the others, the second was aimed at the suspension or annihilation of their otherness." See Zygmunt Bauman, *Liquid Modernity* (Cambridge: Polity Press, 2000), 101.

69. *Relatório do Hospício Nacional de Alienados* (Rio de Janeiro, 1899), Arquivo Nacional.

70. Despite the fact that the first nursing school was established in Brazil in 1890, many historians mark the advent of "modern" nursing with the robust Brazilian public health movement of the 1920s and the arrival of US nurses to Rio de Janeiro. See Ieda de Alencar Barreira, "The Beginning of Nursing in Brazil," *Nursing School Review* 10 (2002): 33–47.

71. F. Lobo, *Relatório apresentado ao Vice-Presidente da República dos Estados Unidos do Brasil, pelo Dr. Fernando Lobo, Ministro de Estado da Justiça e Negócios Interiores, em abril de 1893* (Rio de Janeiro: Imprensa Nácional, 1893), 362.

72. D. L. S. Araújo, *Relatório do Diretor das Colônias de Alienados, Dr. Domingos Lopes da Silva Araújo, apresentado ao diretor geral da Assisência, Dr. João Carlos Teixeira Brandão, em 28 de janeiro de 1895* (Rio de Janeiro: Imprensa Nácional, 1895), 22.

73. Ibid.

74. Ibid., 31–32. To make matters worse, at approximately 10:00 a.m. on October 24, 1893, rebellious troops, under the command of Captain of Sea and War Eliezer Tavares, invaded the Conde de Mesquita Colony taking medicine, clothing, and various animals. Because the approach of troops was feared, all the insane were removed from the São Bento Colony, along with items from the pharmacy and nursing

stations, leaving the establishment under the care of some employees. On the morning of the October 25, the troops ransacked the colony.

75. J. Moreira, "Relatório do diretor do Hospício Nacional de Alienados relativo ao ano de 1905," In *Relatório apresentado ao president da república dos Estados Unidos do Brasil, pelo ministro de estado da justiça e negócios interiores, em março de 1906*, ed. J. J. Seabra (Rio de Janeiro: Imprensa Nácional, 1906), 84. European psychiatry adopted family care in the nineteenth century, inspired by the experience of villagers in Geel, Belgium, where a procession takes place each year dedicated to St. Dynfne for healing the mentally insane. The villagers received the insane and their families in their homes and sometimes even lodged them there until the religious festival of the following year, establishing the coexistence between the sane and the insane. Paulo Amarante, "Psiquiatria Social e Colônias de Alienados no Brasil (1830–1920)" (master's thesis, Programa de Pós-Graduação em Saúde Coletiva da Universidade do Estado do Rio de Janeiro, Rio de Janeiro, 1982), 52.

Chapter Four

1. Michael Mann, *The Sources of Social Power*, 2 vols. (Cambridge: Cambridge University Press, 1993), 2:59.

2. Svetlana Boym, *The Future of Nostalgia* (New York: Basic Books, 2001), xiii.

3. Marco Morel and Mariana Monteiro de Barros, *Palavra, Imagem, e Poder: O Surgimento da Imprensa no Brasil do Século XIX* (Rio de Janeiro: DP&A Editoria Ltda., 2003), 40–42.

4. Popkin, *Press, Revolution, and Social Identities in France*, 9.

5. Leslie Bethell, ed. *Brazil: Empire and Republic, 1822–1930* (Cambridge: Cambridge University Press, 1989), 45. Jorge Padua found that as late as 1960, only 39 percent of the adult population was literate. Jorge Padua, *El Analfabetismo en America Latina: Un Estudio Empirico con Especial Referencia a los Casos de Peru, Mexico y Argentina* (Mexico City: El Colegio de Mexico, 1979): 37.

6. Burns writes, "Somehow the intellectuals communicated to the lower strata of urban society the ideas of which they were brokers." E. Bradford Burns, "The Intellectuals as Agents of Change and the Independence of Brazil 1724–1822," in *Colony to Nation: Essays on the Independence of Brazil*, ed. A. J. R. Russell-Wood (Baltimore: Johns Hopkins University Press, 1975), 245. The transference of printed ideas to illiterate listeners has been explored in other contexts. For example, David Cressy has traced the involvement of illiterate people in the debates of colonial North America. He believes there was a "spillover from the literate to the illiterate." See David Cressy, *Literacy and the Social Order: Reading and Writing in Tudor and Stuart England* (Cambridge: Cambridge University Press, 1980), 14.

7. Robert Walsh, *Notices of Brazil in 1828 and 1829* (Boston: Richardson, Lord & Holbrook, 1831), 240. The practice of reading printed material out loud is well documented for nineteenth-century Latin America. See for example, François Xavier Guerra, *Modernidad e Independencia: Ensayos sobre las Revoluciones Hispánicas* (Madrid: Editorial Mapfere, 1992); Nancy Vogeley, "Mexican Newspaper Culture on the Eve of Mexican Independence," *Institute for the Study of Ideologies and Literature* 2, no. 17 (September–October 1983), 358–77.

8. J. M. Pereira da Silva, *Segundo Periodo do Reinado de Dom Pedro I no Brazil* (Rio de Janeiro: B. L. Garnier, 1871), 24.

9. Ibid.

10. *Anais do Senado,* September 11, 1894, 92.

11. Ibid., 93.

12. Ibid., 97.

13. Ibid.

14. A number of children entered the asylum at approximately age six (*Relatório da Assistencia Médico-Legal de Alienados apresentado pelo diretor geral Dr. João Carlos Teixeira Brandão em março* de 1894," 5), while others were born in the asylum. When families did not accept children (which was often the case), the asylum sheltered them—both before and after declaration of the republic. Children elevated costs, as it was necessary to secure nurses, among other resources, for them.

15. *Anais do Senado,* September 11, 1896, 98.

16. Ibid., 101.

17. Ibid.

18. Ibid., 103.

19. Douglas Coupland, *Generation X: Tales for an Accelerated Culture* (New York: St. Martin's Griffin, 1991), 41.

20. *Anais do Senado,* September 11, 1894, 102.

21. Ibid., 106.

22. Ibid., 107.

23. João Carlos Brandão, *Questões Relativas à Assistência Médico-Legal a Alienados* (Rio de Janeiro: Imprensa Nácional, 1897), 5.

24. Ibid., 10.

25. Ibid., 11.

26. Ibid., 21.

27. Ibid.

28. Ibid., 22.

29. Ibid., 23.

30. Ibid., 43.

31. Ibid., 144.

32. *Anais do Senado,* November 19, 1894, 8.

33. Ibid., 143.

34. Ibid.

35. *O Paiz* and the *Gazeta de Noticias* allowed for a comprehensive debate. Known informally at the time as the "generation of 1870," ardent positivists, who were writers and intellectuals critical of monarchical rule and the encroachment of religion in state affairs, founded the *O Paiz* journal. As staunch supporters of republicanism, they used the journal as an outlet from which to further the socioeconomic, political, and cultural modernization of Brazil.

36. Founded by the lawyer, journalist, and politician Rodolfo de Souza Dantas in 1891.

37. *Jornal do Brasil,* May 29, 1896, 1.

38. Ibid.

39. *Gazeta de Notícias,* May 29, 1896, 1.

40. *Jornal do Brasil,* May 31, 1896, 2.

41. *Diário Official*, May 30, 1896.
42. *Jornal do Brasil*, May 31, 1896, 2.
43. *Gazeta da Tarde*, May 30, 1896.
44. *Diário Official*, May 30, 1896.
45. *O Paiz*, June 5, 1896, 1.
46. Ibid.
47. Ibid.
48. *Jornal do Brasil*, June 7, 1896, 2.
49. Ibid.
50. Ibid.
51. *Jornal do Brasil*, June 9, 1896, 2.
52. Ibid., June 16, 1896, 2.
53. Ibid., June 18, 1896, 2.
54. Ibid.
55. *O Paiz*, June 13, 1896, 1.
56. *Anais do Senado*, July 28, 1896, 255–56.
57. Ibid.
58. Ibid., 256.
59. Ibid., 259.
60. Ibid.
61. Ana Teresa A. Venancio, "Ciência Psiquiátrica e Política Assistencial: A Criação do Instituto de Psiquiatria da Universidade do Brasil," *História, Ciências, Saúde-Manguinhos* 10, no. 3 (2003): 889. In his wake, the succession of directors that followed included Márcio Nery (1898–99), Pedro Dias Carneiro (1900–1901), and Antonio Dias Carneiro (1902–3).
62. To get a sense of this, depreciation in 1890 was only 16.2 percent while in March 1899 it was 74.53 percent. See J. M. Murtinho, *Relatório apresentado ao president da República dos Estados Unidos do Brasil pelo Ministro de Estado dos Negócios da Fazenda, Joaquim Murtinho, no ano de 1899* (Rio de Janeiro: Imprensa Nácional, 1899), 10.
63. Cost-saving measures included increasing the daily costs of pensioners (Decree 2779 of December 1897) by 50 percent.
64. *Ofício do Diretor Geral de Assistência Pública, ao prefeito, sobre o assunto referente à Assistência a alienados no Distrito Federal em 9 de Janeiro de 1899* (Rio de Janeiro: Arquivo Geral da Cidade do Rio de Janeiro, 1899), 1.
65. For example, during January 1900, 758 patients (403 men [53 percent] and 355 women [47 percent]) constituted the asylum population. Over the course of the year, 615 patients entered (351 men [57 percent], 264 women [43 percent]), making a total of 1,373 patients. During the same period, 263 individuals left while 228 died. Similar demographic figures were present in the agricultural colonies. In January there were 246 patients, all men, with 109 entered during the course of the year, totaling 355 patients. Of this number, 11 left while 52 died. Asylum director Pedro Dias Carneiro (1897–1902) sought to explain why the number of deaths was almost the same as the number of releases in the asylum, and higher in the agricultural colonies, noting that "with the body profoundly affected by the use of alcohol" and harmed by the "deprivations that accompany indigence, by the burdensome and constant work that are taken in the struggle for life," the high mortality rate is not surprising. See Epitácio Pessoa, *Relatório apresentado ao presidente da República dos*

Estados Unidos do Brasil pelo ministro da justiça e negócios interiores, Epitácio Pessoa, em março de 1901 (Rio de Janeiro: Imprensa Nácional, 1901), 242–43.

66. *O Paiz*, January 22, 1901, 1. By 1901 the asylum was divided into four sections (two for men and two for women) in addition to the Observation Pavilion.

67. Ibid.

68. Ibid.

69. *Gazeta de Notícias*, February 8, 1902, 1.

70. Ibid.

71. Ibid.

72. Ibid.

73. On December 25, 1902, each worker was sent an office circular requesting "a written exposition, thorough as possible, on the state of the section that he or she directly works," beyond necessary repairs, of the irregularities that occurred and all that could improve the "good functioning of their section." F. M. da Silva Araújo, Relatório da comissão de inquérito sobre as condições da assistência a alienados no Hospício Nacional e colônias da Ilha do Governador, in *Relatório apresentado ao presidente da República dos Estados Unidos do Brasil, pelo ministro de Estado da justice e negócios interiores, J. J. Seabra, em abril de 1903*, ed. J. J. Seabra (Rio de Janeiro: Nácional, 1903), 4.

74. Ibid., 29.

75. Ibid., 36.

Chapter Five

1. Antônio Dias Barros, in T. M. P. Müller, "A Primeira Escola Especial para Creanças Anormaes no Distrito Federal—o Pavilhão Bourneville do Hospício Nacional de Alienados (1903–1920)" (EdD diss., apresentada à Faculdade de Educação da UERJ, 1998), 73.

2. A number of scholars describe the epistemological revolution in Western medical thinking that followed from the studies of several French physicians working in the newly secularized public hospitals of post-revolutionary Paris. See Erwin Ackerknecht, *La Medicine Hospitalière à Paris* (Paris: Payot, 1986); W. F. Bynum, *Science and the Practice of Medicine in the Nineteenth Century* (Cambridge: Cambridge University Press, 1994); Toby Gelfand, *Professionalizing Modern Medicine: Paris Surgeons and Medical Science and Institutions in the Eighteenth Century* (Westport, CT: Greenwood Press, 1980); and Louis Greenbaum, "Medicine in Revolution: An Essay Review," *Journal of the History of Medicine and Allied Sciences* 37, no. 1 (1982): 90–95.

3. Flávio Coelho Edler, "O Debate em Torno da Medicina Experimental no Segundo Reinado," *História, Ciências, Saúde-Manguinhos*, Rio de Janeiro, 3, no. 2 (1996): 284–99. For the US context, see Kenneth Ludmerer, *American Medical Education from the Turn of the Century to the Era of Managed Care* (Oxford: Oxford University Press, 1999).

4. Joanna Bleker, "Medical Students—to the Bedside or to the Laboratory? The Emergence of Laboratory training in German Medical Education, 1870–1900," *Clio Medica* 21 (1987–88): 35–46; Christopher Booth, "Clinical Research," in *Companion*

Encyclopedia of the History of Medicine, ed. W. F. Bynum and Roy Porter, vol. 1 (London: Routledge, 1993), 205–29.

5. See German Berrios and Renate Hauser, "The Early Development of Kraepelin's Ideas on Classification: A Conceptual History," *Psychological Medicine* 18 (1988): 813–21; Henri Ellenberger, *The Discovery of the Unconscious: The History and Evolution of Dynamic Psychiatry* (New York: Basic Books, 1970).

6. Daniel T. Rodgers, "In Search of Progressivism," *Reviews in American History* 10, no. 4 (1982): 122–23.

7. Nisia Trindade Lima and Gilberto Hochman, "Condenado pela Raça, Absolvido pela Medicina: O Brasil descoberto pelo Movimento Sanitarista da Primeira República," in *Raça, Ciência e Sociedade*, ed. Marcos Chor Maio and Ricardo Ventura Santos (Rio de Janeiro, Fiocruz, 1996), 23–40.

8. See Jonathan Toms, "Political Dimensions of 'the Psychosocial': The 1948 International Congress on Mental Health and the Mental Hygiene Movement," *History of the Human Sciences* 25, no. 5 (2012): 91–106, for a compelling examination of how the psychosocial, understood as the "relationship of mind, body and social environment in terms of mental health and ill-health," is a form of politics.

9. Cristiana Facchinetti, "Psicanálise para Brasileiros: História de sua Circulação e sua Apropriação no Entre-Guerras," *Culturas Psi* 1 (2012): 46.

10. Contrary to the dominant historiography, not all psychiatrists and social reformers subscribed to this understanding of degeneracy. Most notably, psychiatrist Renato Kehl understood racial and cultural degeneracy as fixed and argued for negative eugenics. See, for example, Robert Wegner and Vanderlei Sebastião de Souza, "Eugenia 'Negativa,' Psiquiatria e Catolicismo: Embates em torno da Esterilização Eugênica no Brasil," *História, Ciências, Saúde-Manguinhos* 20, no. 1 (January–March 2013): 263–88.

11. In 1925 Einstein visited Brazil, Argentina, and Uruguay within a series of travels around the world in the 1920s in the wake of a suddenly acquired fame. These travels had not only scientific repercussions but also (and in some cases especially) political and ideological purposes. Einstein was the first German with public prominence to visit these nations after World War I. He had the explicit aim of tightening the links among European nations and attempted to illustrate that science, as a transnational endeavor, could not be submitted to divisive issues of nationalism. See Alfredo Tolmasquim and I. C. Moreira, "Einstein in Brazil: the Communication to the Brazilian Academy of Sciences on the Constitution of Light," in *History of Modern Physics, Proceedings of the XXth International Congress of History of Science*, ed. H. Kragh, G. Vanpaemel, and P. Marage (Turnhout, Belgium: Brepols, 2002), 229–42.

12. Nonetheless, there were spontaneous cultural expressions that overshadowed the government-controlled domain.

13. Thomas E. Skidmore, *Black into White: Race and Nationality in Brazilian Thought* (Durham, NC: Duke University Press, 1993), 91.

14. Ibid., 136–37.

15. See Pablo Piccato, *City of Suspects: Crime in Mexico City, 1900–1931* (Durham, NC: Duke University Press, 2001), and Marcos Luiz Bretas, *Ordem na cidade: O Exercício Cotidiano da Autoridade Policial no Rio de Janeiro: 1907–1930* (São Paulo: Rocco, 1997).

16. Christine Ritui, "João do Rio: Ombre et Lumière du Rio de Janeiro de la Belle Époque," in *Littérature et Modernisation au Brésil*, ed. Jacqueline Penon and José Antonio Pasta Jr. (Paris: Sorbonne Nouvelle, 2004), 32.

17. "A favela," *Correio da Manhã*, June 4, 1907, 8.

18. "Os Ladrões do Rio," *Correio da Manhã*, April 27, 1907, 4.

19. "Não Se Pode Viver no Rio: Um Paiz Selvage," *Correio da Manhã*, August 14, 1907, 7.

20. "Colonia Correccional," *Correio da Manhã*, January 9, 1903, 13.

21. Alexandre Passos, *Juliano Moreira (Vida e Obra)* (Rio de Janeiro: Livraria São José, 1975), 17–18.

22. Ibid.

23. While the confluence of his intelligence and precociousness clearly made his meteoric rise to professional success deserved, he also benefited from the influence of a wealthy godfather as a steadfast patron.

24. Franklin Henry Martin, *South America from a Surgeon's Point of View* (Austin: Fleming H. Revell, 1922), 201.

25. Ibid.

26. Passos, *Juliano Moreira (vida e obra)*, 18–19.

27. Twelve members of the medical staff resided in the Wurzburg asylum, and most took months out of their clinical work to conduct research. Juliano Moreira, "A Clínica Psiquiátrica da Universidade de Wursburg," *Revista do Grêmio dos Internos dos Hospitais* 3, no. 2 (April 15, 1902): 18–21; no. 3 (May 15, 1902): 40–43.

28. France was model and inspiration for scientists and technicians in Brazil. The examples of École Polytecnique and Baron de Haussmann and the influence of Auguste Comte were constitutive elements in a larger background of Gallic influence in the arts, sciences, and elite culture in Brazil.

29. *Jornal do Brasil*, September 8, 1904, quoted in *O Rio de Janeiro de Pereira Passos: Uma Cidade em Questão II*, ed. Giovanna Rosso del Brenna (Rio de Janeiro: Index, 1985), 216.

30. Nicolau Sevcenko, *A Revolta da Vacina: Mentes Insanas em Corpos Rebeldes* (São Paulo: Cosac Naify, 2010), 80.

31. Jaime L. Benchimol, "Reforma Urbana e Revolta da Vacina na Cidade do Rio de Janeiro," in *O Brasil Republicano: O Tempo do Liberalismo Excludente: Da Proclamação da República à Revolução de 1930*, vol. 1, ed. Jorge Ferreira and Lucília de Almeida Neves Delgado (Rio de Janeiro: Civilização Brasileira, 2006), 265.

32. The frequent yellow fever outbreaks, especially during 1849–50, and smallpox outbreaks in 1834, 1836, and 1844, as well as a political recentralization of the imperial administration after 1840, led to the creation of a permanent public health infrastructure to replace temporary methods such as hospitalization and isolation. In 1846 the Imperial Vaccination Institute (Instituto Vacínico do Império) was established; it was incorporated, together with the health service of the ports, into the Public Hygiene Central Command (Junta Central de Higiene Pública) in 1850. This was Brazil's first attempt to standardize and nationalize its sanitary administration. The main epidemic diseases in Rio de Janeiro were yellow fever and smallpox, which made the imperial capital unsafe for passengers and freighters. After a decrease in epidemics in the 1860s, the city saw almost annual outbreaks of smallpox with high

rates of mortality during the 1870s. The 1887 epidemic, in particular, devastated Rio and stimulated the most important innovation at the end of the empire as animal vaccine production was at last begun that year. See Gilberto Hochman, *A Era do Saneamento: As Bases da Política de Saúde Pública no Brasil*, 3rd ed. (São Paulo: Hucitec, 1998).

33. In 1908, under the new name of *Arquivos Brasileiros de Psiquiatria, Neurologia e Medicina Legal*, it became the journal of the Society of Psychiatry, Neurology, and Forensic Medicine. Starting in 1919, it was published under the title *Arquivos Brasileiros de Neuriatria e Psiquiatria*. This psychiatric journal was the second one published in Latin America, after Argentina's *Archivos de Psiquiatria Criminologia*. See Paulo Dalgalarrondo, "As primeiras Revistas Psiquiátricas no Brasil e no Mundo," *Revista Brasileira de Psiquiatria* 21, no. 4 (December 1999): 237–38.

34. Nota Editorial, *Archivos Brasileiros de Psychiatria e Sciencias Affins* 1 (1905), 7.

35. Ibid.

36. Brasil, Ministério da Justiça e Negócios Interiores, *Relatório apresentado ao Presidente da República dos Estados Unidos do Brasil pelo Dr. Rivadavia da Cunha Corrêa* (Rio de Janeiro: Imprensa Nácional, 1912), 62. The Seabra Pavilion was where mentally ill men engaged in occupational therapy. They were engaged in works such as electrical mechanics, carpentry, woodwork, printing and bookbinding, shoemaking, bedmaking, and painting.

37. Ede Conceição Bispo Cerqueira, "A Sociedade Brasileira de Neurologia, Psiquiatria e Medicina Legal e o seu Papel na Institucionalização da Psiquiatria (1907–1928)," in ANPUH Anais do XXVII Simpósio Nacional de História, Natal, Rio Grande do Norte, 2013.

38. Juliano Moreira, "Quais os Melhores Meios de Assistência aos Alienados?" *Arquivos Brasileiros de Psiquiatria, Neurologia e Medicina Legal* 6, no. 2 (1910): 374.

39. Ibid., 374–75.

40. Max Nonne, "Impressiones de mi Viaje a la América del Sur," *Revista Médica de Hamburgo* 3, no. 3 (1923): 98.

41. *Archivos Brasileiros de Neuriatria e Psychiatria* 5, no. 1 (1923): 50.

42. Wilhelm Weygandt, "Juliano Moreira," trans. Inaldo de Lyra Neves-Manta. *Semanário de Psiquiatria e Neurologia* 25 (June 24, 1933): n.p.

43. *Deutsche Rio-Zeitung*, July 16, 1925, 1.

44. Ibid., July 18, 1925, 2.

45. Paulo Dalgalarrondo, "Cartas de Juliano Moreira a Emil Kraepelin," 1905, in *Civilização e Loucura: Uma Introdução à História da Ethnopsiquiatria* (São Paulo: Lemos, 1996), 117–24.

46. Karl Jaspers, *General Psychopathology*, trans. J. Hoenig and M. W. Hamilton (Manchester: Manchester University Press, 1963). Originally published in 1913 as *Allgemeine Psychopathologie*.

47. H. S. Decker, "The Psychiatric Works of Emil Kraepelin: A Many-Faceted Story of Modern Medicine," *Journal of the History of Neuroscience* 13 (2004): 248–76. Many scholars have pointed to his anti-Semitism and antisocialist biases. For example, he often claimed to "observe" a host of genetic predispositions for psychiatric disorders in Jews. See E. J. Engstrom, "Psychiatric Observations on Contemporary Issues," *History of Psychiatry* 3 (1992): 253–69.

48. Juliano Moreira, "Ligeira Vista sobre a Evolução da Assistência a Alienados na Alemanha, a Clínica Psiquiátrica de Munique," *Archivos Brasileiros de Psychiatria, Neurologia e Medicina Legal* 4, nos. 1–2 (1908): 184.

49. Juliano Moreira and Afrânio Peixoto, "Classificação das Moléstias Mentais do Prof. Emil Kraepelin," *Archivos Brasileiros de Psychiatria e Sciencias Affins* 1, no. 2 (1905): 205.

50. Paul Hoff, "Kraepelin and Degeneration Theory," *European Archives of Psychiatry and Clinical Neuroscience* 258, no. 2 (June 2008): 12–17.

51. Dain Borges, "'Puffy, Ugly, Slothful and Inert': Degeneration in Brazilian Social Thought, 1880–1940," *Journal of Latin American Studies* 25 (1993): 235. On classical texts that focus on degeneration, see J. Edward Chamberlain and Sander Gilman, eds., *Degeneration: The Dark Side of Progress* (New York: Columbia University Press, 1985); Robert Nye, *Crime, Madness, and Politics in Modern France: The Medical Concept of National Decline* (Princeton, NJ: Princeton University Press, 1984).

52. Borges, "'Puffy, Ugly, Slothful and Inert,'" 235.

53. Mariza Corrêa, *As Ilusões da Liberdade: A Escola Nina Rodrigues e a Antropologia no Brasil* (São Paulo: Edusp, 1998), 26.

54. One of his most often-cited works is *Os Africanos no Brasil* (São Paulo: Companhia Editora Nacional, 1932).

55. Nonetheless, he remained uncertain about mulattos and provided them with more agency by dividing them into typologies ranging from superior to degenerate. His uncertain classification of the mulatto may have reflected his own ambivalence about his mixed-race identity as well as many Brazilian elites, many of whom could be classified as mulatto.

56. Juliano Moreira, *Relatório do diretor do Hospício Nacional de Alienados relativo ao ano de 1905* (Rio de Janeiro: Imprensa Nácional, 1905), 65–66.

57. Ibid.

58. Juliano Moreira, "As Diretrizes da Higiene Mental entre Nós," *Revista de Medicina e Higiene Militar* (1922).

59. Juliano Moreira and A. Peixoto, "Les Maladies Mentales dans les Climats Tropicaux," *Archivos Brasileiros de Psychiatria, Neurologia e Sciencias Affins* 2, no. 1 (1906): 238.

60. Juliano Moreira and A. Peixoto, "A Paranóia e as Síndromes Paranoids," *Revista Latinoamericana de Psicopatologia Fundamental* 4, no. 2 (June 2001): 137. Originally published in 1905.

61. Ibid.

62. Afrânio Peixoto, *Elementos de Medicina Legal* (Rio de Janeiro: Francisco Alves, 1914), 77–78.

63. Afrânio Peixoto, *Clima e Saúde Introdução Bio-Geográfica à Civilização Brasileira* (São Paulo: Companhia Editora Nacional, 1938), 42, 140, 167; emphasis added.

64. Lilia Moritz Schwarcz, *O Espetáculo das Raças: Cientistas, Instituições e Pensamento Racial no Brasil: 1870–1930* (São Paulo: Companhia das Letras, 1993).

65. Nancy Leys Stepan, *The Hour of Eugenics: Race Gender, and Nation in Latin America* (Ithaca, NY: Cornell University Press, 1991), 73.

66. Ibid., 87.

67. Alcoholism went through various medical iterations that included alcoholic madness, alcoholic psychosis, and dipsomania. "Beginning in the early 19th century,

a series of medical writers began to lay the groundwork for what would eventually become the disease concept of alcoholism. Among these early contributors was Bruhl-Cramer, who in 1819 introduced the concept of drink seeking, or dipsomania. Esquirol (1845) was the first to give drunkenness or monomania a place in psychiatric nomenclatures, and Huss (1849) was first to use the term alcoholism. By the latter part of the nineteenth century, Carpenter (1850), Crothers (1893), Kerr (1888), and McBride (1910) had promulgated the disease concept of inebriety, which resembles what doctors now call dependence. In this formulation, inebriety and dipsomania were diseases, and their presumed origin was biological or possibly genetic." Bridget F. Grant and Debora A. Dawson, "Alcohol and Drug Use, Abuse, and Dependence: Classification, Prevalence, and Comorbidity," in Barbara McCrady and Elizabeth E. Epstein *Addictions: A Comprehensive Guidebook* (New York: Oxford University Press, 1999), 10. Also see Russil Durrant and Jo Thakker, *Substance Use and Abuse: Cultural and Historical Perspectives* (Thousand Oaks, CA: Sage, 2003).

68. Henrique Roxo, "Causas de Reinternação de Alienados no Hospício Nacional," *Arquivos Brasileiros de Psiquiatria, Neurologia e Medicina Legal.* Rio de Janeiro, ano VI, nos. 1 and 2, 406.

69. Lima Barreto, *Diário do Hospício*, 85.

70. A. A. Bandeira, *Gangrena social* (Rio de Janeiro: Typ. Jornal do Commercio, 1904).

71. Afrânio Peixoto, "Defesa Social Contra o Alcoolismo no Brasi," Actas do IV Congresso Medico Latino-Americano, Buenos Aires, 1904, in *Brazil-Medico, Revista Semanal de Medicina e Cirurgia* 18, no. 35 (September 15, 1904): 355–57.

72. Juliano Moreira, Hospital Nacional de Alienados (relatório), in *Arquivos Brasileiros de Psiquiatria, Neurologia e Ciências Afins*, 3, nos. 3–4 (1907): 274. Also Juliano Moreira, Relatório do Ministério da Justiça e Negócios Interiores (Rio de Janeiro: Imprensa Nácional, 1915), 76.

73. Brasil, Decreto nº 4.294, de 6 de julho de 1921. For example, segments of Decreto-Lei nº 4.294 (1921) called for the compulsory detainment of narcotics users (Article 6) in addition to the creation of specialized establishments of the cases.

74. He was also director of the Colônia de Psycopathas do Engenho do Dentro.

75. Liga Brasileira de Hygiene Mental, A Campanha Pró-Hygiene Mental: A Mais Relevante de Todas as Obras Medico-Sociaes em Nosso Paiz, *Archivos Brasileiros de Hygiene Mental* 7, no. 1 (1934): 65.

76. The *Archivos Brasileiros de Hygiene Mental* was the organization's primary publication. Due to federal funding cuts, the journal suspended publication from 1925 to 1929. *Archivos Brasileiros de Hygiene Mental* 2 (1929): 48–56; 5: 1–3.

77. *Archivos Brasileiros de Hygiene Mental* 2 (1929): 39–47; 13 (1941): 91–95.

78. M. Caldas, editorial, Os Archivos Brasileiros de Hygiene Mental, *Archivos Brasileiros de Hygiene Mental* 2, no. 1 (1929): 2.

79. Julia Kristeva, *Revolution in Poetic Language*, trans. Margaret Waller (1974; repr., New York: Columbia University Press, 1984), 84.

80. See Jean-Michel Quinodoz, *Reading Freud: A Chronological Exploration of Freud's Writings* (New York: Routledge, 2005).

81. The history of psychoanalysis in Brazil primarily chronicles its evolution from the 1930s to the 1970s. Notable recent works include C. Lucia M. Valladres de Oliveira, "Psychoanalysis in Brazil during Vargas' Time," and Jane A. Russo, "The

Social Diffusion of Psychoanalysis during the Brazilian Military Regime: Psychological Awareness in an Age of Political Repression," in *Psychoanalysis and Politics: Histories of Psychoanalysis Under Conditions of Restricted Freedom*, ed. Joy Damousi and Mariano Ben Plotkin (Oxford: Oxford University Press, 2012), 113–35, 165–84.

82. Richard G. Parker, *Bodies, Pleasures, and Passions: Sexual Culture in Contemporary Brazil* (Boston: Beacon Press, 1991), 33–34.

83. Franco da Rocha, *A Doutrina de Freud* (São Paulo: Cia Edit. Nacional, 1930), 169.

84. For example, Roxo, professor of psychiatry at the Rio de Janeiro School of Medicine, introduced Freudian doctrines in his courses, while Austregésilo, a doctor at the asylum and the first professor of neurology at the School of Medicine, featured psychoanalysis prominently in his self-help books for "nervous personalities." Arthur Ramos, a noted disciple of Raimundo Nina Rodrigues (a key figure in forensic medicine), made use of psychoanalytic theory in his anthropological studies on Afro-Brazilian culture. Further, sexuality features prominently in four iconic authors of Brazilian historiography during the 1920s and 1930s: Paulo Prado, Gilberto Freyre, Sérgio Buarque de Hollanda, and Caio Prado Júnior.

85. If not the most influential, he was second only to Arthur Ramos.

86. J. Porto-Carrero, *Ensaios de Psychanalyse* (Rio de Janeiro: Flores e Mano, 1929), 39–40.

87. J. Porto-Carrero, *Psicanálise de uma Civilização* (Rio de Janeiro: Guanabara, 1933), 226.

88. Porto-Carrero, *Ensaios de Psicanálise*, 73.

89. Sigmund Freud, *The Standard Edition of the Complete Psychological Works of Sigmund Freud*, ed. and trans. J. Strachey, 24 vols. (London: Hogarth Press, 1961), 14:94. The psychoanalytic literature even has some tendency to at least implicitly identify sublimation as a species of repression. For example, in his book *Sublimation: Inquiries into Theoretical Psychoanalysis* (New Haven, CT: Yale University Press, 1988), Hans Loewald posits that "traditionally sublimation is classified in psychoanalysis as a defense" (3), and in fact Freud's earliest reference to sublimation in his 1892 letter to Fliess refers to sublimations as "protective structures." In this sense, sublimations are another manifestation of the phenomenon that Freud calls "the return of the repressed." Sublimations undo the repressing of the energetic component; they steer it to an outlet, an aim that deviates from its original aim. See Ken Gemes, "Freud and Nietzsche on Sublimation," *Journal of Nietzche Studies* 38 (Autumn 2009): 38–59.

90. J. Porto-Carrero, *Grandezas e Misérias do Sexo* (Rio de Janeiro: Irmãos Pongetti, 1934), 35–36.

91. Ibid., 116.

92. For analysis of the construction of the bourgeois family in Brazilian medical and psychological discourse, see Roberto Machado, Ângela Loureiro, Rogério Luz, and Kátia Muricy, *Danação da Norma* (Rio de Janeiro: Graal, 1978); Jurandir Freire Costa, *Ordem Médica e Norma Familiar* (Rio de Janeiro: Graal, 1979); and Magali Engel, *Meretrizes e Doutores: O Saber Médico e a Prostituição na Cidade do Rio de Janeiro, 1845–1890* (São Paulo: Brasiliense, 1990).

93. Paulo Augusto de Figueiredo, "O Estado Novo e o Homem Novo," *Cultura Política* 1, no. 1 (March–April 1941): 133–38.

94. With the advent of the Estado Novo in 1937, all organs of the Ministry of Education and Public Health (from the then Ministry of Education and Health) related to health care became part of the Departamento Nacional de Saúde (DNS; National Department of Health). Among the four sections, the Care for the Mentally Ill was responsible for the "services relating to care for psychopaths and mental prophylaxis of national character, as well as those of local character that are run by the State, being further responsible for promoting the cooperation of the State on local services by means of federal grants and assistance to monitor the use of funds granted" (Brazil Constitution, 1937, Article 17). The National Department of Health was composed of four divisions: Public Health Division, Hospital Care Division, Support to Maternity and Child Division, and the Psychopath Care Division.

95. Cristina M. Fonseca, *Saúde no Governo* Vargas *(1930–1945): Dualidade Institucional de um Bem Público* (Rio de Janeiro: Editora Fiocruz, 2007).

96. Located in São Paulo and managed by Durval Marcondes, the other notable national institution during the 1930s was the Clínica de Orientação Infantil (1938). These clinics were some of the many institutions founded during the administration of Getúlio Vargas as part of an effort of widespread social reform. See Jerry Dávila, *Diploma of Whiteness: Race and Social Policy in Brazil, 1917–1945* (Durham, NC: Duke University Press, 2003), and Daryle Williams, *Culture Wars in Brazil: The First Vargas Regime, 1930–1945* (Durham, NC: Duke University Press, 2001).

97. The term was coined by psychiatrist Mirandolino Caldas. See M. Caldas, "A euphrenia: a Sciencia da Bôa Cerebração," *Archivos Brasileiros de Hygiene Mental* 5, no. 2 (December 1932).

98. *Archivos Brasileiros de Hygiene Mental* 5, no. 2 (October–December 1932): 68.

99. *Archivos Brasileiros de Hygiene Mental* 6, no. 1 (January–March 1933): 36–42.

100. "A Clínica de Euphrenia," *Archivos Brasileiros de Hygiene Mental* 5, no. 2 (March 1932).

101. Dávila, *Diploma of Whiteness*, 39.

102. Arthur Ramos, *A Familia e a Escola* (Conselhos de Higiene Mental aos Pais), Série D-Vulgarização (Rio de Janeiro: Oficina Gráfica do Departamento de Educação, 1934), 7.

103. Gilberto Freyre, "O Afro-Brasileiro," *Diário de Pernambuco* (November 3, 1934), 3. For a review of the conference, see Robert M. Levine, "The First Afro-Brazilian Congress: Opportunities for the Study of Race in the Brazilian Northeast," *Race and Class* 15, no. 2 (1973): 185–93. For an analysis of Arthur Ramos and racial thought in the 1930s, see Brad Lange, "Importing Freud and Lamarck to the Tropics: Arthur Ramos and the Transformation of Brazilian Racial Thought, 1926–1939," *The Americas*, 65, no. 1 (July 2008): 9–34, and Dávila, *Diploma of Whiteness*, 39–41.

104. In 1931 Prefect Pedro Ernesto invited him to become director general of public education for the Federal District. The post later became known as the Directorate General of the Department of Education of the Federal District, and in 1935, the General Secretariat for Education and Culture.

105. Arthur Ramos, *A Criança Problema*, 4th ed. (São Paulo: Casa do Estudante do Brasil, 1950), 20.

106. Ibid., 8.

107. Ibid., 23–25.

108. Dávila, *Diploma of Whiteness*, 49.

109. Arthur Ramos, *Saúde do Espírito—Higiene Mental* (Rio de Janeiro: Serviço de propaganda e educação sanitária, 1939), 51. The work bore the influence of the studies he had undertaken in *A Criança Problema.*

110. Ramos, *A Criança Problema,* 13. Ramos's condemnation of genetic determinism in particular reflects the influence of both Lévy-Bruhl and Neo-Lamarckian eugenics: "The action of the cultural environment is immense. Man is the product of his civilization and his society. This study is the specific result of sociology and cultural anthropology. . . . Human behavior varies in time and space. Opinions, attitudes, desires, and human logic vary historically and geographically. 'Culture' impregnates the individual, giving him his characteristic façade." See ibid., 40.

111. Ibid., 8.

112. Ibid.

113. Brazil Constitution, 1937, Article 17. Brasil. Lei no 378 de 13 de janeiro de 1937. Dá Nova Organização ao Ministério da Educação e Saúde Pública. Diário Oficial da União, Rio de Janeiro, January 15, 1937, 1210.

114. *Archivos Brasileiros de Hygiene Mental* 7, no. 3 (1934): 261.

115. See Jeffrey D. Needell, "The *Revolta Contra Vacina* of 1904: The Revolt Against 'Modernization' in Belle-Époque Rio de Janeiro," *Hispanic American Historical Review,* 67, no. 2 (May 1987): 233–69.

116. Maria Alice Rezende de Carvalho, *Quatro Vezes Cidade* (Rio de Janeiro: Sette Letras, 1994), 42.

Chapter Six

1. Antonio Xavier de Oliveira, *Espiritismo e Loucura, Contribuição ao Estudo do Factor Religioso em Psychiatria* (Rio de Janeiro: Alba, 1931), 192.

2. Raymundo Nina Rodrigues, *O Animismo Fetichista dos Negros Baianos* (Rio de Janeiro: Civilização Brasileira, 1935), 81.

3. Ibid., 36.

4. Lee Clarke and Caron Chess, "Elites and Panic: More to Fear than Fear Itself," *Social Forces* 87, no. 2 (2008): 993–1014. As the authors note, definitions of panic have been inconsistent, 996.

5. Neil J. Smelser, *Theory of Collective Behavior* (New York: Free Press, 1962), 131.

6. Janet Roitman, *Anti-crisis* (Durham, NC: Duke University Press, 2014), 3–4.

7. Lucien Febvre, "History and Psychology," 1938, in *A New Kind of History,* ed. Peter Burke (London: Harper & Row, 1973), 9.

8. Lucien Febvre, "Sensibility and History: How to Reconstitute the Emotional Life of the Past," 1941, in *A New Kind of History,* ed. Peter Burke (London: Harper & Row, 1973), 24.

9. Steven Lukes, Michael Carrithers, and Steven Collins, eds., *The Category of the Person: Anthropology, Philosophy, History* (Cambridge: Cambridge University Press, 1985), 299.

10. David J. Hess, *Spirits and Scientists: Ideology, Spiritism, and Brazilian Culture* (University Park: Penn State University Press, 1991), and Emerson Giumbelli, *O Cuidado dos Mortos: Uma História da Condenção e Legitimação do Espiritismo* (Rio de Janeiro: Arquivo Nacional, 1997).

11. See Alexander Moreira-Almeida, Angélica A. Silva de Almeida, and Francisco Lotufo Neto, "History of 'Spiritist Madness' in Brazil," *History of Psychiatry* 16, no. 1 (2005): 5–25.

12. See Roger Bastide, *O Candomblé da Bahia* (1958; repr., São Paulo: Companhia das Letras, 2001), in addition to his edited work, *Estudos Afro-Brasileiros* (São Paulo: Perspectiva, 1973). R. Lewis-Fernández and A. Kleinman, "Cultural Psychiatry: Theoretical, Clinical, and Research Issues, *Psychiatric Clinics of North America* 18 (1995): 433–48.

13. Agenor Miranda Rocha, *Os Candomblés Antigos do Rio de Janeiro: A Naçao Ketu: Origens, Ritos, e Crenças* (Rio de Janeiro: Faculdade da Cidade, Topbooks, 1995), 31–34.

14. Teresa A. Meade, *'Civilizing' Rio: Reform and Resistance in a Brazilian City, 1889–1930* (University Park: Penn State University Press, 1997), 34.

15. Clovis Moura, *Brasil: Raizes do Protesto Negro* (São Paulo: Global Editora, 1983), 90.

16. Holloway, *Policing Rio de Janeiro.*

17. Yvonne Maggie, *Medo do Feitiço: Relações entre Magia e Poder no Brasil* (Rio de Janeiro: Arquivo Nacional, Orgão do Ministério da Justiça, 1992), 22.

18. Ibid.

19. Another national attempt at mediating the new religious liberty came just shortly thereafter with the addition of Law 173 of 1893, which regulated religious associations. It granted juridic rights only to associations that declared their existence in civil registers and that did not promote "illicit" and "immoral" ends. Maggie, *Medo do Feitiço,* 43–44. The terminology of these measures, as those of 1890, remained ominously vague with its reference to some acts as "illegal medicine" or "illicit ends."

20. Jurandir Freire Costa, *Ordem Medica e Norma Familiar* (Rio de Janeiro: Graal, 1989).

21. Ibid., 57.

22. Dain Borges, "The Recognition of Afro-Brazilian Symbols and Ideas, 1890–1940," *Luso-Brazilian Review* 32, no. 2 (1995): 59–78, 63.

23. Maggie, *Medo do Feitiço,* 43.

24. Paulo (João do Rio) Barreto, *As Religiões no Rio* (1906; repr., Rio de Janeiro: Edição da Organização Simões, 1951).

25. Ibid., 35.

26. Ibid., 200.

27. Most studies of spiritism in Brazil have focused on the national context. Apart from David J. Hess, *Spirits and Scientists: Ideology, Spiritism, and Brazilian Culture* (University Park: Penn State University Press, 1991), and Emerson Giumbelli, *O Cuidado dos Mortos: Uma História da Condenção e Legitimação do Espiritismo* (Rio de Janeiro: Arquivo Nacional, 1997), see Angélica Aparecida Silva de Almeida, Ana Maria Galdini Raimundo Oda, and Paulo Dalgalarrondo, "O Olhar dos Psiquiatrias Brasileiros sobre Os Fenômenos de Transe e Possessão," *Revista de Psiquiatria Clínica* (São Paulo) 34: suppl. 1 (2007): 34–41, and Yvonne Maggie, *Medo do Feitiço: Relações entre Magia e Poder no Brasil* (Rio de Janeiro: Arquivo Nacional, 1992). Most studies give a perfunctory nod to spiritism's international presence. Some scholars, however, have gestured toward transnational spiritism and spiritualism or offered multisited studies. See, for example, Bridget Bennett, *Transatlantic Spiritualism and*

Nineteenth-century American Literature (New York: Palgrave Macmillan, 2007); Alex Owen, *The Darkened Room: Women, Power and Spiritualism in Late Victorian England*, New Cultural Studies Series (Philadelphia: University of Pennsylvania Press, 1990); Cristina Rocha, "A Globalização Do Espiritismo: Fluxos Do Movimento Religioso de João de Deus Entre a Austrália e o Brasil," *Revista de Antropologia* 52, no. 2 (July 1, 2009): 571–603; and Reinaldo Roman, *Governing Spirits: Religion, Miracles, and Spectacles in Cuba and Puerto Rico, 1898–1956* (Chapel Hill: University of North Carolina Press, 2008).

28. Allan Kardec, in *Qu'est-ce que le Spiritisme? Préambule of Le Livre des Esprits* (Paris: E. Dentu, 1857). Translated from the original French.

29. Catherine L. Albanese, *A Republic of Mind and Spirit: A Cultural History of American Metaphysical Religion* (New Haven, CT: Yale University Press, 2007), 180. As Albanese notes, Quakers had flirted with spirit communication prior to the sisters' séances, and Kate and Margaret Fox's spirit demonstrations appealed to their belief in "an unbroken chain of communication" between "the Infinite and all beings." 181.

30. Ibid.

31. Ibid., 266, 260.

32. The term *codification* refers to the set of books written by Allan Kardec. The books are a compilation of questions made by Allan Kardec and the answers that allegedly stemmed from spirits between the years 1857 and 1868. The books included *The Spirits' Book* (Le Livre des Esprits) (1857); *The Mediums' Book* (Le Livre des Médiums) (1861); *The Gospel According to Spiritism* (L'Évangile Selon le Spiritisme) (1864); *Heaven and Hell* (Le Ciel et L'Enfer) (1865); and *The Genesis According to Spiritism* (La Genèse) (1868). Lynn Sharp, *Secular Spirituality: Reincarnation and Spiritism in Nineteenth-century France* (Plymouth, MA: Lexington Books, 2006), 73–81.

33. Ibid., 54, 65.

34. Ibid., 100. Note, however, that Kardec's emphasis on individual responsibility stands at odds with what Sharp identifies as French spiritists' interest in socialism.

35. Ibid.

36. According to Kardec, "It is easy to distinguish between advanced and less advanced spirits. The language of higher spirits is dignified, high-minded, and free from every trace of human passion. . . . On the other hand, remarks by less advanced spirits make use of commonplace, sometimes coarse, language and often contain substantial inconsistencies." See Allan Kardec, *The Spirits' Book* (1857; repr., New York: Studium, 1980), 13.

37. Artur César Isaia, "A República e a Teleologia Histórica do Espiritismo," in *Espiritismo e Religiões Afro-Brasileiras*, ed. Artur César Isaia, Ivan Aparecido Manoel (São Paulo: Ed. Unesp., 2012), 103–17, 110.

38. Ubiratan Machado, *Os Intelectuais e o Espiritismo: De Castro Alves a Machado de Assis* (Rio de Janeiro: Publicações Lachâtre, 1996), 103.

39. Garnier editors published the books. *The Spirits' Book, The Mediums' Book*, and *Heaven and Hell* were published in 1875; *The Gospel According to Spiritism* was published in 1876. The homeopathic doctor Joaquim Carlos Travassos translated all works to Portuguese.

40. Syliva Damazio, *Da elite ao Povo: Advento e Expansão do Espiritismo no Rio de Janeiro* (Rio de Janeiro: Bertrand Brasil, 1994).

41. See John Warne Monroe, *Laboratories of Faith: Mesmerism, Spiritism, and Occultism in Modern France* (Ithaca, NY: Cornell University Press, 2008).

42. Machado, *Os Intelectuais e o Espiritismo,* 210.

43. Barreto, *As Religiões no Rio,* 72.

44. Machado, *Os Intelectuais e o Espiritismo,* 227.

45. Ibid., 25.

46. By the turn of the twentieth century, the O Centro Espírita Redemptor (1911) would join the FEB and together they would eclipse other organizations as the de facto public representatives of spiritism. However, they differed in ideological orientation, as the FEB followed the teachings of Kardec and the Redemptor rejected them.

47. Reformador, January 1884.

48. The organization's newspaper, *The Reformador,* noted that all were welcome to visit the open assistance clinic located on Rua da Alfandega, 34, second floor, and attend sessions at two o'clock. *Reformador,* May 15, 1890.

49. See Robert Henry Moser, *The Carnivalesque Defunto: Death, and the Dead in Modern Brazilian Literature* (Athens: Ohio University Press, 2008), 10–41. Menezes Cavalcanti is also known as the Brazilian Freud. See G. Reginald Daniel, *Machado de Assis: Multiracial Identity and the Brazilian Novelist* (University Park: Penn State University Press, 2012), 249.

50. Adolfo Bezerra de Menezes Cavalcanti, *A Loucura Sob Novo Prisma,* 12th ed. (Rio de Janeiro: FEB, 2005), 110.

51. Ibid., 148.

52. Ibid., 157.

53. Carlos Aguirre and Ricardo D. Salvatore, "Writing the History of Law, Crime, and Punishment in Latin America," in *Crime and Punishment in Latin America: Law and Society since Late Colonia Times,* ed. Ricardo D. Salvatore, Carlos Aguirre, and Gilbert M. Joseph (Durham, NC: Duke University Press, 2001), 4.

54. Jacques Derrida, "Force of Law: The 'Mystical Foundation of Authority,'" trans. Mary Quaintance, *Cardozo Law Review* 2, nos. 5–6 (July–August 1990): 929.

55. Maggie, *Medo do Feitiço.*

56. *O Reformador,* December 15, 1890, 1–2.

57. Isaia, "A República e a Teleologia Histórica do Espiritismo," 109.

58. *O Reformador,* November 1, 1890, 1.

59. Ibid., November 15, 1890, 1.

60. *Jornal do Commércio,* December 23, 1890, 2.

61. Ibid.

62. Ibid.

63. Ibid., January 16, 1891, 2.

64. Smith's book, *Conjuring Culture: Biblical Formations of Black America,* investigates "how black Americans have attempted to render American law as a social curative or pharmakon (Greek: medicine and poison) for transforming the destructive reality of slavery." See Theopus H. Smith, *Conjuring Culture: Biblical Formations of Black America* (New York: Oxford University Press, 1994), 82.

65. Francisco da Rocha (1864–1933) was the founder of the Juquery Hospital Asylum, a landmark institution in the history of psychiatry in the state of São Paulo.

He was also founder of the first psychoanalytic society in South America (1927). In 1918 he became university professor at today's University of São Paulo.

66. Francisco da Rocha, *Hospício de Alienados de São Paulo—Estatística* (São Paulo: Typographia do Diario Oficial, 1896), 33.

67. *O Paulista,* October 14, 1885, in Rocha, *Hospício de Alienados de São Paulo,* 22.

68. Nina Rodrigues, *O Animismo Fetichista dos Negros Bahianos* (1896; repr., Rio de Janeiro: Civilização Brasileira, 1935), 99, 116–17.

69. Paul C. Johnson, *Spirited Things: The Work of "Possession" in Afro-Atlantic Religions* (Chicago: University of Chicago Press, 2014), 42.

70. O. S. Pimentel, "Em torno do Espiritismo" (MD thesis, Faculdade de Medicina do Rio de Janeiro, 1919); A. Guimarães Filho, "Da hygiene mental e sua importância em nosso meio" (MD thesis, FMSP, São Paulo, 1926); C. Marques, "Espiritismo e idéias delirantes" (MD thesis FMRJ, Rio de Janeiro, 1929"; P. Cavalcanti, "Estado mental dos médiuns" (MD thesis, Faculdade de Medicina, Recife, 1934).

71. Although the session occurred in 1909, details of its account were not published until 1939. See *Diário da Noite,* 1939; *Annaes da Academia de Medicina,* 1911, 326.

72. Ibid.

73. *Annaes da Academia de Medicina,* 1911, p. 328.

74. I. Ferreira, *Têm Razão?* (Uberaba, Brazil: Gráfica Mundo Espírita, 1946), 51.

75. Ibid., 49.

76. Ibid., 54.

77. The poet Oswald de Andrade developed this concept of cultural cannibalism (Manifesto Antropófago, 1928).

78. They included one engineer and eleven distinguished doctors and professors from the colleges of Medicine and Law based out of Rio de Janeiro, São Paulo, and Bahia. There were five psychiatrists (Henrique Roxo, Franco da Rocha, Julio Porto-Carrero, Pacheco e Silva, and Silva Pernambuco Filho), two neurologists (Antônio Austregésilo and Faustino Esposel), one pathologist (Raul Leitão da Cunha), one legal scholar (Tanner de Abreu), two public health investigators (João Froes and Carlos Seidl), and an engineer (Everardo Backeuser).

79. L. Ribeiro and M. Campos, *O Espiritismo no Brasil: Contribuição ao seu Estudo Clínico e Medico-Legal* (São Paulo: Companhia Editora Nacional, 1931), 153.

80. Ibid.

81. It was characterized by auditory hallucinations and kinesthetic hallucinations, with secondary deliriums, that emerge after a session. See H. Roxo, "Delirio espirita episodico nas classes populares do Rio de Janeiro," *Archivos Brasileiros de Medicina* 28, no. 2 (1938): 60–61.

82. Rocha, *Hospício de Alienados de São Paulo,* 168.

83. See ibid. and Roxo, "Delirio espirita." Also see A. C. Pacheco e Silva, "A Higiene Mental e o Espiritismo," in his *Palavras de Psiquiatria* (São Paulo: Pacheco e Silva, 1950); A. C. Pacheco e Silva, "O Espiritismo e As Doenças Mentais no Brasil," *Anais Portugueses de Psiquiatria* 2, no. 2 (1950): 1–6; and L. Ribeiro, *De Médico a Criminalista* (Rio de Janeiro: Livraria São José, 1967).

84. Rocha, *Hospício de Alienados de São Paulo.*

85. Ribeiro and Campos, *O Espiritismo no Brasil*; X. de. Oliveira, *Espiritismo e Loucura* (Rio de Janeiro: A. Coelho Franco Filho, 1931).

86. M. Caldas, "As Causas e a Prophylaxia do Suicidio," *Archivos Brasileiros de Hygiene Mental*, 2, no. 3 (1929): 158–59.

87. A. Peixoto, "Violencia Carnal e Mediunidade," *Archivos Brasileiros de Psychiatria, Neurologia e Medicina Legal* 5, nos. 1–2 (1909): 78–94.

88. Emerson A. Giumbelli, "Heresia, Doença, Crime ou Religião: O Espiritismo no Discurso de Médicose Cientistas Sociais," *Revista de Antropologia* 40, no. 2 (1997): 31–82.

89. Quoted in Maggie, *Medo do Feitiço*, 44–45 (author's translation).

90. A. L. Nobre de Mello, *Diário da Noite*, June 2, 1939.

91. S. O., "O Espiritismo Atacado por ter Feito 1.372 Loucos em dez annos, responde com a assistência gratuita de 10.000 enfermos em 24 mezes," *Diário da Noite* 1–2 (June 1939).

92. The program lasted until 1942.

93. Artur Cesar Isaia, "João do Rio: O Flâneur e O Preconceito: Um Olhar Sobre o Transe Mediúnico na Capital Federal de Inícios do Século XX," in *Religiões, Religiosidades e Diferenças Culturais*, ed. J. R. Marin (Campo Grande, Brazil: UCDB, 2005), 112.

94. Peixoto in Ribeiro and Campos, *O Espiritismo no Brasil*, 6.

95. Oliveira, *Espiritismo e Loucura*, 241.

96. Odilon Galloti, "O Espiritismo," *O Globo* (Rio de Janeiro), October 23, 1935, 1.

97. Osório César, "Fenomenologia Supranormal," *Revista Paulista de Medicina* 195 (1941): 60.

98. Ibid., 49–50.

99. José Leme Lopes, "Psiquiatria e Antropologia," *Neurobiologia, Recife*, 42, no. 1 (1979): 3–12. Bastide affirmed that possession trance was foremost a sociological rather than a pathological phenomenon. See Roger Bastide, *O Candomblé da Bahia* (São Paulo: Companhia Editora Nacional, 1978).

100. René Ribeiro, *Antropologia da Religião e outros Estudos* (Recife: Editora Massangana, 1982), and C. Martins, "Psiquiatria Transcultural e Países em Desenvolvimento, *Revista Brasileira de Psiquiatria*, 3, no. 1 (1969): 31–62.

101. Birgit Meyer and Peter Pels, eds., *Magic and Modernity: Interfaces of Revelation and Concealment* (Stanford, CA: Stanford University Press, 2003), 3.

102. Michael Saler, "Modernity and Enchantment: A Historiographical Review," *American Historical Review* 111, no. 3 (2006): 692–716.

103. Robert Levine, *The Vargas Regime: The Critical Years, 1934–1938* (New York: Columbia University Press, 1970).

104. Ibid.

105. Williams, *Culture Wars in Brazil*, 83–85.

106. E. Bradford Burns, ed., *A Documentary History of Brazil* (New York: Alfred A. Knopf, 1966), 352.

107. James C. Scott, *Seeing like a State: How Certain Schemes to Improve the Human Condition Have Failed* (New Haven, CT: Yale University Press, 1998), 2.

108. Maggie, *Medo do Feitiço*, 46.

109. This did not so much resolve the issue, though, as simply push it into a different arena. Although the law indirectly affirmed that some forms of traditional candomblé could constitute a legitimate religion and ought to be protected, the article simultaneously implied that most terreiros are not traditional, legitimate, or worthy

of state protection; they were not, in other words, a religion. Vargas's acts left the issue of religion versus magic open to interpretation as a valid distinction.

Conclusion

1 See "A Assistencia do Governo aos Enfermos: Visita do Presidente da Republica á Colonia Juliano Moreira," *Jornal do Brasil*, September 1, 1940, 8.

2. Charles H. Long, *Significations: Signs, Symbols and Images in the Interpretation of Religion* (1986; Reprint., Aurora, CO: Davies Group Publishers, 1999), 7.

3. Unlike earlier philosophical and religious definitions of being human, Freud transformed ideas of what it means to be a person through the psychoanalytic method, replacing the moral or religious view of man with a scientific view. From this perspective, Albert Borgmann posits that Freud extended modernism to the study of man in that he elaborated the principles developed by Bacon, Descartes, and Locke, which incorporated man's dominations of nature, the primacy of method, and the sovereignty of the individual. See Albert Borgmann, *Crossing the Postmodern Divide* (Chicago: University of Chicago Press, 1992).

Bibliography

Archives

Academia Nacional de Medicina, Rio de Janeiro.
Arquivo do Instituto Histórico e Geográfico Brasileiro, Rio de Janeiro.
Arquivo Geral da Cidade do Rio de Janeiro.
Arquivo Nacional do Rio de Janeiro.
Arquivo Público do Estado do Rio de Janeiro.
Biblioteca Nacional do Rio de Janeiro, Seção de Periódicos & Seção de Manuscritos.
Juliano Moreira Municipal Institute of Assistance and Health (Rio de Janeiro).
Nise da Silveira Municipal Institute (Rio de Janeiro).
Philippe Pinel Institute (Rio de Janeiro).

Published Primary Sources

Anais da Câmara dos Deputados: 1852; 1896; 1897; 1903; 1906; 1920; 1926.

Anais do Senado: 1882; 1894; 1896; 1898; 1903; 1926.

Araújo, D. L. S. *Relatório do Diretor das Colônias de Alienados, Dr. Domingos Lopes da Silva Araújo, apresentado ao diretor geral da Assisência, Dr. João Carlos Teixeira Brandão, em 28 de janeiro de 1895*. Rio de Janeiro: Imprensa Nacional, 1895.

Azevedo, Manuel Duarte Moreira de. "A Faculdade de Medicina do Rio de Janeiro: Notícia Histórica." *Revista do Instituto Histórico e Geográfico Brasileiro* 30, no. 4 (1867): 397–418.

———. *O Rio de Janeiro: Sua História, Monumentos, Home ns Notáveis, Usos e Curiosidades*. Vol. 1. Rio de Janeiro: Garnier, 1877.

Barbosa, M. J. *Relatório e estatística do Hospício de Pedro II*, de 09/12/1852 até 30/07/1853. Rio de Janeiro: Tip. Dois de Dezembro, 1853.

———. "Relatório e estatística do Hospital de Pedro II, desde 1 de Julho de 1854 até 30 de Julho de 1855." *Anais Brasilienses de Medicina* 10, no. 4 (1856): 98–104, 118–21.

Beviláqua, Clóvis. *Esboços e Fragmentos*. Rio de Janeiro: Laemmert, 1899.

Bilac, Olavo. "No Hospicio Nacional—Uma Visita á Secção das Creanças." *Revista Kosmos* 2, no. 2 (1905).

Brandão, João Carlos Teixeira. *Os Alienados no Brasil*. Rio de Janeiro: Imprensa Nácional, 1886.

———. *Questões Relativas à Assistência Médico-Legal a Alienados.* Rio de Janeiro: Imprensa Nácional, 1897.

———. *Relatório da Assistência Médico Legal de Alienados apresentado ao Ministro de Estado Negócios do Interior, Fernando Lobo Leite Pereira, pelo Dr. João Carlos Teixeira Brandão, Diretor Geral.* Rio de Janeiro: Imprensa Nacional, 1892.

Brasil. *Decreto nº 4.294, de 6 de julho de 1921.*

Brasil, Ministério da Justiça e Negócios Interiores. *Relatório apresentado ao Presidente da República dos Estados Unidos do Brasil pelo Dr. Rivadavia da Cunha Corrêa.* Rio de Janeiro: Imprensa Nácional, 1912.

Brasil, 1937, Article 17. Brasil. Lei no 378 de 13 de janeiro de 1937. *Dá Nova Organização ao Ministério da Educação e Saúde Pública.* Diário Oficial da União, Rio de Janeiro, pg. 1210. 15 jan. 1937.

Caldas, Mirandolino. "A euphrenia: a Sciencia da Bôa Cerebração." *Archivos Brasileiros de Hygiene Mental* 5, no. 2 (December 1932).

———. "As Causas e a Prophylaxia do Suicidio." *Archivos Brasileiros de Hygiene Mental* 2, no. 3 (1929): 158–59.

———. "Os Archivos Brasileiros de Hygiene Mental." *Archivos Brasileiros de Hygiene Mental* 2, no. 1 (1929).

Cavalcanti, Pedro. "Estado mental dos médiuns." PhD thesis, Faculdade de Medicina, Recife, 1934.

César, Osório. "Fenomenologia Supranormal." *Revista Paulista de Medicina* 19, no. 5 (1941): 49–73.

de Oliveira, Antonio Xavier. *Espiritismo e Loucura.* Rio de Janeiro: Alba, 1931.

De Simoni, Luís Vicente. "Importância e necessidade da criação de um manicômioo ou estabelecimento especial para o tratamento de alienados." *Revista Médica Fluminense* 5, no. 6 (September 1839): 241–62.

Eiras, M. J. F. "Questões Sociais: A Nova Cadeira de Psychiatria-Hospício de Pedro II-organização de novos asylos de alienados e uma legislação apropriada." Parts I, II, III, IV, V. *Jornal do Commércio,* February 17, 18, 21, 23 and March 1, 1883.

Ferreira, Inácio. *Têm Razão?* Uberaba, Brazil: Gráfica Mundo Espírita, 1946.

Figueiredo, Paulo Augusto de. "O Estado Novo e o Homem Novo." *Cultura Política* 1, no. 1 (March–April 1941): 133–38.

Filho, A. Guimarães. "Da hygiene mental e sua importância em nosso meio." MD thesis, FMSP, São Paulo, 1926.

Freyre, Gilberto. "O Afro-Brasileiro." *Diário de Pernambuco,* November 3, 1934.

Kardec, Allan. *Qu'est-ce que le Spiritisme? Préambule of Le Livre des Esprits.* Paris: E. Dentu, 1857.

———. *The Spirits' Book.* 1857. Reprint, New York: Studium, 1980.

Liga Brasileira de Hygiene Mental. "A campanha pró-hygiene mental: A mais relevante de todas as obras medico-sociaes em nosso paiz." *Archivos Brasileiros de Hygiene Mental* 7, no. 1 (1934): 63–72.

Lobo, Fernando. *Relatório apresentado ao Vice-Presidente da República dos Estados Unidos do Brasil, pelo Dr. Fernando Lobo, Ministro de Estado da Justiça e Negócios Interiores, em Abril de 1893.* Rio de Janeiro: Imprensa Nacional, 1893.

Machado de Assis, Joaquim M. *Crônica de 02/12/1894,* in *Obra Complete: Poesia, Crônica, Miscelânea e Epistolário.* Rio de Janeiro: Edior José Aguilar, 1959.

Marques, João Coelho. "Espiritismo e idéias delirantes." MD thesis, FMRJ, Rio de Janeiro, 1929.

Martin, Franklin Henry. *South America from a Surgeon's Point of View.* New York: Fleming H. Revell Company, 1922.

McDowall, T. W. "Part Three: Psychological Retrospect." *Journal of Mental Science* 22 (1877): 614–28.

Moreira, Juliano. "As Diretrizes da Higiene Mental entre Nós." *Revista de Medicina e Higiene Militar* (1922): n.p.

———. "Hospital Nacional de Alienados (relatório)." *Arquivos Brasileiros de Psiquiatria, Neurologia e Ciências Afins* 3, nos. 3–4 (1907): 429–35.

———. "Ligeira Vista sobre a Evolução da Assistência a Alienados na Alemanha, a Clínica Psiquiátrica de Munique." *Archivos Brasileiros de Psychiatria, Neurologia e Medicina Legal* 4, nos. 1–2 (1908): 172–86.

———. "Quais os Melhores Meios de Assistência aos Alienados?" *Arquivos Brasileiros de Psiquiatria, Neurologia e Medicina Legal* 6, nos. 1–2 (1910): 373–96.

———. *Relatório do diretor do Hospício Nacional de Alienados relativo ao ano de 1905.* Rio de Janeiro: Imprensa Nácional, 1905.

Moreira, Juliano, and Afrânio Peixoto. "A Paranóia e as Síndromes Paranoids." 1905. *Revista Latinoamericana de Psicopatologia Fundamental* 4, no. 2 (June 2001): 134–67.

———. "Classificação das Moléstias Mentais do Prof. Emil Kraepelin." *Archivos Brasileiros de Psychiatria e Sciencias Affins* 1, no. 2 (1905): 204–16.

———. "Les Maladies Mentales dans les Climats Tropicaux." *Archivos Brasileiros de Psychiatria, Neurologia e Sciencias Affins* 2, no. 1 (1906): 222–41.

Nonne, Max. "Impressiones de mi Viaje a la América del Sur." *Revista Médica de Hamburgo* 3, no. 3 (1923): 97–100.

Nota Editorial. *Archivos Brasileiros de Psychiatria e Sciencias Affins* 1 (1905): n.p.

Peixoto, Afrânio. *Clima e Saúde Introdução Bio-Geográfica à Civilização Brasileira.* São Paulo: Companhia Editora Nacional, 1938.

———. "Defesa Social Contra o Alcoolismo no Brasil." Actas do IV Congresso Medico Latino-Americano, Buenos Aires, April 1904. In *Brazil-Medico, Revista Semanal de Medicina e Cirurgia* 18, no. 35 (September 15, 1904): 355–57.

———. *Elementos de Medicina Legal.* Rio de Janeiro: Francisco Alves, 1914.

———. "Violencia Carnal e Mediunidade." *Archivos Brasileiros de Psychiatria, Neurologia e Medicina Legal* 5, nos. 1–2 (1909): 78–94.

Pimentel, Oscar dos Santos. *Em Torno do Espiritismo.* MD thesis, Faculdade de Medicina do Rio de Janeiro, 1919.

Porto-Carrero, Júlio. *Ensaios de Psicanálise.* Rio de Janeiro: Flores e Mano, 1929.

———. *Ensaios de Psychanalyse.* Rio de Janeiro: Flores e Mano, 1929.

———. *Grandezas e Misérias do Sexo.* Rio de Janeiro: Irmãos Pongetti, 1934.

———. *Psicanálise de uma Civilização.* Rio de Janeiro: Guanabara, 1933.

Ramos, Arthur. *A Criança Problema.* 4th ed. São Paulo: Casa do Estudante do Brasil, 1950.

———. *A Familia e a Escola* (Conselhos de Higiene Mental aos Pais), Série D-Vulgarização. Rio de Janeiro: Oficina Gráfica do Departamento de Educação, 1934.

———. *Saúde do Espírito—Higiene Mental.* Rio de Janeiro: Serviço de propaganda e educação sanitária, 1939.

Relatórios do Ministério do Império, 1833–42; 1852–60; 1863; 1865–71. *A Santa Casa de Misericórdia do Rio de Janeiro e o Hospício de Pedro II (Documentos)*. Rio de Janeiro: Tip. de J. Villenuve e C., 1882.

Républica do Estados Unidos dos Brasil, Recenseamento do Rio de Janeiro (Distrito Federal). Rio de Janeiro: Officina da Estatística, 1930.

Rey, Phillipe-Marius. *L'Hospice Pédro II et les Aliénés au Brésil*. Paris: Imprimerie de E. Donnaud, 1875.

Ribeiro, L., and M. Campos. *O Espiritismo no Brasil: Contribuição ao seu estudo clínico e medico-legal*. São Paulo: Companhia Editora Nacional, 1931.

Rocha, Francisco da. *Hospício de Alienados de São Paulo—Estatística*. São Paulo: Typographia do Diario Oficial, 1896.

Rocha, Franco da. *A Doutrina de Freud*. São Paulo: Cia Edit. Nacional, 1930.

Rodrigues, Raymundo Nina. *As Raças Humanas e a Responsabilidade Penal*. 1894. Reprint, Salvador, Brazil: Livraria Progresso, 1957.

———. *O Animismo Fetichista dos Negros Baianos*. Rio de Janeiro: Civilização Brasileira, 1935.

———. *Os Africanos no Brasil*. São Paulo: Companhia Editora Nacional, 1932.

Roxo, Henrique. "Causas de Reinternação de Alienados no Hospício Nacional." *Arquivos Brasileiros de Psiquiatria, Neurologia e Medicina Legal* 6, nos. 1–2 (1910): 403–15.

———. "Delirio espirita episodico nas classes populares do Rio de Janeiro." *Archivos Brasileiros de Medicina* 28, no. 2 (1938): 59–72.

Sigaud, José Francisco Xavier. "Reflexões acerca do trânsito livre dos doidos pelas ruas da cidade do Rio de Janeiro." *Diário de Saúde* 1, no. 1. Rio de Janeiro: Tip. Imp. E Const. De Seignot-Plancher e Comp., 1835.

Silva, J. J. L. da. "Relatório apresentado ao Provedor da Santa Casa da Misericórdia do Rio de Janeiro, de julho de 1866 a junho de 1867." *Gazeta Médica da Bahia* 40, nos. 42–43 (1868): 186–90, 214–15, 225–27.

Silva, J. M. Pereira da. *Segundo Periodo do Reinado de Dom Pedro I no Brazil*. Rio de Janeiro: B. L. Garnier, 1871.

Walsh, Robert. *Notices of Brazil in 1828 and 1829*. Boston: Richardson et al., 1831.

Weygandt, Wilhelm. "Juliano Moreira." Translated in Portugese in abbreviated form by Inaldo de Lyra Neves-Manta. *Semanário de Psiquiatria e Neurologia* 25 (June 24, 1933): n.p.

Secondary Works

Abel, Christopher. *Hygiene and Sanitation in Latin America c. 1870–1950*. London: Institute of Latin American Studies, University of London, 1996.

Ablard, Jonathan. *Madness in Buenos Aires: Patients, Psychiatrists, and the Argentine State, 1880–1983*. Calgary, Canada: Calgary University Press, 2009.

Ackerknecht, Erwin. *La médecine hospitalière à Paris*. Paris: Payor, 1986.

———. *A Short History of Psychiatry*. New York: Hafner, 1968.

Agamben, Giorgio. *Homo Sacer: Sovereign Power and Bare Life*. Stanford, CA: Stanford University Press, 1998.

Aguirre, Carlos, and Ricardo D. Salvatore. "Writing the History of Law, Crime, and Punishment in Latin America." In *Crime and Punishment in Latin America: Law and Society since Late Colonia Times*, edited by Ricardo D. Salvatore, Carlos Aguirre, and Gilbert M. Joseph. Durham, NC: Duke University Press, 2001.

Albanese, Catherine L. *A Republic of Mind and Spirit: A Cultural History of American Metaphysical Religion*. New Haven, CT: Yale University Press, 2007.

Alves, Lourence Cristine. *O Hospício Nacional de Alienados: Terapêutica ou Higiene Social?* Rio de Janeiro: Tese, 2010.

———. "Quem Eram os Habitantes do 'Cemitério dos Vivos': Uma Análise Quantitativa dos Prontuários dos Pacientes do Hospício Nacional de Alienados (1883–1910)." Unpublished paper, 2011.

Amarante, Paulo. "Psiquiatria Social e Colônias de Alienados no Brasil (1830–1920)." Master's thesis, Programa de Pós-Graduação em Saúde Coletiva da Universidade do Estado do Rio de Janeiro, 1982.

Andrews, George Reid. *Blacks and Whites in São Paulo, Brazil 1888–1988*. Madison: University of Wisconsin Press, 1991.

Arantes, Marco Antonio. "Hospício de doutores." *História, Ciências, Saúde-Manguinhos* 15, no. 1 (March 2008): 49–63.

Araújo, Achilles Ribeiro, de. *A Assistênca Médica Hospitalar no Rio de Janeiro no Século XIX*. Rio de Janeiro: Conselho Federal de Cultura, 1982.

Araujo, Ana Lucia. *Public Memory of Slavery: Victims and Perpetrators in the South Atlantic*. Amherst, NY: Cambria Press, 2010.

Arrom, Silvia Marina. *Containing the Poor: The Mexico City Poor House, 1774–1871*. Durham, NC: Duke University Press, 2000.

Bachelard, Gaston. *The Poetics of Space*. Translated by Maria Jolas. Boston: Beacon Press, 1994.

Barman, Roderick J. *Citizen Emperor, Pedro II and the Making of Brazil, 1825–1891*. Stanford, CA: Stanford University Press, 2000.

Barreira, Ieda de Alencar. "The Beginning of Nursing in Brazil." *Nursing School Review* 10 (2002): 33–47.

Barreto, Paulo (João do Rio). *As Religiões no Rio*. 1906. Reprint, Rio de Janeiro: Edição da Organização Simões, 1951.

Bastide, Roger. *Estudos Afro-Brasileiros*. São Paulo: Perspectiva, 1973.

———. *O Candomblé da Bahia*. São Paulo: Companhia Editora Nacional, 1978.

Bauman, Zygmunt. *Liquid Modernity*. Cambridge, UK: Polity Press.

Beattie, Peter M. *The Tribute of Blood: Army, Honor, Race, and Nation in Brazil, 1864–1945*. Durham, NC: Duke University Press, 2001.

Beirne, Piers. *Inventing Criminology: Essays on the Rise of "Homo Criminalis."* Albany: State of New York Press, 1993.

Benchimol, Jaime L. "Reforma Urbana e Revolta da Vacina na Cidade do Rio de Janeiro." In *O Brasil Republicano: O Tempo do Liberalismo Excludente: da Proclamação da República à Revolução de 1930*. Vol. 1, edited by Jorge Ferreira and Lucília de Almeida Neves Delgado, 233–77. Rio de Janeiro: Civilização Brasileira, 2006.

Benedict, Ruth. "Anthropology and the Abnormal." *Journal of General Psychology* 10 (1934): 59–82.

———. *Patterns of Culture*. Boston: Houghton, Mifflin and Company, 1934.

Bennett, Bridget. *Transatlantic Spiritualism and Nineteenth-century American Literature.* New York: Palgrave Macmillan, 2007.

Berrios, German, and Renate Hauser. "The Early Development of Kraepelin's Ideas on Classification: A Conceptual History." *Psychological Medicine* 18, no. 4 (1988): 813–21.

Besse, Susan K. *Restructuring Patriarchy: The Modernization of Gender Inequality in Brazil, 1914–1940.* Chapel Hill: University of North Carolina Press, 1996.

Bethell, Leslie. *Brazil: Empire and Republic, 1822–1930.* New York: Cambridge University Press, 1989.

Bhugra, Dinesh, and Kamaldeep Bhui. "Racism in Psychiatry: Paradigm Lost, Paradigm Regained." *International Review of Psychiatry* 11, nos. 2–3 (1999): 236–43.

Bishop, Peter. "Surveying 'The Waiting Room.'" *Architectural Theory Review* 18, no. 2 (2013): 135–49.

Bleker, Joanna. "Medical Students—to the Bedside or to the Laboratory? The Emergence of Laboratory Training in German Medical Education, 1870–1900." *Clio Medica* 21 (1987–88): 35–46.

Booth, Christopher. "Clinical Research." In *Companion Encyclopedia of the History of Medicine.* Vol. 1. Edited by W. F. Bynum and Roy Porter, 205–29. London: Routledge, 1993.

Borges, Dain. *The Family in Bahia, Brazil, 1870–1945.* Stanford, CA: Stanford University Press, 1994.

———. "'Puffy, Ugly, Slothful and Inert': Degeneration in Brazilian Social Thought, 1880–1940." *Journal of Latin American Studies* 25, no. 2 (May 1993): 235–50.

———. "The Recognition of Afro-Brazilian Symbols and Ideas, 1890–1940." *Luso-Brazilian Review* 32, no. 2 (1995): 59–78.

Borgmann, Albert. *Crossing the Postmodern Divide* (Chicago: University of Chicago Press, 1992).

Bourdieu, Pierre. *The Field of Cultural Production.* Cambridge, UK: Polity Press, 1993.

Boym, Svetlana. *The Future of Nostalgia.* New York: Basic Books, 2001.

Bretas, Marcos Luiz. *Ordem na cidade: O exercício cotidiano da autoridade policial no Rio de Janeiro 1907–1950.* Rio de Janeiro: Rocco, 1997.

Burns, E. Bradford, ed. *A Documentary History of Brazil.* New York: Alfred A. Knopf, 1966.

———. *A History of Brazil.* 2nd ed. New York: Columbia University Press, 1980.

———. "The Intellectuals as Agents of Change and the Independence of Brazil 1724–1822." In *Colony to Nation: Essays on the Independence of Brazil,* edited by A. J. R. Russell-Wood, 211–46. Baltimore: Johns Hopkins University Press, 1975.

Butler, Kim D. *Freedoms Given, Freedoms Won: Afro-Brazilians in Post-Abolition São Paulo and Salvador.* New Brunswick, NJ: Rutgers University Press, 1998.

Bynum, W. F. *Science and the Practice of Medicine in the Nineteenth Century.* Cambridge: Cambridge University Press, 1994.

Calmon, Pedro. *O Palácio da Praia Vermelha.* Rio de Janeiro: Universidade do Brasil, 1952.

Campos, Paulo Fernando de Souza, Taka Oguisso, and Genival Fernandes de Freitas. "Cultura dos Cuidados: Mulheres Negras e Formação da Enfermagem Profissional Brasileira." *Cultura de los Cuidados Año* 11, no. 22 (2007): 33–39.

Canguilhem, Georges. *The Normal and the Pathological.* Translated by Carolyn R. Fawcett. 1978. Reprint, New York: Zone Books, 1989.

Carlos, Luiz. "Os escravos de ganho no Rio de Janeiro século XIX," *Revista Brasileira de História* 8, no. 16 (1988): 107–42.

Caulfield, Sueann. *In Defense of Honor: Sexual Morality, Modernity, and Nation in Early-Twentieth-Century Brazil.* Durham, NC: Duke University Press, 2000.

Cavalcanti, Adolfo Bezerra de Menezes. *A Loucura sob novo Prisma (estudo psíquico-fisiológico).* Rio de Janeiro: Bohemia, 1920.

Cerqueira, Ede Conceição Bispo. "A Sociedade Brasileira de Neurologia, Psiquiatria e Medicina Legal e o seu Papel na Institucionalização da Psiquiatria (1907–1928)." In *ANPUH Anais do XXVII Simpósio Nacional de História,* Federal University of Rio Grande do Norte in Rio Grande do Norte, Brazil, July 22–26, 2013.

Chalhoub, Sidney. *Cidade Febril: Cortiços e Epidemias na Corte Imperial.* São Paulo: Companhia das Letras, 1996.

———. *Trabalho, Lar e Botequim: O Cotidiano dos Trabalhadores no Rio de Janeiro da Belle* Époque. São Paulo: Brasiliense, 1986.

———. "Vadios e Barões no Ocaso do Império: O Debate sobre a Repressão da Ociosidade na Câmara dos Deputados em 1888." *Estudos Ibero-Americanos* 9, nos. 1–2 (1983): 53–67.

———. *Visões da liberdade: Uma História das Ultima Décadas da Escravidão na Corte.* São Paulo: Companhia das Letras, 1990.

Chamberlain, J. Edward, and Sander Gilman, eds. *Degeneration: The Dark Side of Progress.* New York: Columbia University Press, 1985.

Clarke, Lee, and Caron Chess. "Elites and Panic: More to Fear than Fear Itself." *Social Forces* 87, no. 2 (2008): 993–1014.

Cohen, Stanley. *Folk Devils and Moral Panics: The Creation of the Mods and Rockers.* London: MacGibbon and Kee, 1972.

Conrad, Robert. *The Destruction of Brazilian Slavery, 1850–1888.* Berkeley: University of California Press, 1972.

Conrad, Peter. *The Medicalization of Society: On the Transformation of Human Conditions into Treatable Disorders.* Baltimore: Johns Hopkins University Press, 2007.

Corrêa, Mariza. *As Ilusões da Liberdade: A Escola Nina Rodrigues e a Antropologia no Brasil.* Bragança Paulista: EDUSF, 1998.

Costa, Jurandir Freire. *História da Psiquiatria no Brasil: Um Corte Ideológico.* Rio de Janeiro: Venou, 1974.

———. *Ordem Medica e Norma Familiar.* Rio de Janeiro: Graal, 1989.

Coupland, Douglas. *Generation X: Tales for an Accelerated Culture.* New York: St. Martin's Griffin, 1991.

Cressy, David. *Literacy and the Social Order: Reading and Writing in Tudor and Stuart England.* Cambridge: Cambridge University Press, 1980.

Crossley, Ceri. "Using and Transforming the French Countryside: The 'Colonies Agricoles' (1820–1850)." *French Studies* 45, no. 1 (1991): 36–54.

Cruikshank, Barbara. *The Will to Empower: Democratic Citizens and Other Subjects.* Ithaca, NY: Cornell University Press, 1999.

Cueto, Marcos. *El Regreso de las Epidemias: Salud y Sociedad en el Perú del Siglo XX.* Lima, Peru: Instituto de Estudios Peruanos, 1997.

———. *Missionaries of Science: The Rockefeller Foundation in Latin America.* Bloomington: Indiana University Press, 1994.

———. *Saberes andinos: Ciencia y tecnología en Bolivia, Ecuador, y Perú.* Lima, Peru: Instituto de Estudios Peruanos, 1995.

———. *Salud, Cultura y Sociedad en América Latina.* Lima, Peru: Instituto de Estudios Peruanos, 1996.

Cunha, Maria Clementina Pereira. *O Espelho do Mundo—Juquery, A História de um Asilo.* Rio de Janeiro: Paz e Terra, 1986.

Curtin, Philip. *The Atlantic Slave Trade.* Madison: University of Wisconsin Press, 1969.

Dalgalarrondo, Paulo. "As primeiras Revistas Psiquiátricas no Brasil e no Mundo." *Revista Brasileira de Psiquiatria* 21, no. 4 (December 1999): 237–38.

———. "Cartas de Juliano Moreira a Emil Kraepelin." 1905. In *Civilização e Loucura: Uma Introdução à História da Ethnopsiquiatria,* edited by Paulo Dalgalarrondo, 117–24. São Paulo: Lemos, 1996.

DaMatta, Roberto, and David J. Hess, eds. *The Brazilian Puzzle.* New York: Columbia University Press, 1995.

Damazio, Syliva. *Da elite ao Povo: Advento e Expansão do Espiritismo no Rio de Janeiro.* Rio de Janeiro: Bertrand Brasil, 1999.

Daniel, G. Reginald. *Machado de Assis: Multiracial Identity and the Brazilian Novelist.* University Park: Pennsylvania State University Press, 2012.

Dávila, Jerry. *Diploma of Whiteness: Race and Social Policy in Brazil, 1917–1945.* Durham, NC: Duke University Press, 2003.

Decker, Hannah S. "The Psychiatric Works of Emil Kraepelin: A Many-Faceted Story of Modern Medicine." *Journal of the History of the Neurosciences* 13, no. 3 (2004): 248–76.

Del Brenna, Giovanna Rosso, ed. *O Rio de Janeiro de Pereira Passos: Uma Cidade em Questão II.* Rio de Janeiro: Index, 1985.

Derrida, Jacques. "Force of Law: The 'Mystical Foundation of Authority.'" Translated by Mary Quaintance. *Cardozo Law Review* 11, nos. 5–6 (July–August 1990): 921–1045.

Didi-Huberman, Georges. *Invention of Hysteria: Charcot and the Photographic Iconography of the Salpêtrière.* Translated by Alisa Hartz. Cambridge, MA: MIT Press, 2003.

Digby, Anne. *Madness, Morality and Medicine: A Study of the York Retreat, 1796–1914.* Cambridge: Cambridge University Press, 1985.

Downs, Laura Lee. *Childhood in the Promised Land: Working-Class Movements and the Colonies de Vacances in France, 1880–1960.* Durham, NC: Duke University Press, 2002.

Drouard, Alain. *L'Eugénisme en Questions: L'Exemple de l'Eugénisme Français.* Paris: Ellipses, 1999.

Duarte, Luiz Fernando, Jane Russo, and Ana Teresa Venancio, eds. *Psicologização no Brasil, Atores e Autores.* Rio de Janeiro: Contracapa, 2005.

Durrant, Russil, and Jo Thakker. *Substance Use and Abuse: Cultural and Historical Perspectives.* Thousand Oaks, CA: Sage, 2003.

Edington, Claire. "Beyond the Asylum: Colonies Agricoles and the History of Psychiatry in French Indochina, 1918–1945." *Proceedings of the Western Society for French History* 39 (2011): 267–77.

Edler, Flávio Coelho. "O Debate em Torno da Medicina Experimental no Segundo Reinado." *História, Ciências, Saúde-Manguinhos* 3, no. 2 (1996): 284–99.

Ellenberger, Henri. *The Discovery of the Unconscious: The History and Evolution of Dynamic Psychiatry*. New York: Basic Books, 1970.

Engel, Magali Gouveia. *Meretrizes e Doutores: O Saber Médico e a Prostituição na Cidade do Rio de Janeiro, 1845–1890*. São Paulo: Brasiliense, 1990.

———. *Os Delírios da Razão: Médicos, Loucos e Hospícios Rio de Janeiro, 1830–1930*. Rio de Janeiro: Editora Fiocruz, 2001.

Engstrom, E. J. "Psychiatric Observations on Contemporary Issues." *History of Psychiatry* 3 (1992): 253–56.

Ernst, Waltraud, and Thomas Mueller, eds. *Transnational Psychiatries: Social and Cultural Histories of Psychiatry in Comparative Perspective, c. 1800–2000*. Cambridge: Cambridge University Press, 2010.

Evaristo de Morais, Antonio. *Reminiscencias de um Rábula Criminalista*. Rio de Janeiro: Editora Briguiet, 1989.

Facchinetti, Cristiana. "Psicanálise para Brasileiros: História de sua Circulação e sua Apropriação no Entre-Guerras." *Culturas Psi* 1 (2012): 45–62.

Facchinetti, Cristiana, Andréa Ribeiro, and Pedro Felipe Neves de Muñoz. "As insanas do Hospício Nacional de Alienados 1900–1939." *História, Ciências, Saúde-Manguinhos* 15 (2008): 231–42.

Facchinetti, Cristiana, and Pedro Felipe Neves de Muñoz, "Emil Kraepelin na Ciência Psiquiátrica do Rio de Janeiro, 1903–1933." *História, Ciências, Saúde-Manguinhos* 20, no. 1 (2013): 239–62.

Failer, Judith Lynn. *Who Qualifies for Rights? Homelessness, Mental Illness, and Civil Commitment*. Ithaca, NY: Cornell University Press, 2002.

Febvre, Lucien. "History and Psychology." 1938. In *A New Kind of History*, edited by Peter Burke, 1–11. London: Harper & Row, 1973.

———. "Sensibility and History: How to Reconstitute the Emotional Life of the Past." 1941. In *A New Kind of History*, edited by Peter Burke, 12–26. London: Harper & Row, 1973.

Filho, Adolfo de Morales de los Rios. *O Rio de Janeiro Imperial*. 1946. Reprint, Rio de Janeiro: Topbooks Editora, 2000.

Filho, Lycurgo de Castro Santos. *História Geral d a Medicina Brasileira*, vol. 1. São Paulo: Editora Humanismo, Ciencia e Tecnologia, 1977.

Florentino, Manoel. "Alforrias e Ethnicidade No Rio de Janeiro Oitocentista: Notas de Pesquisa." *Topoi* 3, no. 5 (2002): 9–40.

———. "Slave Trading and Slave Traders in Rio de Janeiro, 1790–1830." In *Enslaving Connections: Changing Cultures of Africa and Brazil during the Era of Slavery*, edited by José C. Curto and Paul E. Lovejoy, 57–80. Amherst, NY: Humanity Books, 2004.

Fonseca, Cristina M. *Saúde no Governo Vargas (1930–1945): Dualidade Institucional de um Bem Público*. Rio de Janeiro; Editora Fiocruz, 2007.

Forty, Adrian. *Discipline and Punish: The Birth of the Prison*. Translated by Alan Sheridan. 2nd ed. New York: Vintage Press, 1995.

———. "The Modern Hospital in England and France." In *Buildings and Society: Essays on the Social Development of the Built Environment*, edited by Anthony D. King, 32–50. London: Routledge, 1980.

Foucault, Michel. *Discipline and Punish: The Birth of the Prison.* Translated by Alan Sheridan. Harmondsworth, UK: Penguin, 1979.

———. *History of Madness.* Edited by Jonathan Murphy and Jean Khalfa. New York: Routledge Press, 2006.

———. *Madness and Civilization: A History of Insanity in the Age of Reason.* New York: Pantheon Books, 1965.

———. "Questions of Method." In *The Foucault Effect: Studies in Governmentality,* edited by Graham Burchell, Colin Gordon, and Peter Miller, 73–86. Chicago: University of Chicago Press, 1991.

Freud, Sigmund. *The Uncanny.* London: Penguin Books, 2003.

———. *The Standard Edition of the Complete Psychological Works of Sigmund Freud.* Edited and translated by J. Strachey. Vol. 14. London: Hogarth Press, 1961.

Freyre, Gilberto. *The Masters and the Slaves.* New York: Alfred A. Knopf, 1956.

———. *Tempo Morto e Outros: Trechos de um Diário de Adolescência e Primeira Mocidade, 1915–1930.* Rio de Janeiro: José Olympio, 1975.

Gandelman, Luciana Mendes. "A Santa Casa da Misericórdia do Rio de Janeiro nos Séculos XVI a XIX." *História, Ciências, Saúde-Manguinhos* 8, no. 3 (2001): 613–30.

Garland, David. "On the Concept of Moral Panic." *Crime, Media, Culture* 4, no. 1 (2008): 9–30.

———. "The Limits of the Sovereign State: Strategies of Crime Control in Contemporary Society." *British Journal of Criminology* 36, no. 4 (1996): 452–55.

Gelfand, Toby. *Professionalizing Modern Medicine: Paris Surgeons and Medical Science and Institutions in the Eighteenth Century.* Westport, CT: Greenwood Press, 1980.

Gemes, Ken. "Freud and Nietzsche on Sublimation." *Journal of Nietzche Studies* 38 (Autumn 2009): 38–59.

Giumbelli, Emerson. "Heresia, Doença, Crime ou Religião: O Espiritismo no Discurso de Médicose Cientistas Sociais." *Revista de Antropologia* 40, no. 2 (1997): 31–82.

———. *O Cuidado dos Mortos: Uma História da Condenção e Legitimação do Espiritismo.* Rio de Janeiro: Arquivo Nacional, 1997.

Goldberg, Ann. *Sex, Religion, and the Making of Modem Madness: The Eberbach Asylum and German Society, 1815–1849.* New York: Oxford University Press, 1999.

Goldstein, Jan. *Console and Classify: The French Psychiatric Profession in the Nineteenth Century.* Cambridge: Cambridge University Press, 1987.

Gomes da Cunha, Olivia Maria, and Flávio dos Santos Gomes, eds. *Quase-cidadão: Histórias e Antropologias da Pós-Emancipação no Brasil.* Rio de Janeiro: FGV Editora, 2007.

Gonçalves, Monique de Siqueira, and Flávio Coelho Edler, "Os Caminhos da Loucura na Corte Imperial: Um Embate Historiográfico Acerca do Funcionamento do Hospício Pedro II de 1850 a 1889." *Revista Latinoamericana de Psicopatologia Fundamental* 12, no. 2 (June 2009): 393–410.

Goode, Erich, and Nachman Ben-Yehuda. *Moral Panics: The Social Construction of Deviance.* 2nd ed. Chichester, UK: Wiley-Blackwell, 2009.

Gordon, Colin, ed. *Power/Knowledge: Selected Interviews and Other Writings 1972–1977.* New York: Pantheon Books, 1980.

———. "Psychiatry as a Problem of Democracy." In *The Power of Psychiatry*, edited by Peter Miller and Nikolas S. Rose, 267–315. Cambridge, UK: Polity Press, 1986.

Graham, Sandra Lauderdale. *House and Street: The Domestic World of Servants and Masters in Nineteenth-Century Rio de Janeiro.* New York: Cambridge University Press, 1988.

Grant, Bridget F., and Debora A. Dawson. "Alcohol and Drug Use, Abuse, and Dependence: Classification, Prevalence, and Comorbidity." In *Addictions: A Comprehensive Guidebook*, edited by Barbara McCrady and Elizabeth E. Epstein, 9–29. New York: Oxford University Press, 1999.

Greenbaum, Louis. "Medicine in Revolution: An Essay Review." *Journal of the History of Medicine and Allied Sciences* 37, no. 1 (1982): 90–95.

Grob, Gerald. *The Mad Among Us: A History of the Care of America's Mentally Ill.* New York: Free Press, 1994.

Guerra, François Xavier. *Modernidad e Independencia: Ensayos sobre las Revoluciones Hispánicas.* Madrid: Editorial Mapfere, 1992.

Guimarães, Antônio Sérgio. *Racismo e Anti-Racismo no Brasil.* São Paulo: Editora 34, 1999.

Guy, Donna J. Introduction to "Rise of the Welfare State in Latin America." *Americas* 58, no. 1 (July 2001): 1–6.

Hall, Stuart, Chas Critcher, Tony Jefferson, John Clarke et al. *Policing the Crisis: Mugging, the State, and Law and Order.* London: Macmillan, 1978.

Harding, Rachel E. *A Refuge in Thunder: Candomblé* and *Alternative Spaces of Blackness.* Bloomington: Indiana University Press, 2000.

Hess, David. *Spirits and Scientists: Ideology, Spiritism, and Brazilian Culture.* University Park: Pennsylvania State University Press, 1991.

Hochman, Gilberto. *A Era do Saneamento: As Bases da Política de Saúde Pública no Brasil.* São Paulo: HUSITEC, 1998.

Hoff, Paul. "Kraepelin and Degeneration Theory." *European Archives of Psychiatry and Clinical Neuroscience* 258, no. 2 (June 2008): 12–17.

Holloway, Thomas H. *Policing Rio de Janeiro: Repression and Resistance in a 19th-Century City.* Stanford, CA: Stanford University Press, 1993.

Holston, James. *Insurgent Citizenship: Disjunctions of Democracy and Modernity in Brazil.* In-Formation Series. Princeton, NJ: Princeton University Press, 2009.

Hoornaert, Eduardo. "The Church in Brazil." In *The Church in Latin America, 1492–1992*, edited by Enrique Dussel, 185–201. Maryknoll, NY: Orbis, 1992.

Hothersall, David. *History of Psychology.* Philadelphia: Temple University Press, 1984.

Imbassahy, Carlos. *Espiritismo e Loucura.* São Paulo: Livraria Allan Kardec Editora, 1949.

Ingleby, David. "The Social Construction of Mental Illness." In *The Problem of Medical Knowledge: Examining the Social Construction of Medicine*, edited by Peter Wright and Andrew Treacher, 123–43. Edinburgh: Edinburgh University Press, 1982.

Isaia, Arthur Cesar. "A República e a Teleologia Histórica do Espiritismo." In *Espiritismo e Religiões Afro-Brasileiras*, edited by Artur César Isaia and Ivan Aparecido Manoel, 103–17. São Paulo: UNESP, 2012.

———. "João do Rio: O Flâneur e O Preconceito: Um Olhar Sobre o Transe Mediúnico na Capital Federal de Inícios do Século XX." In *Religiões, Religiosidades e Diferenças Culturais,* edited by Jérri Roberto Marin, 100–115. Campo Grande, Brazil: UCDB, 2005.

Jaspers, Karl. *General Psychopathology*. Translated by J. Hoenig and M. W. Hamilton. Manchester: Manchester University Press, 1963.

Johnson, Paul C. *Spirited Things: The Work of "Possession" in Afro-Atlantic Religions*. Chicago: University of Chicago Press, 2014.

Jouin, François. "Uma Visita ao Asilo de Pedro II no Rio de Janeiro, Brasil." *Rev. Latinoam. Psicopat. Fund* 15, no. 2 (2012): 404–12.

Karasch, Mary C. *Slave Life in Rio de Janeiro, 1808–1850.* Princeton, NJ: Princeton University Press, 1987.

Kardec, Allan. *Introduction to the Spiritist Philosophy*. 1959. Reprint, Philadelphia: Allan Kardec Educational Society, 1999.

Keller, Richard. *Colonial Madness: Psychiatry in French North Africa*. Chicago: University of Chicago Press, 2007.

Klein, Herbert S. *The Atlantic Slave Trade*. Cambridge: Cambridge University Press, 1999.

Klein, Herbert S., and Francisco Vidal Luna. *Slavery in Brazil*. New York: Cambridge University Press, 2010.

Kristeva, Julia. *Revolution in Poetic Language*. Translated by Margaret Waller. 1974. Reprint, New York: Columbia University Press, 1984.

Lange, Brad. "Importing Freud and Lamarck to the Tropics: Arthur Ramos and the Transformation of Brazilian Racial Thought, 1926–1939." *The Americas* 65, no. 1 (July 2008): 9–34.

Lefebvre, Henri. *Production of Space*. Oxford, UK: Blackwell, 1991.

Levine, Robert M. "The First Afro-Brazilian Congress: Opportunities for the Study of Race in the Brazilian Northeast." *Race and Class* 15, no. 2 (1973): 185–93.

———. *The Vargas Regime: The Critical Years, 1934–1938*. New York: Columbia University Press, 1970.

Levy, Maria Bárbara. *História da Bolsa de Valores do Rio de Janeiro*. Rio de Janeiro: IBMEC, 1977.

Lewis-Fernández, Roberto, and Arthur Kleinman. "Cultural Psychiatry: Theoretical, Clinical, and Research Issues. *Psychiatric Clinics of North America* 18, no. 3 (1995): 433–48.

Lima, Nisia Trindade, and Gilberto Hochman. "Condenado pela Raça, Absolvido pela Medicina: O Brasil descoberto pelo Movimento Sanitarista da Primeira República." In *Raça, Ciência e Sociedade,* edited by Marcos Chor Maio and Ricardo Ventura Santos, 23–40. Rio de Janeiro: Fiocruz, 1996.

Lima Barreto, Afonso Henriques de. *O Diário do Hospício: O Cemitério dos Vivos*. Rio de Janeiro: Secretaria Municipal de Cultura, Dep. Geral de Doc. E Inf. Cultural, 1988. Reprint, 1993.

Lira, Heitor. *História de Dom Pedro II (1825–1891): Declínio (1880–1891)*. Belo Horizonte: Itatiaia, 1977.

Lobo, Eulalia Maria Lahmeyer. *História do Rio de Janeiro: Do capital federal ao capital industrial financeiro*. Vol. 2. Rio de Janeiro: IBMEC, 1978.

Locke, John. *Two Treatises of Government.* 2nd ed. London: Cambridge University Press, 1967.

Loewald, Hans. *Sublimation: Inquiries into Theoretical Psychoanalysis.* New Haven, CT: Yale University Press, 1988.

Long, Charles H. *Significations: Signs, Symbols and the Interpretation of Religion.* Aurora, CO: The Davies Group Publishers, 1999.

Lopes, José Leme. "Psiquiatria e Antropologia." *Neurobiologia, Recife* 42, no. 1 (1979): 3–12.

Ludmerer, Kenneth. *American Medical Education from the Turn of the Century to the Era of Managed Care.* Oxford: Oxford University Press, 1999.

Lukes, Steven, Michael Carrithers, and Steven Collins, eds. *The Category of the Person: Anthropology, Philosophy, History.* Cambridge: Cambridge University Press, 1985.

Machado, Roberto, Ángela Loureiro, Rogério Luz, and Kátia Muricy. *Danação DaNorma: Medicina Social e Constituição da Psiquiatria no Brasil.* Rio de Janeiro: Graal, 1978.

Machado, Ubiratan. *Os Intelectuais e o Espiritismo: De Castro Alves a Machado de Assis.* Rio de Janeiro: Publicações Lachâtre, 1996.

Maggie, Yvonne. *Medo do Feitiço: Relações entre Magia e Poder no Brasil.* Rio de Janeiro: Arquivo Nacional, 1992.

Mahone, Sloane, and Megan Vaughan, *Psychiatry and Empire.* Basingstoke, UK: Palgrave Macmillan 2008.

Mann, Michael. *The Sources of Social Power.* 2 vols. Cambridge: Cambridge University Press, 1993.

Martins, Clóvis. "Psiquiatria Transcultural e Países em Desenvolvimento." *Revista Brasileira de Psiquiatria* 3, no. 1 (1969): 31–62.

Meade, Teresa A. *"Civilizing" Rio: Reform and Resistance in a Brazilian City, 1889–1930.* University Park: Pennsylvania State University Press, 1997.

Mehta, Uday Singh. "Liberal Strategies of Exclusion." *Politics and Society* 18, no. 4 (December 1990): 427–54.

———. *Liberalism and Empire: A Study in Nineteenth-Century British Liberal Thought.* Chicago: University of Chicago Press, 1999.

Melo, Cristiane Silva, and Maria Cristina Gomes Machado. "Notas para a História da Educação: Considerações acerca do Decreto N° 7.247, de 19 de Abril de 1879, de Autoria de Carlos Leôncio de Carvalho," *Revista HISTEDBR On-line* 34 (June 2009): 294–305.

Meyer, Birgit, and Peter Pels, eds. *Magic and Modernity: Interfaces of Revelation and Concealment.* Stanford, CA: Stanford University Press, 2003.

Mill, John Stuart. *On Liberty.* Northbrook, IL: AHM Publishing, 1947.

Monroe, John Warne. *Laboratories of Faith: Mesmerism, Spiritism, and Occultism in Modern France.* Ithaca, NY: Cornell University Press, 2008.

Moreira, Martha Cristina Nunes. "A Fundação Rockefeller e a Construção da Identidade Profissional de Enfermagem no Brasil na Primeira República." *História, Ciências, Saúde-Manguinhos* 5, no. 3 (November 1998–February 1999): 621–45.

Moreira-Almeida, Alexander, Angélica A. Silva de Almeida, and Francisco Lotufo Neto. "History of 'Spiritist Madness' in Brazil." *History of Psychiatry* 16, no. 1 (2005): 5–25.

Morel, Marco, and Mariana Monteiro de Barros. *Palavra, Imagem, e Poder: O Surgimento da Imprensa no Brasil do Século XIX.* Rio de Janeiro: DP&A Editoria Ltda., 2003.

Moser, Robert Henry. *The Carnivalesque Defunto: Death, and the Dead in Modern Brazilian Literature.* Athens: Ohio University Press, 2008.

Mott, Maria Lucia. "Midwifery and the Construction of an Image in Nineteenth-Century Brazil." *Nursing History Review* 11 (2003): 31–49.

Moura, Clovis. *Brasil: Raizes do Protesto Negro.* São Paulo: Global Editora, 1983.

Müller, T. M. P. "A Primeira Escola Especial para Creanças Anormaes no Distrito Federal—O Pavilhão Bourneville do Hospício Nacional de Alienados (1903–1920)." EdD diss., State University of Rio de Janeiro, 1998.

Needell, Jeffrey D. *A Tropical Belle Epoque: Elite Culture and Society in Turn-of-the-Twentieth-Century Rio de Janeiro.* Cambridge: Cambridge University Press, 1987.

———. "The *Revolta Contra Vacina* of 1904: The Revolt Against 'Modernization' in *Belle-Époque* Rio de Janeiro." *Hispanic American Historical Review* 67, no. 2 (May 1987): 233–69.

———. "The State and Development under the Brazilian Monarchy, 1822–1889." In *State and Nation Making in Latin America and Spain: Republics of the Possible,* edited by Miguel A. Centeno and Augustin E. Ferraro, 79–99. New York: Cambridge University Press, 2013.

Nelson, Sioban. *Say Little, Do Much: Nursing, Nuns, and Hospitals in the Nineteenth Century.* Philadelphia: University of Pennsylvania Press, 2001.

Nye, Robert A. *Crime, Madness, and Politics in Modern France: The Medical Concept of National Decline.* Princeton, NJ: Princeton University Press, 1984.

Oda, Ana Maria Galdini Raimundo, and Paulo Dalgalarrondo. "História das primeiras instituições para alienados no Brasil." *História, Ciências, Saúde-Manguinhos* 12, no. 3 (December 2005): 983–1010.

Ong, Aihwa. "Making the Biopolitical Subject: Cambodian Immigrants, Refugee Medicine, and Cultural Citizenship in California." *Social Science and Medicine* 40, no. 9 (1995): 1243–57.

Owen, Alex. *The Darkened Room: Women, Power, and Spiritualism in Late Victorian England.* New Cultural Studies Series. Philadelphia: University of Pennsylvania Press, 1990.

Pacheco e Silva, Antônio Carlos. "O Espiritismo e As Doenças Mentais no Brasil." *Anais Portugueses de Psiquiatria* 2, no. 2 (1950): 1–6.

Padua, Jorge. *El Analfabetismo en America Latina: Un Estudio Empirico con Especial Referencia a los Casos de Peru, Mexico y Argentina.* Mexico City: El Colegio de Mexico, 1979.

Parker, Richard G. *Bodies, Pleasures, and Passions: Sexual Culture in Contemporary Brazil.* Boston: Beacon Press, 1991.

Passos, Alexandre. *Juliano Moreira (vida e obra).* Rio de Janeiro: Livraria São José, 1975.

Paula, Richard Negreiro. "Um Doutor contra Doutos Leigos: Teixeira Brandão e suas Opiniões quanto ao Poder de Decisão sobre a Custódia Médica." *Revista de História (USP)* 1 (2009): 169–94.

Peard, Julyan. *Race, Place, and Medicine: The Idea of the Tropics in Nineteenth-Century Brazilian Medicine.* Durham, NC: Duke University Press, 1999.

Peres, M. A. A. "A ordem no Hospício: Primórdios da Enfermagem Psiquiátrica no Brasil (1852–1890)." PhD diss., Universidade Federal do Rio de Janeiro, Escola de Enfermagem Anna Nery, Programa de Pós-Graduação em Enfermagem, 2008.

Piccato, Pablo. *City of Suspects: Crime in Mexico City, 1900–1931.* Durham, NC: Duke University Press, 2001.

Pinel, Philippe. *A Treatise on Insanity.* Translated by D. D. Davis. New York: Hafner, 1962.

Pinto, Luiz de Aguiar Costa. *O Negro no Rio de Janeiro: Relações de Raça numa Sociedade em Mudança.* 2nd ed. Rio de Janeiro: Editora Universidade Federal do Rio de Janeiro, 1998.

Plotkin, Mariano Ben. *Freud in the Pampas: The Emergence and Development of a Psychoanalytic Culture in Argentina.* Stanford, CA: Stanford University Press, 2002.

Popkin, Jeremy D. *Press, Revolution, and Social Identities in France, 1830–1835.* University Park: Pennsylvania State University Press, 2002.

Porter, Roy. *A Social History of Madness: Stories of the Insane.* London: Phoenix Giants, 1996.

Porter, Roy, and David Wright, eds. *The Confinement of the Insane: International Perspectives, 1800–1965.* Cambridge: Cambridge University Press, 2003.

———. *Madness: A Brief History.* Oxford: Oxford University Press, 2002. Roy Porter, *A Social History of Madness: Stories of the Insane* (London: Phoenix Giants, 1996).

Preziosi, Donald. *Architecture, Language and Meaning: The Origins of the Built World and its Semiotic Organization.* The Hague: De Gruyter Mouton, 1979.

Prior, Lindsay. "The Architecture of the Hospital: A Study of Spatial Organization and Medical Knowledge." *British Journal of Sociology* 39, no. 1 (1988): 86–113.

Quétel, Claude. *Histoire de la Folie: De l'Antiquité à Nos Jours.* Paris: Tallendier, 2009.

Quinodoz, Jean-Michel. *Reading Freud: A Chronological Exploration of Freud's Writings.* New York: Routledge, 2005.

Ramos, Arthur. *As Collectividades Anormaes.* Rio de Janeiro: Civilização Brasileira, 1939.

———. *Le Métissage au Brésil.* Paris: Hermann et Cie Éditeurs, 1952.

Rapoport, Amos. *The Meaning of The Built Environment: A Nonverbal Communication Approach.* Tucson: University of Arizona Press, 1990.

Resende, Heitor. "Política de Saúde Mental no Brasil: Uma Visão Histórica." In *Cidadania e Loucura: Políticas de Saúde Mental no Brasil,* edited by Silvério Almeida Tundis and Nilson do Rosário Costa, 15–73. Petrópolis, Brazil: Editora Vozes, 1990.

Rey, Philippe-Marius. "O Hospício e os Alienados No Brasil." *Rev. Latinoam. Psicopat. Fund* 15, no. 2 (June 2012): 382–403.

Rezende de Carvalho, Maria Alice. *Quatro Vezes Cidade.* Rio de Janeiro: Sette Letras, 1994.

Ribeiro, Leonidio. *De Médico a Criminalista.* Rio de Janeiro: Livraria São José, 1967.

Ribeiro, René. *Antropologia da Religião e Outros Estudos.* Recife: Editora Massangana, 1982.

Ritui, Christine. "João do Rio: Ombre et Lumière du Rio de Janeiro de la Belle Époque." In *Littérature et Modernisation au Brésil,* edited by Jacqueline Penon and José Antonio Pasta Jr. Paris: Sorbonne Nouvelle, 2004.

Rivera-Garza, Cristina. "Dangerous Minds: Changing Psychiatric Views of the Mentally Ill in Porfirian Mexico, 1876–1911." *Journal of the History of Medicine and Allied Sciences* 56, no. 1 (2001): 36–67.

———. *La Castañeda: Narrativas dolientes desde el Manicomio General, México 1910–1930.* Mexico City: Tusquests, 2010.

———. *Nadie Me Verá Llorar.* Mexico City: Tusquets Editores, 2003.

———. "'She Neither Respected nor Obeyed Anyone': Inmates and Psychiatrists Debate Gender and Class at the General Insane Asylum La Castañeda, Mexico, 1910–1930." *Hispanic American Historical Review* 81, no. 3 (2001): 653–88.

Rocha, Agenor Miranda. *Os Candomblés Antigos do Rio de Janeiro: A Naçao Ketu: Origens, Ritos, e Crenças.* Rio de Janeiro: Faculdade da Cidade, Topbooks, 1995.

Rocha, Cristina. "A Globalização Do Espiritismo: Fluxos Do Movimento Religioso de João de Deus Entre a Austrália e o Brasil." *Revista de Antropologia* 52, no. 2 (July 1, 2009): 571–603.

Rodgers, Daniel T. "In Search of Progressivism." *Reviews in American History* 10, no. 4 (December 1982): 113–32.

Rodriguez, Julia. *Civilizing Argentina: Science, Medicine and the Modern State.* Chapel Hill: University of North Carolina Press, 2006.

Roitman, Janet. *Anti-crisis.* Durham, NC: Duke University Press, 2014.

Roman, Reinaldo. *Governing Spirits: Religion, Miracles, and Spectacles in Cuba and Puerto Rico, 1898–1956.* Chapel Hill: University of North Carolina Press, 2008.

Roos, Neil. "Work Colonies and South African Historiography." *Journal of Social History* 36, no. 1 (2011): 54–76.

Rose, Nikolas. "Governing 'Advanced' Liberal Democracies," In *Foucault and Political Reason: Liberalism, Neo-liberalism and Rationalities of Government,* edited by Andrew Barry, Thomas Osborne, and Nikolas Rose, 50–62. Chicago: University of Chicago Press, 1996.

Rose, Nikolas, and Peter Miller. "Political Power Beyond the State: Problematics of Government," *British Journal of Sociology* 43, no. 2 (1992): 173–205.

Rothman, David J. *The Discovery of the Asylum: Social Order and Disorder in a New Republic.* Boston: Little, Brown, 1971.

Rubin, Miri. *Charity and Community in Medieval Cambridge.* Cambridge: Cambridge University Press, 1987.

Russell-Wood, A. J. R. *Fidalgos and Philanthropists: The Santa Casa da Misericórdia of Bahia, 1550–1755.* Berkeley: University of California Press, 1968.

Russo, Jane A. "The Social Diffusion of Psychoanalysis during the Brazilian Military Regime: Psychological Awareness in an Age of Political Repression." In *Psychoanalysis and Politics: Histories of Psychoanalysis under Conditions of Restricted Freedom,* edited by Joy Damousi and Mariano Ben Plotkin, 165–84. Oxford: Oxford University Press, 2012.

Sá, Isabel dos Guimarães. *As Misericórdias Portuguesas de D. Manuel I a Pombal.* Lisbon: Livros Horizonte, 2001.

———. "Assistance to the Poor on a Royal Model: The Example of the Misericórdias in the Portuguese Empire from the Sixteenth to the Eighteenth Century." *Confraternitas* 13, no. 1 (2002): 3–14.

———. "Catholic Charity in Perspective: The Social Life of Devotion in Portugal and Its Empire 1450–1700." *E-Journal of Portuguese History* 2, no. 1 (Summer 2004): 1–19.

Sadowsky, Jonathan. *Imperial Bedlam: Institutions of Madness and Colonialism in Southwest Nigeria.* Berkeley: University of California Press, 1999.

———. "The Reality of Mental Illness and the Social World: Lessons from Colonial Psychiatry." *Harvard Review of Psychiatry* 11, no. 4 (July 2003): 91–112.

Saler, Michael. "Modernity and Enchantment: A Historiographical Review." *American Historical Review* 111, no. 3 (2006): 692–716.

Santos Filho, Lycurgo de Castro. *História Geral da Medicina Brasileira,* 2 vols. São Paulo: Hucitec, 1991.

Schorske, Carl. *Fin de Siècle Vienna: Politics and Culture.* New York: Alfred A. Knopf, 1979.

Schrauwers, Albert. "The 'Benevolent' Colonies of Johannes van den Bosch: Continuities in the Administration of Poverty in the Netherlands and Indonesia." *Comparative Studies in Society and History* 43, no. 2 (2001): 298–328.

Schultz, Kirsten. *Tropical Versailles: Empire, Monarchy, and the Portuguese Royal Court in Rio de Janeiro, 1808–1821.* New York: Routledge, 2001.

Schwarcz, Lilia Moritz. *O Espectáculo das Raça: Cientistas, Instituições e Questão Racial No Brasil, 1870–1930.* São Paulo: Companhia das Letras, 1993.

Scott, James C. *Seeing like a State: How Certain Schemes to Improve the Human Tradition Have Failed.* New Haven, CT: Yale University Press, 1998.

Scull, Andrew, ed. *The Asylum as Utopia: W. A. F. Browne and the Mid-Nineteenth Century Consolidation of Psychiatry.* London: Routledge Press, 1991.

———. *The Most Solitary of Afflictions: Madness and Society in Britain, 1700–1900.* New Haven, CT: Yale University Press, 1993.

———. *Museums of Madness: The Social Organization of Insanity in Nineteenth-Century England.* New York: St. Martin's Press, 1979.

Scull, Andrew, Charlotte MacKenzie, and Nicholas Hervey. *Masters of Bedlam: The Transformation of the Mad-Doctoring Trade.* Princeton, NJ: Princeton University Press, 1996.

Sevcenko, Nicolau. *A Revolta da Vacina: Mentes Insanas em Corpos Rebeldes.* São Paulo: Cosac Naify, 2010.

Sharp, Lynn. *Secular Spirituality: Reincarnation and Spiritism in Nineteenth-Century France.* Plymouth, UK: Lexington Books, 2006.

Silva de Almeida, Angélica Aparecida, Ana Maria Galdini Raimundo Oda, and Paulo Dalgalarrondo. "O Olhar dos Psiquiatrias Brasileiros sobre Os Fenômenos de Transe e Possessão." *Revista de Psiquiatria Clínica* 34, no. 1 (2007): 34–41.

Skidmore, Thomas E. *Black into White: Race and Nationality in Brazilian Thought.* Durham, NC: Duke University Press, 1993.

———. *Brazil: Five Centuries of Change.* New York: Oxford University Press, 1999.

———. "Racial Ideas and Social Policy in Brazil 1870–1940." In *The Idea of Race in Latin America,* edited by Richard Graham, 7–36. Austin, TX: University of Texas Press 1990.

Smelser, Neil J. *Theory of Collective Behavior.* New York: Free Press, 1962.

Smith, Joseph. *A History of Brazil.* New York: Pearson Education Limited, 2002.

Smith, Theopus H. *Conjuring Culture: Biblical Formations of Black America.* New York: Oxford University Press, 1994.

Sommers, Doris. *Foundational Fictions: The National Romances of Latin America.* Berkeley: University of California Press, 1991.

Steiner, Michael J. *A Study of the Intellectual and Material Culture of Death in Nineteenth-Century America.* Lewiston, NY: Edwin Mellen Press, 2004.

Stepan, Nancy Leys. *"The Hour of Eugenics": Race, Gender and Nation in Latin America.* Ithaca, NY: Cornell University Press, 1991.

Stoler, Ann Laura. *Along the Archival Grain.* Princeton, NJ: Princeton University Press, 2009.

———. *Carnal Knowledge: Race and the Intimate in Colonial Rule.* Berkeley: University of California Press, 2002.

Taylor, Jeremy. *The Architect and the Pavilion Hospital: Dialogue and Design Creativity in England, 1850–1914.* London: Leicester University Press, 1997.

Tolmasquim, Alfredo, and Ildeu de Castro Moreira. "Einstein in Brazil: the Communication to the Brazilian Academy of Sciences on the Constitution of Light." In *History of Modern Physics, Proceedings of the XXth International Congress of History of Science,* edited by Helge Kragh, Geert Vanpaemel, and Pierre Marage, 229–42. Turnhout, Belgium: Brepols, 2002.

Tomes, Nancy. *A Generous Confidence: Thomas Story Kirkbride and the Art of Asylum-Keeping, 1840–1883.* Cambridge: Cambridge University Press, 1984.

Toms, Jonathan. "Political Dimensions of 'the Psychosocial': The 1948 International Congress on Mental Health and the Mental Hygiene Movement." *History of the Human Sciences* 25, no. 5 (2012): 91–106.

Toth, Stephen. *Beyond Papillon: The French Overseas Penal Colonies, 1854–1952.* Lincoln: University of Nebraska Press, 2006.

Valladres de Oliveira, Carmen Lucia M. "Psychoanalysis in Brazil during Vargas' Time." In *Psychoanalysis and Politics: Histories of Psychoanalysis,* edited by Joy Damousi and Mariano Ben Plotkin, 113–35. Oxford: Oxford University Press, 2012.

Vaz de Oliveira, William. *A Assistência a Alienados na Capital Federal da Primeira República: Discursos e Práticas entre Rupturas e Continuidades.* Rio de Janeiro: Universidade Federal Fluminense (Niterói), 2012.

Venancio, Ana Teresa A. "Ciência Psiquiátrica e Política Assistencial: A Criação do Instituto de Psiquiatria da Universidade do Brasil." *História, Ciências, Saúde-Manguinhos* 10, no. 3 (2003): 883–900.

———. "From the Agricultural Colony to the Hospital-Colony: Configurations for Psychiatric Care in Brazil in the First Half of the Twentieth Century." *História, Ciências, Saúde-Manguinhos* 18, no. 1 (2011): 35–52.

Vidler, Anthony. *Architectural Uncanny: Essays in the Modern Unhomely.* Cambridge, MA: MIT Press, 1992.

Viotti da Costa, Emilia. *The Brazilian Empire: Myths and Histories.* Belmont, CA: Wadsworth Publishing, 1985.

Warner, John Harley. "Grand Narrative and Its Discontents: Medical History and the Social Transformation of American Medicine." *Journal of Health Politics, Policy, and Law* 29, nos. 4–5 (2004): 757–80.

Weber, Max. "Science as a Vocation (1917/1919)." In *From Max Weber: Essays in Sociology*. Translated, edited, and with an introduction by H. H. Gerth and C. Wright Mills. 1917. New York: Oxford University Press, 1946.

Wegner, Robert, and Vanderlei Sebastião de Souza. "Eugenia 'Negativa,' Psiquiatria e Catolicismo: Embates em torno da Esterilização Eugênica no Brasil." *História, Ciências, Saúde-Manguinhos* 20, no. 1 (January–March 2013): 263–88.

Weiner, Dora B. "The Madman in the Light of Reason: Enlightenment Psychiatry, Part I. Custody, Therapy, Theory and the Need for Reform." In *History of Psychiatry and Medical Psychology*, edited by Edwin R. Wallace and John Gach, 255–77. New York: Springer Press, 2010.

———. "The Madman in the Light of Reason: Enlightenment Psychiatry, Part II. Alienists, Treatises, and the Psychologic Approach in the Era of Pinel." In *History of Psychiatry and Medical Psychology*, edited by Edwin R. Wallace and John Gach, 281–303. New York: Springer Press, 2010.

Whyte, William. "How Do Buildings Mean? Some Issues on the Interpretation in the History of Architecture." *History and Theory Journal* 45 (2006): 153–77.

Williams, Daryle. *Culture Wars in Brazil: The First Vargas Regime, 1930–1945*. Durham, NC: Duke University Press, 2001.

Yanni, Carla. *The Architecture of Madness: Insane Asylums in the United States*. Minneapolis: University of Minnesota Press, 2007.

Zilboorg, Gregory. *A History of Medical Psychology*. New York: W. W. Norton, 1967.

Zulawski, Ann. *Unequal Cures: Public Health and Political Change in Bolivia, 1900–1950*. Durham, NC: Duke University Press, 2007.

Index

An italicized page number indicates a figure or table.